Haematology

FOURTH EDITION

AN ILLUSTRATED COLOUR TEXT

Martin R Howard

MBChB MD FRCP FRCPath
Consultant Haematologist
York Teaching Hospital NHS Foundation Trust
Clinical Senior Lecturer
Hull York Medical School
York, UK

Peter J Hamilton

MA BM BCh FRCP FRCPath (retired)
Formerly Consultant Haematologist
Royal Victoria Infirmary
Lecturer in Medicine
University of Newcastle-upon-Tyne
Newcastle-upon-Tyne, UK

Illustrated by Robert Britton and Antbits Ltd.

CHURCHILL LIVINGSTONE

ELSEVIER

EDINBURGH   LONDON   NEW YORK   OXFORD   PHILADELPHIA   ST LOUIS   SYDNEY   TORONTO   2013

CHURCHILL
LIVINGSTONE
ELSEVIER

© 2013 Elsevier Ltd. All rights reserved.

First edition 1997
Second edition 2002
Third edition 2008
Fourth edition 2013

ISBN 978-0-7020-5139-5
ebook ISBN 978-0-7020-5415-0

British Library Cataloguing in Publication Data
A catalogue record for this book is available from the British Library

Library of Congress Cataloging in Publication Data
A catalog record for this book is available from the Library of Congress

ELSEVIER your source for books, journals and multimedia in the health sciences
www.elsevierhealth.com

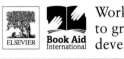

Working together to grow libraries in developing countries

www.elsevier.com • www.bookaid.org

The publisher's policy is to use **paper manufactured from sustainable forests**

Printed in China

Preface to the fourth edition

The principles that guided the first edition of this book sixteen years ago still apply. In the era of whole genome sequencing and targeted therapies, the proper clinical management of patients with blood disorders relies very heavily on traditional skills: history taking, clinical examination and careful selection of laboratory investigations.

This edition has been considerably updated to acknowledge recent developments in the understanding and treatment of benign and malignant diseases of the blood. The addition of a section addressing 'Haematology in the Elderly' reflects the increasing age of the population. A number of case histories have been added to allow the enthusiastic student to test their learning. These are intended to be enjoyed. Although it can seem complicated, haematology remains a fascinating specialty which well repays attempts at understanding.

MRH

Preface to the first edition

Blood is a 'hot, temperate, red humour whose office is to nourish the whole body to give it strength and colour, being dispersed by the veins through every part of it,' wrote Richard Burton in 1628. Studying the red humour can be hard work. Complex nomenclature and classifications make haematology seem tedious and unintelligible to the uninitiated. The object of this book is to give a basic grounding in the biology and diseases of the blood. We hope that the format, with double page spreads and extensive colour illustration, will allow information to be absorbed painlessly and with enjoyment! The text is designed to be suitable for medical students, junior hospital doctors, general practitioners, biomedical scientists, and nurses with a special interest in haematology. Those taking higher medical examinations should find it a useful revision aid.

We have stressed recent advances in technology in the laboratory and newer treatment strategies on the ward. However, if this book has a 'message' it is that best practice and management of blood diseases still relies heavily on traditional skills – history taking, clinical examination, and careful selection of laboratory investigations.

MRH, PJH

Acknowledgements

We are grateful to the following colleagues for their advice and help with illustrations: Dr A Anderson, Dr L Bond, Dr A Clarke, Dr I N Reid, Dr R. Mannion, Dr A Turnbull, Dr H Wilkinson (York); Dr A Hall, Dr A Lennard, Dr M Reid, Dr P W G Saunders (Newcastle-upon-Tyne); Mr M Cullen, Mrs H Dickinson, Dr D Norfolk, Mrs S Ricketts, Dr A Scarsbrook (Leeds); Prof D Grimwade, Dr E Letsky, Dr J Marsh (London); Prof E Preston (Sheffield); Dr P Bolton-Maggs, Mrs H Jones (SHOT); Haematology Laboratories at York Teaching Hospital and The Royal Victoria Infirmary, Newcastle-upon-Tyne; the Medical Illustration Department at York Teaching Hospital. Thanks to all involved at Elsevier.

Contents

Preface to the fourth edition **v**

Preface to the first edition **v**

Acknowledgements **v**

1 Anatomy and physiology 2

1 The bone marrow **2**

2 Red cells **4**

3 Neutrophils, eosinophils, basophils and monocytes **6**

4 Lymphocytes **8**

5 The spleen **10**

6 Haemostasis **12**

2 The haematology patient 14

7 History taking **14**

8 Examining the patient **16**

9 Laboratory haematology I – Blood and bone marrow **18**

10 Laboratory haematology II – Coagulation and the acute phase response **20**

3 Anaemia 22

11 Introduction and classification **22**

12 Iron deficiency anaemia **24**

13 Megaloblastic anaemia **26**

14 Haemolytic anaemia I – General features and inherited disorders **28**

15 Haemolytic anaemia II – Acquired disorders **30**

16 The thalassaemias **32**

17 Sickle cell syndromes **34**

18 Anaemia of chronic disease **36**

4 Leukaemia 38

19 Introduction **38**

20 Acute myeloid leukaemia **40**

21 Acute lymphoblastic leukaemia **42**

22 Chronic myeloid leukaemia **44**

23 Chronic lymphocytic leukaemia **46**

24 Other leukaemias **48**

25 The myelodysplastic syndromes **50**

26 Aplastic anaemia **52**

27 Chemotherapy and related treatments **54**

28 Stem cell transplantation **56**

5 Lymphoma and myeloma 58

29 Hodgkin's lymphoma **58**

30 Non-Hodgkin's lymphoma **60**

31 Myeloma **62**

6 Myeloproliferative neoplasms 64

32 Polycythaemia **64**

33 Essential thrombocythaemia and myelofibrosis **66**

7 Haemostasis and thrombosis 68

34 Thrombocytopenia **68**

35 Disorders of platelet function and vascular purpuras **70**

36 Haemophilia **72**

37 Von Willebrand disease and other inherited coagulation disorders **74**

38 Acquired disorders of coagulation **76**

39 Thrombophilia **78**

40 Anticoagulation and thrombolytic therapy **80**

8 Blood transfusion 82

41 Blood groups and blood testing **82**

42 Clinical practice **84**

9 Special situations 86

43 The immunosuppressed patient **86**

44 Pregnancy **88**

45 Paediatric haematology **90**

46 Haematology in the elderly **92**

47 Palliative care in haematological malignancy **94**

48 Systemic disease **96**

49 The developing world **98**

10 Recent advances in haematology 100

50 Molecular biology **100**

51 Potential advances in treatment **102**

11 Practical procedures 104

52 Venepuncture and venous access **104**

53 Bone marrow aspiration and trephine biopsy **106**

Appendices 108

Case histories 110

Index 115

1 The bone marrow

In early fetal life, blood is produced in the mesoderm of the yolk sac. During the second to seventh months the liver and spleen take over. Only in the last 2 months of fetal development does the bone marrow become the predominant site of blood formation. During childhood, marrow in the more peripheral bones becomes gradually replaced by fat, so that in adult life over 70% is located in the pelvis, vertebrae and sternum (Fig 1.1). This explains the sites used for bone marrow sampling (see p. 106).

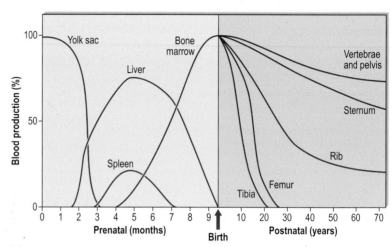

Fig 1.1 **Sites of blood production in the fetus and after birth.**

The structure of the bone marrow

A trephine biopsy allows a two-dimensional view of the bone marrow down the light microscope (Fig 1.2). Haematopoietic cells of varying lineage and maturity are packed between fat spaces and bony trabeculae. Ultrastructural studies reveal clusters of haematopoietic cells surrounding vascular sinuses which allow eventual discharge of mature cells into the blood. Different lineages are compartmentalised; for example, the most immature myeloid precursors lie deep in the marrow parenchyma while more mature forms migrate towards the sinus wall. Lymphocytes tend to surround small radial arteries while erythrocytes form islands around the sinus walls.

Blood precursor cells in the marrow exist in close proximity to stromal cells. Stromal cells are those cells which do not mature into the three main types of peripheral blood cells – thus they include macrophages, fat cells, endothelial cells and reticulum cells.

Immature blood cells are attached to these stromal cells by multiple cellular adhesion molecules (e.g. fibronectin and collagen). Adhesive molecules have specific receptors on stromal and haematopoietic cells. As blood cells mature, the receptors down-regulate and the cells become less adherent and commence the journey through the sinus wall and into the bloodstream.

Fig 1.2 **Normal bone marrow.** Light microscopy of bone marrow trephine biopsy.

Haematopoiesis: the stem cell hierarchy

Haematopoiesis means the formation of blood. A number of transcription factors (e.g. GATA-1, MLL) are critical both for stem cell formation and function and lineage-specific differentiation.

The first adult haematopoietic stem cells (HSCs) are generated in the aorto-gonad-mesonephros (AGM) region of the embryo. The classical hierarchy diagram (Fig 1.3) where all cells arise in orderly fashion from a HSC is helpful but simplified; in reality, HSCs are groups of cells with diverse potentials depending on transcription factors and the local microenvironment. HSCs are not detectable by microscopic techniques but their existence can be inferred from cell cultures. Culture of these early cells on agar generates groups of more mature and thus recognisable progenitor cells known as colony-forming units (CFUs). For myeloid development the earliest

detectable precursor cell creates granulocytes, erythrocytes, monocytes and megakaryocytes and is thus called CFU$_{GEMM}$. HSCs may also be identified and separated from more committed progenitors by the use of flow cytometry as they have a characteristic immunophenotype.

HSCs have the capacity for self-renewal as well as differentiation and the system allows enormous amplification. A lifetime of human haematopoiesis with the generation of incalculable numbers of mature cells may rely on only a few thousand stem cells present at birth. These cells depend on their micoenvironment, the 'niche', for regulation of self-renewal and differentiation. Both haematopoietic and stromal stem cells have the capacity to produce cells associated with other tissues such as bone, liver, lung and muscle. This concept of 'plasticity' has therapeutic implications as stem cells are used to repair a variety of damaged tissues.

Regulators of haematopoiesis

Control of haematopoiesis is mediated via regulatory molecules (or 'growth factors' – Table 1.1). These are generally glycoproteins produced by stroma and differentiated blood cells. They may act on more than one cell lineage and frequently show additive and synergistic interactions with each other. Their actions are multiple, including the promotion of proliferation, differentiation and maturation, as well as changing functional activity. Proliferative regulators alter the behaviour of cells by interacting with specific receptors on the cell surface (Fig 1.4).

Receptors for haematopoietic regulators have been molecularly cloned and many are related in structure (haematopoietic receptor superfamily). The combination of regulator and membrane receptor leads to a structural change in the receptor and the triggering of a complex sequence of biochemical events (signal transduction). The end result is the generation of intracellular regulators in the cell cytoplasm which have the capacity to activate genes, which in turn encode proteins essential in cell activation.

Under normal circumstances regulators circulate in the plasma at virtually unidentifiable levels. The activities of many factors are likely to be localised and transient so that systemic levels are of limited significance. For instance, in the marrow, regulators acting at the earliest stages of haematopoiesis (e.g. c-kit ligand) are released from stromal cells in close proximity to haematopoietic precursor cells.

The colony-stimulating factors (CSFs) were originally defined by their ability to stimulate blood progenitor cells while the interleukins (ILs) were defined by their effects on mature lymphocytes. Subsequent discoveries have rendered this dual nomenclature unhelpful – thus IL-3 is a key stem cell growth factor. The term cytokine incorporates all growth factors.

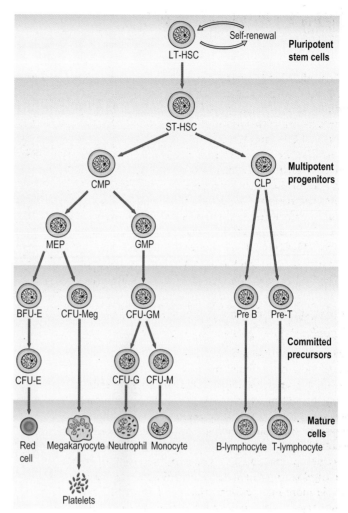

Fig 1.3 **The stem cell hierarchy.** LT-HSC, long-term haematopoietic stem cell; ST-HSC, short-term haematopoietic stem cell; CMP, common myeloid progenitor; CLP, common lymphoid progenitor; MEP, megakaryocyte/erythroid progenitor; GMP, granulocyte/macrophage progenitor; CFU, colony-forming unit; BFU, burst-forming unit; G, granulocyte; E, erythroid; M, monocyte; Meg, megakaryocyte.

Table 1.1 **Key actions of some haematopoietic regulators**

Growth factor	Key actions
Interleukin-1	Mediates acute phase responses; cofactor for other growth factors
Interleukin-2	Growth factor for activated T-lymphocytes
Interleukin-3	Supports early haematopoiesis by promoting growth of stem cells
c-kit ligand (stem cell factor)	Interacts with other factors to stimulate pluripotent stem cells
Erythropoietin	Lineage-specific growth factor promoting production of red cells
GM-CSF	Growth factor promoting production of neutrophils, monocytes, macrophages, eosinophils, red cells and megakaryocytes
G-CSF	Lineage-specific growth factor promoting production of neutrophils
M-CSF	Lineage-specific growth factor promoting monocyte and macrophage production
Thrombopoietin (Mpl ligand)	Lineage-specific growth factor promoting platelet production

CSF, colony-stimulating factor; G, granulocyte; M, macrophage.

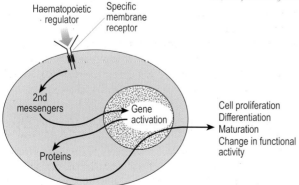

Fig 1.4 **Schematic view of action of regulator on haematopoietic cell.** Second messengers include protein kinase C and calcium ions.

The bone marrow

- The bone marrow is the site of blood formation (haematopoiesis) after birth.

- The cells recognisable in the blood are ultimately all derived from haematopoietic stem cells (HSCs) which reside in a bone marrow 'niche'.

- Immature blood cells in the marrow are attached to stromal cells by multiple cellular adhesion molecules. Maturing blood cells are eventually released through vascular sinus walls into the bloodstream.

- Control of haematopoiesis is mediated via transcription factors and haematopoietic regulators.

2 Red cells

The mature red cells of the blood transport the respiratory gases, oxygen and carbon dioxide (CO_2). Oxygen is carried from the lungs to the tissues, where it is exchanged for CO_2. Red cells are equipped to perform this function for 120 days during which they make a 300 mile journey around the microcirculation.

Prior to discharge from marrow sinuses into the peripheral blood, red cells shed their nuclei. This gives the advantages of reduced weight and transformation into a biconcave disc with increased deformability compared with the more rigid spheroidal nucleated precursor (Fig 2.1).

The blood volume comprises the mass of red cells and the plasma. Plasma volume is regulated by stretch receptors in the heart and kidney which influence secretion of antidiuretic hormone (ADH) and aldosterone. Erythropoiesis is regulated chiefly by the growth factor erythropoietin.

Erythropoietin

Unlike other growth factors, erythropoietin is mainly synthesised by the peritubular endothelial cells of the kidney. Production is triggered by tissue hypoxia (lack of oxygen). Cells can sense hypoxia via mediators such as the transcription factor HIF (hypoxia-inducible factor). HIF activates genes vital in the adaptive response to hypoxia including the erythropoietin gene. Erythropoietin molecules bind to specific membrane receptors on primitive erythroid cells in the bone marrow and induce maturation. The increase in red cells released into the blood stops when normal oxygen transport is restored – this feedback circuit is illustrated in Figure 2.2.

Structure

The mature red cell is around 7.8 μm across and 1.7 μm thick. Its biconcave shape allows maximum flexibility and an umbrella shape is adopted to traverse the smallest capillaries which have diameters of only 5 μm. The ability of red cells to recover from the recurrent stresses of the turbulent circulation hinges on the design of the membrane.

The red cell membrane is composed of a collapsible lattice of specialised proteins (the 'cytoskeleton') and an outer lipid bilayer (Fig 2.3). The protein skeleton is responsible for maintaining red cell shape while the lipid bilayer provides a hydrophobic skin. The main skeletal proteins are spectrin, actin, proteins 4.1 and 4.2, and ankyrin. Spectrin is the most abundant and consists of alpha and beta chains wound around each other. Spectrin heterodimers can align at the ends to form tetramers (i.e. four chains). Spectrin tetramers are joined together by actin in association with protein 4.1. This flexible skeleton is attached to the rest of the membrane by ankyrin, which interacts with protein 4.2 to link the spectrin beta chain to the cytoplasmic end of the transmembrane protein band 3. The lipid bilayer consists mainly of a mixture of phospholipids and cholesterol. Cholesterol molecules are inserted between phospholipid molecules in such a way that they stiffen the membrane while still allowing a degree of fluidity between the bilayers.

Defects of both the red cell membrane proteins and lipids may lead to changes in red cell shape and premature destruction.

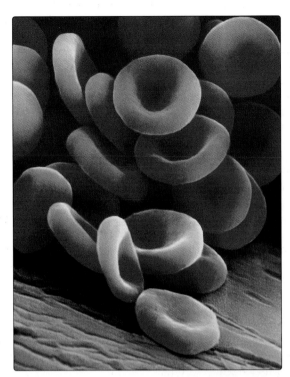

Fig 2.1 **Scanning electron microscope picture of mature red cells showing clearly the characteristic biconcave shape.** (Copyright Dennis Kunkel Microscopy Inc.)

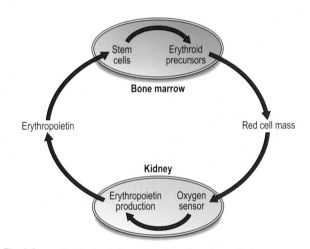

Fig 2.2 **Feedback circuit in production of erythropoietin.**

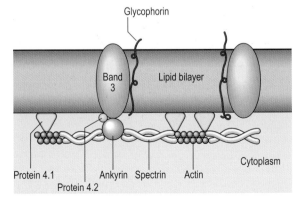

Fig 2.3 **The red cell membrane.**

Metabolism

Red cells require an energy source to maintain their structure and also a mechanism for detoxification of oxidants. Energy is provided by the *Embden–Meyerhof pathway*, a sequence of biochemical reactions in which glucose is metabolised to lactate with the generation of two molecules of adenosine triphosphate (ATP). ATP maintains the osmotic pressure of the cell by driving sodium and calcium pumps in the membrane. It also provides energy for the cytoskeletal changes needed for recovery of cell shape. The Embden–Meyerhof pathway does not require oxygen as a substrate but a small amount of oxidative glycolysis occurs by the *hexose monophosphate shunt* (pentose phosphate pathway) in which glucose-6-phosphate is metabolised to generate nicotinamide adenine dinucleotide phosphate (NADPH). The hexose monophosphate shunt plays a vital role in oxygen detoxification and when oxidised substrates accumulate in the cell it increases activity several fold. Inherited deficiencies of red cell enzymes in either the Embden–Meyerhof pathway (e.g. pyruvate kinase) or the hexose monophosphate shunt (e.g. glucose-6-phosphate dehydrogenase) can lead to shortened red cell survival and haemolytic anaemia (see p. 29).

Haemoglobin and oxygen transport

The key function of red cells, to carry oxygen to the tissues and return CO_2 from the tissues to the lungs, depends on the specialised protein haemoglobin which is present in large amounts in mature cells. The normal adult haemoglobin molecule (HbA) contains four polypeptide chains ('globin' chains): the two alpha chains and two beta chains are often notated as $\alpha_2\beta_2$. Combined with each of the polypeptide chains is a 'haem' molecule which contains ferrous iron (Fe^{2+}) and protoporphyrin (Fig 2.4). The iron combines reversibly with oxygen and thus haem forms the oxygen-carrying part of the molecule. Other globin chains are formed by the fetus and the change from fetal to adult haemoglobin occurs in the first 3–6 months of life. However, the subunits designated γ and δ persist into later life and small amounts of fetal haemoglobin (HbF; $\alpha_2\gamma_2$) and HbA_2 ($\alpha_2\delta_2$) are found in adults.

Haemoglobin is more than an inert carrier molecule. The individual globin chains interact with each other to facilitate the offloading of oxygen at lower oxygen saturations. The metabolite 2,3-diphosphoglyceride (2,3-DPG) generated in a side-arm of the Embden–Meyerhof pathway has an important role in the process, which results in a sigmoid-shaped oxygen dissociation curve (Fig 2.5). In anatomical terms haemoglobin has a high affinity for oxygen in the lungs and a much lower affinity in the tissues. The oxygen dissociation curve moves to the left when oxygen affinity increases; this occurs when H^+ ion concentration is reduced or haemoglobin F (which cannot bind 2,3-DPG) raised. The curve moves to the right when oxygen affinity decreases; for instance when 2,3-DPG concentration rises or the abnormal sickle haemoglobin (HbS) is present. The P_{50} level is defined as the partial pressure of oxygen at which haemoglobin is half saturated.

Ageing and death

Beyond 100 days red cells start to show features of ageing including a declining rate of glycolysis, reduced levels of ATP and membrane lipid, and a loss of flexibility. The terminal event is unclear but effete cells are removed from the circulation by the macrophages of the liver and spleen.

Most of the catabolised haemoglobin, particularly the iron, is reused (see also p. 24). The protoporphyrin of haem is metabolised to the yellow pigment bilirubin which is bound to albumin in the plasma. Bilirubin is conjugated in the liver to a water-soluble diglucuronide that is converted to stercobilin and stercobilinogen and excreted in the faeces. Some stercobilin and stercobilinogen are reabsorbed from the intestine and excreted in the urine as urobilin and urobilinogen.

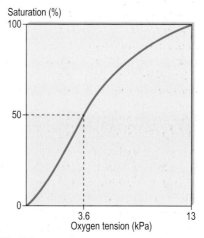

Fig 2.5 **The oxygen dissociation curve.** The P_{50} is 3.6 kPa in normal red cells.

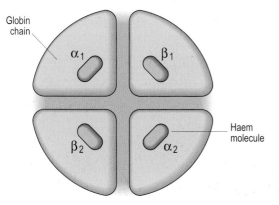

Fig 2.4 **The essential elements of the haemoglobin molecule.** In reality each globin chain has a complex helical structure. The α chain has 141 amino acids and the β chain 146. The haem molecule consists of four pyrrole rings arranged around a ferrous ion.

> ### Red cells
>
> - Erythropoiesis (the formation of red cells) is regulated by the growth factor erythropoietin.
>
> - Mature red cells have a biconcave disc shape and no nucleus.
>
> - The red cell membrane consists of a lattice of specialised proteins and an outer lipid bilayer.
>
> - Red cells derive energy principally from the metabolism of glucose to lactate (Embden–Meyerhof pathway).
>
> - Red cells contain a specialised protein, haemoglobin, which allows carriage of oxygen to the tissues and return of CO_2 from the tissues to the lungs.

3 Neutrophils, eosinophils, basophils and monocytes

The term 'white cells' or 'leucocytes' refers to the nucleated cells of the blood – the neutrophils, lymphocytes, monocytes, eosinophils and basophils. All these cells play a role in defending the host against infection and other insults. Neutrophils, monocytes, eosinophils and basophils are phagocytes. They engulf and destroy foreign material and damaged cells. The term 'granulocytes' may be used to particularly describe neutrophils, eosinophils and basophils.

Neutrophils

The blood neutrophil (Fig 3.1a) is the end-product of an orchestrated sequence of differentiation in the myeloid cells of the bone marrow. The mature cell has a multi-lobed nucleus and four different types of granules in the cytoplasm. Neutrophils have a limited lifespan of around 5–6 days in the blood. Approximately half the cells are included in a normal blood count (the circulating pool), the remainder being in the 'marginal pool'. The essential function of all these cells is to enter the tissues and combat infection. This requires both migration to the site of infection or tissue injury (chemotaxis) and the destruction of foreign material (phagocytosis). Normal chemotaxis is dependent on the release of chemotactic factors generated by bacteria and leucocytes already present at the infection site. Neutrophils may migrate intravascularly as they navigate healthy tissues to reach the site of tissue injury.

Neutrophil mobility is imbued both by the presence of adhesion molecules on the cell surface and by an actin–myosin assembly in the cell membrane, the latter mediating the movement necessary for locomotion and phagocytosis. Once the cell is at the target site the foreign antigen or particle is recognised via cell surface receptors and engulfed within a phagocytic vacuole. There are various methods of killing; key mechanisms are the generation of nitric oxide and antimicrobial proteins, and oxidative metabolism in which antimicrobial oxidants are formed (the 'respiratory burst'). Cytokines such as G-CSF and GM-CSF (see p. 3) not only increase neutrophil production but also promote chemotaxis and phagocytosis.

In clinical practice an increase in neutrophils in the blood ('neutrophil leucocytosis' or 'neutrophilia') is a common

Fig 3.1 **Leucocytes in the blood. (a)** Neutrophils; **(b)** neutrophil with phagocytosed bacteria; **(c)** eosinophil; **(d)** basophil; **(e)** monocyte.

accompaniment to infection and tissue injury (Table 3.1). The strain on the neutrophil compartment often leads to younger 'band forms' being discharged from the marrow into the bloodstream and the appearance of toxic changes, including coarsened granulation and vacuolation. Occasionally, phagocytosed bacteria are visible (Fig 3.1b).

Reduced neutrophils in the blood (neutropenia) is seen in a wide range of inherited and acquired disorders. Serious infection is not seen regularly until the count falls below 0.5×10^9/L. Neutropenia may be an isolated abnormality or associated with a pancytopenia. Some causes of an isolated neutropenia are listed in Table 3.2. In general, neutropenia may be caused by underproduction from the marrow (e.g. leukaemia), reduced neutrophil lifespan (e.g. immune neutropenia), or pooling of neutrophils in a large spleen. It is important to remember that drugs may be responsible. The term *chronic benign neutropenia* is generally used in patients who have an isolated moderate neutropenia with no clear aetiology and a benign course. There may be an associated monocytosis. There is some ethnic variation in neutrophil counts with black people having a lower normal reference range than white people. In the rare genetic disorder *cyclical neutropenia*, the neutrophil count falls every 15–35 days and recurrent infections occur.

In addition to quantitative abnormalities, neutrophils can be functionally abnormal. There are several rare inherited diseases characterised by impaired neutrophil adherence, chemotaxis or bactericidal activity. In *chronic granulomatous disease*, neutrophils are able to phagocytose but not kill catalase-positive microorganisms. Inheritance is autosomal or X-linked and patients suffer recurrent purulent infections and associated granuloma formation. Diagnosis is made in the nitroblue tetrazolium test where the patient's neutrophils fail to reduce the dye.

Eosinophils

Eosinophils (Fig 3.1c) are characterised by their two-lobed nucleus and red-orange staining granules. They have significant proinflammatory and cytotoxic activity and play a role in the pathogenesis of various allergic, parasitic and neoplastic disorders. Interleukin 5 is a key mediator of eosinophil differentiation and activation.

Table 3.1 **Causes of a neutrophil leucocytosis**
■ Physiological (e.g. pregnancy)
■ Bacterial infections
■ Inflammatory diseases (e.g. vasculitis, inflammatory bowel disease)
■ Trauma/surgery
■ Malignancy
■ Acute haemorrhage
■ Severe metabolic disorders (e.g. diabetic ketoacidosis)
■ Myeloproliferative diseases (e.g. chronic myeloid leukaemia)
■ Iatrogenic (e.g. treatment with growth factors, corticosteroids)

Table 3.2 **Causes of an isolated neutropenia**[1]
■ Drugs[2]
■ Idiopathic/benign/constitutional
■ Congenital (Kostmann's syndrome)
■ Cyclical neutropenia
■ Autoimmune (sometimes with a connective tissue disorder)
■ Infections (e.g. viral, typhoid, tuberculosis)

[1] Most bone marrow diseases (e.g. leukaemia, aplastic anaemia) cause a pancytopenia.
[2] Some drugs are well-documented causes (e.g. penicillin, co-trimoxazole, carbimazole, phenothiazines) but in practice any agent the patient is taking should be viewed with suspicion.

The most common causes of eosinophilia in the Western world are allergic disorders such as asthma, eczema and hay fever. In developing countries, parasitic infections are frequently implicated. Other relatively common aetiologies are drug hypersensitivity, malignancy, various skin diseases and connective tissue disorders. *Hypereosinophilic syndrome* is characterised by a marked sustained eosinophilia and associated tissue damage. The disorder is very variable with several subtypes. The myeloproliferative variant is associated with a *FIP1L1-PDGFRA* fusion gene and often responds to imatinib (see p. 45).

Basophils

Basophils are the least numerous of the blood leucocytes. They are easily recognised by their abundant dark purple cytoplasmic granules (Fig 3.1d). The granules contain mediators of acute inflammation, including heparin and histamine. Basophils and their tissue equivalent, mast cells, have receptors for the Fc portion of IgE. They play a central role in immediate hypersensitivity reactions. Basophilia is usually associated with myeloproliferative disorders (e.g. chronic myeloid leukaemia). However, it may be reactive to a range of systemic diseases including inflammatory bowel disease and hypothyroidism. It sometimes occurs during the recovery phase from acute infection.

Monocytes

Monocytes circulate in the blood before entering the tissues where they undergo transformation into macrophages. Monocyte colony-stimulating factor (M-CSF) is vital for monocyte and macrophage development and activation. The 'mononuclear phagocyte' system consisting of monocytes and macrophages is a potentially confusing concept as macrophages subserve different functions and adopt discrete nomenclature in different tissues (e.g. osteoclasts in bone, Kuppfer cells in liver). Macrophages are phagocytic cells but unlike neutrophils are able to survive the phagocytic event. They also act as accessory cells in the immune response by presenting antigens to T-lymphocytes (see p. 8) and secreting a wide range of cytokines involved in inflammation, immunity and haematopoiesis.

Blood monocytes typically have a kidney-shaped nucleus (Fig 3.1e). A monocytosis in the blood occurs in chronic bacterial infections such as tuberculosis and may accompany a wide range of infective, inflammatory and malignant disorders. Monocytopenia is less frequently noted but can be severe in patients receiving corticosteroid treatment.

Neutrophils, eosinophils, basophils and monocytes

■ The white cells of the blood (leucocytes) play a key role in defending the host against infection and other insults.

■ Neutrophils, monocytes, eosinophils and basophils are phagocytes.

■ These phagocytic cells may perform other functions; monocytes act as accessory cells presenting antigens to T-lymphocytes.

■ Each cell has a characteristic morphological appearance in the blood film.

■ Changes in leucocyte numbers (e.g. neutrophil leucocytosis) are common accompaniments of various disease states.

4 Lymphocytes

Lymphocytes are found in large numbers in blood, lymph (the clear fluid of the lymphatic vessels) and in lymphoid organs such as the thymus, lymph nodes and spleen. They are essential for immunity. B-lymphocytes produce antibody against a specific antigen (humoral immunity) while T-lymphocytes are the cells of the cell-mediated response. Primary lymphoid organs (bone marrow, thymus) are the sites of lymphoid development. In the secondary lymphoid organs (lymph nodes, spleen), mature lymphocytes meet antigens and the immune response is triggered.

Most mature lymphocytes appear under the light microscope as cells with round nuclei and a thin rim of agranular cytoplasm (Fig 4.1). Although B- and T-cells are not distinguishable by their morphology, there are major differences in their mode of maturation and function.

T-lymphocytes

T-cells make up 75% of the lymphocytes of the blood and form the basis of cell-mediated immunity. They are less autonomous than their B-cell companions, needing the cooperation of antigen-presenting cells expressing self-histocompatibility molecules (human leucocyte antigens (HLA)) for the recognition of the antigen by the T-cell receptor (TCR) (Fig 4.2).

T-cells originate in the marrow but many are destroyed in subsequent processing by the thymus, the objective being to select the minority of cells which will recognise self-HLA but not react with self-tissue antigens. The maturation sequence is characterised by changing patterns of cell surface molecules (Fig 4.3). Mature T-cells are divisible into two basic types. About two-thirds of blood T-cells are 'helper' cells expressing the surface marker CD4, while the remainder express CD8 and are mostly of 'cytotoxic' type.

It appears that helper cells recognise the combination of antigen and self-HLA class II molecules on the antigen-presenting cell, and cytotoxic cells bind with antigen in conjunction with HLA class I molecules on the target cell (Fig 4.2). TCR genes, like Ig genes, are subject to rearrangement of germ-line DNA. Following triggering of T-cells by specific antigen reacting with the TCR, the clonal proliferation of activated T-cells is sustained by the secretion of cytokines. Interleukin-2 is the main T-cell growth factor.

Fig 4.1 **Mature lymphocytes in the blood.**

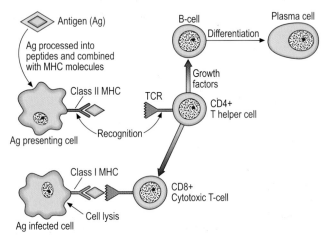

Fig 4.2 **Interaction of T-lymphocyte and antigen-presenting cells.** The T-cell receptor complex (TCR) recognises the combination of processed antigen and major histocompatibility complex (MHC) molecule and the immune response is initiated.

B-lymphocytes

B-lymphocytes are responsible for humoral immunity. Following an appropriate antigenic stimulus they transform into plasma cells and secrete antibody specific to that antigen.

B-cells are derived from the stem cells of the bone marrow. Unlike T-cells it is not clear whether they are subject to further

PC : plasmacytoid   Ig : immunoglobulin
(a)

TCR : T-cell receptor
(b)

Fig 4.3 **Maturation of B- and T-lymphocytes. (a)** B-lymphocyte maturation in the bone marrow. **(b)** T-lymphocyte development in the bone marrow and thymus.

processing at a site outside the marrow in humans. The various stages of B-cell maturation are illustrated in Figure 4.3. Each cell can be defined by its expression of membrane and cytoplasmic antigens in addition to the stage of immunoglobulin gene rearrangement. Within the lymphoid tissues, such as the lymph nodes and spleen, mature unactivated or virgin B-cells can be stimulated by antigen to undergo a morphological transformation into immunoblasts and, ultimately, plasma cells.

Stimulation of a single B-cell by antigen combining with its cell surface immunoglobulin variable region leads to a sequence of proliferation and differentiation resulting in a clone of immunoglobulin-secreting plasma cells. This adaptive immune response is antigen-specific and is facilitated by helper T-cells and cytokine-secreting macrophages. Memories of particular antigens are immortalised by 'memory' B-cells, allowing a prompt response to reinfection. The *immunoglobulins* secreted by lymphocytes and plasma cells are heterogeneous proteins, each designed to interact with a specific antigen in the defence of the body against infection (Fig 4.4). There are five subclasses of immunoglobulin (Ig), dependent on the type of heavy chain (IgG, IgA, IgM, IgD and IgE), with some further division of subclasses (e.g. IgG_{1-4}). IgM is generally produced as the initial response to infection, followed by a more prolonged production of IgG.

IgA is found in secretions, while IgE plays a role in delayed hypersensitivity reactions.

The genes encoding the heavy and light chains of immunoglobulin are rearranged from their germ-line configuration during early B-cell maturation. The variable (V), diverse (D), joining (J) and constant (C) region exons undergo a complex sequence of DNA splicing, deletions and juxtapositions. The rationale of this frenetic activity prior to transcription is to allow the totality of B-cells to produce an enormously diverse population of immunoglobulins (antibodies) targeting a vast number of potential antigens. Lymphocytes that can react against self-molecules are usually functionally inactivated or deleted so that the adaptive immune system normally only targets foreign antigens (natural immunological tolerance).

Natural killer (NK) cells

NK cells are a subset of lymphocytes which share many of the characteristics of cytotoxic T-cells. However, NK cells do not rearrange or express TCR genes. They particularly kill target cells that poorly express class I MHC and are less able to signal viral infection to cytotoxic T-cells. NK cells express two classes of receptors which either activate or inhibit their killing role. Activating receptors bind to a variety of ligands on the target cell whereas the inhibitory receptors generally bind to HLA class I molecules.

In the blood film, NK cells appear as large lymphocytes with abundant cytoplasmic granules.

Changes in disease

An increase in lymphocytes in the blood (lymphocytosis) is generally a reaction to infection or is part of a malignancy. A polyclonal T-cell lymphocytosis is a common response to viral infection, particularly in childhood. Lymphocytes may be morphologically abnormal with variable changes including increased size and cytoplasmic basophilia. These heterogeneous atypical lymphocytes are seen in numerous viral infections but they are a particular feature of infectious mononucleosis (see p. 97).

A number of lymphoid malignancies are associated with lymphocytosis (Table 4.1). In acute lymphoblastic leukaemia and 'spill-over' of non-Hodgkin's lymphoma cells into the blood, the malignant lymphocytes are usually morphologically distinctive and confusion with a reactive lymphocytosis rarely occurs. In chronic lymphocytic leukaemia (CLL), the lymphocytes often appear unremarkable although the presence of disrupted forms, termed 'smear cells', is characteristic.

Lymphocyte counts are often transiently low after surgery and trauma. A more chronic lymphopenia is a feature of ongoing cytotoxic drug treatment and late HIV infection when CD4 counts fall to low levels.

V = variable (antibody binding) region
C = constant region

Fig 4.4 **Basic immunoglobulin structure.** The 'Fab' portion is involved in antigen binding and the 'Fc' portion attaches to macrophages or lymphocytes expressing the relevant 'Fc' receptor.

Table 4.1 **Common causes of a lymphocytosis**	
Infections	Acute viral infections (e.g. pertussis, infectious mononucleosis, rubella)
	Chronic infections (e.g. tuberculosis, toxoplasmosis)
Malignancy	Chronic lymphocytic leukaemia and variants
	Non-Hodgkin's lymphoma (minority)
	Acute lymphoblastic leukaemia

Lymphocytes

- Lymphocytes are essential for normal immunity.

- B-lymphocytes respond to an appropriate antigen by transforming into plasma cells and secreting specific antibody (humoral immunity).

- T-lymphocytes cooperate with antigen-presenting cells in the recognition of antigen; recognition triggers a clonal proliferation of activated T-cells (cell-mediated immunity).

- The genes encoding immunoglobulin chains and the T-cell receptor are subject to rearrangement of germ-line DNA.

- Various disease states lead to an increase in blood lymphocyte numbers (lymphocytosis): in those over 50 years, chronic lymphocytic leukaemia is a common cause.

5 The spleen

Although the spleen has been known of since ancient times, its function has remained obscure until relatively recently. Hippocrates thought it was the source of 'black bile'. Galen suggested it might be a filter, in view of its spongy consistency. Our current understanding of the spleen is dependent on a detailed appreciation of its vascular supply and the organisation of its main component parts: the lymphoid white pulp, the blood-containing red pulp and the intervening marginal zone.

Structure

The spleen is derived from condensation of the mesoderm in the dorsal mesogastrium of the embryo. It plays a modest haematopoietic role in the middle part of fetal life, but in the adult haematopoiesis is usually only seen in pathological states. An average adult spleen weighs about 150 g and it has to become enlarged to at least three times its normal size before becoming palpable on clinical examination (p. 17).

The splenic artery penetrates the thick capsule which invests the organ (Fig 5.1). Branches of the splenic artery are surrounded by a highly organised aggregate of lymphoid tissue which is termed the 'white pulp' (Fig 5.2). Intimate to the central arteriole is the 'periarteriolar lymphatic sheath' – an area mainly populated by T-lymphocytes. Among these T-lymphocytes are non-phagocytic, antigen-presenting cells known as 'interdigitating cells'. Spaced at intervals in the periarteriolar lymphatic sheath are lymphoid follicles ('Malpighian bodies'). In an inactive state these follicles are composed of recirculating B-lymphocytes intertwined with cytoplasmic processes of follicular dendritic cells. The latter cells may play a role in long-term antibody production. When contact with antigen stimulates B-cell activation, a germinal centre of rapidly dividing cells forms in the follicle. This is a key area in the normal B-lymphocyte proliferative response and development of B-cell memory (see p. 8 for discussion of lymphocytes).

The periarteriolar lymphatic sheath and B-lymphocyte follicles are separated from the red pulp by a 'marginal zone' constituted mainly of non-circulating B-cells. The marginal zone also contains specialised macrophages able to take up carbohydrate antigens. The red pulp is composed of two alternating structures: the splenic sinuses and the splenic cords (the 'cords of Billroth'). The cords are a reticular meshwork packed with macrophages and antibody-secreting plasma cells. The sinuses are broad channels lined with fusiform endothelial cells.

Most of the central arterioles open into the marginal zone. As alluded to already, circulating T-lymphocytes move into the periarteriolar lymphatic sheath and B-lymphocytes migrate to the follicles. Other blood cells move slowly through the complex meshwork of the red pulp, and cells which are sufficiently deformable and compliant squeeze between the endothelial cells in the sinus wall into the lumen of the sinus and back into the circulation. The organisation of the spleen into the different compartments is under the control of various cytokines and adhesion molecules.

Function

The spleen has two key functions. It removes older red cells, blood-borne microorganisms and cellular debris from the blood. It also plays a vital role in the body's response to bacterial and fungal infections.

It clears unwanted red cells and particles from the blood in three ways. Firstly, they can be removed by phagocytes. Bacteria, particularly encapsulated organisms that are not opsonised by antibodies and complement, are cleared from the circulation. The spleen is probably the site of the initial immune response to these organisms. Phagocytic cells in the spleen also remove red cells coated with IgG antibody.

The second mechanism at work is the removal of red cells which are not sufficiently deformable to pass through the sinus wall. Pathological states where red cells lose deformability and are destroyed prematurely in the spleen include sickle cell anaemia, hereditary spherocytosis and malaria.

Finally, the spleen can remove debris or organisms from within cells. Howell–Jolly bodies (fragments of nucleus) and malarial parasites are removed when most of the cell passes through the inter-endothelial slit with the intracellular particle abandoned on the cord side.

The spleen has the capacity to mount complex innate and adaptive immune responses. Both types of response occur in the marginal zone, rich in macrophages and marginal zone B-cells, while the white pulp is limited to adaptive immunity.

Abnormal splenic states

Asplenism and hyposplenism

Surgical removal of the spleen (splenectomy) may be indicated in a variety of haematological disorders and following trauma. The spleen may also be absent as a congenital anomaly, often associated with transpositions or malformations of the great vessels and viscera ('asplenia syndrome'). Reduced splenic function can result from splenic atrophy in disorders such as sickle cell anaemia,

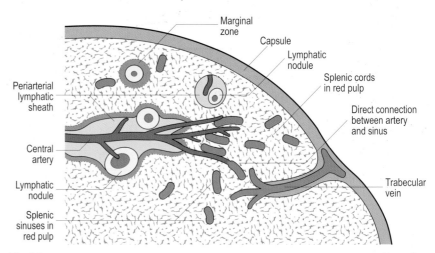

Fig 5.1 **Structure of the spleen.** The white pulp is composed of the periarteriolar lymphatic sheath and lymphatic nodules. The red pulp contains the splenic cords and sinuses and is separated from the white pulp by the marginal zone. See text for full discussion.

Fig 5.2 **Light microscopy of the spleen clearly showing the distribution of red and white pulp.**

Fig 5.3 **The blood film in hyposplenism.** A Howell–Jolly body is seen within a red cell. There are target cells and acanthocytes.

adult coeliac disease and essential thrombocythaemia (Table 5.1).

Hyposplenism leads to characteristic changes in the blood film (Fig 5.3). Changes in red cell appearance include the presence of Howell–Jolly bodies, Pappenheimer (siderotic) granules and target cells. Other less regular red cell features are lipid-rich acanthocytes and circulating nucleated cells. There is often a moderate rise in the lymphocyte, monocyte and platelet count. Approximately one-third of circulating platelets are pooled in the normal spleen. The increase in platelets post-splenectomy is frequently impressive (greater than $1000 \times 10^9/L$) but the count usually falls to a lower level in the longer term. Quantitation of splenic function is not straightforward. Methods include the measurement of the percentage of pitted erythrocytes using interference phase microscopy, various immunological parameters and scintigraphy.

The clinical significance of an absent spleen is the associated increased risk of life-threatening infection. The risk is greatest in children under 5 years of age and where there is a serious underlying medical disorder such as Hodgkin's lymphoma or thalassaemia. Most infections occur within 2 years of splenectomy but fulminating infection can strike at any stage. In most cases infection is with encapsulated bacteria, notably *Streptococcus pneumoniae*, *Haemophilus influenzae* and *Neisseria meningitidis*. In temperate regions more than half of serious infections are caused by the pneumococcus, with high mortality. Splenectomised patients have an increased susceptibility to severe malaria. Prophylaxis against such infections is the best approach and recommendations for the management of asplenic patients are shown in Table 5.2.

Table 5.1 **Causes of hyposplenism**

- Congenital absence of spleen
- Splenectomy
- Sickle cell anaemia
- Coeliac disease
- Essential thrombocythaemia
- Dermatitis herpetiformis
- Inflammatory bowel disease
- Amyloidosis
- Advanced age

Hypersplenism

Hypersplenism is usually defined as a depression of one or more of the cell counts in the blood which can be wholly attributed to splenic enlargement. Other criteria such as the presence of a normal bone marrow, or correction of cytopenia by splenectomy may be appended. Although the definition only requires an isolated anaemia, leucopenia or thrombocytopenia, there is frequently a moderate pancytopenia.

Splenomegaly is not always associated with hypersplenism, and hypersplenism can occur irrespective of the degree of splenic enlargement. Thus, it may be seen in the modest splenomegaly of liver cirrhosis.

The pancytopenia of hypersplenism is probably induced by three contributory mechanisms:

Table 5.2 **Management recommendations in the asplenic patient**

Immunisation[1]	Pneumococcus, *Haemophilus influenzae* type B, group C meningococcus, influenza
Antibiotic prophylaxis[2]	Oral phenoxymethylpenicillin or erythromycin
Prompt treatment of infection	Patients need systemic antibiotics and urgent admission to hospital
Medicalert disc or card	Detailing asplenic state and medical contacts
Avoid travel to high-risk malarial areas	

[1]*Where possible at least 2 weeks prior to splenectomy. Reimmunisation is usually required, the timing determined by measurement of specific antibody levels.*
[2]*The duration of antibiotic prophylaxis is controversial but should generally be 'lifelong'.*

- Hypervolaemia consequent upon a disproportionately expanded plasma volume filling the vascular space of the enlarged spleen and the splanchnic bed.
- Intrasplenic pooling of red cells which is increased from the normal 5–15% to 40% in moderate splenomegaly. This is accompanied by pooling of neutrophils and platelets.
- Premature destruction of circulating blood cells.

The spleen

- The spleen is organised into three main components: the white pulp, the red pulp and the intervening marginal zone.
- The spleen acts as a filter, removing unwanted red cells and particles from the blood.
- The spleen can mount complex adaptive immune responses.
- An absent or poorly functioning spleen leads to characteristic blood changes and an increased risk of overwhelming infection, including fulminating malaria.
- An enlarged spleen (splenomegaly) may cause 'hypersplenism' with reduced cell counts in the blood.

6 Haemostasis

Blood clotting is a critical defence mechanism which, in conjunction with inflammatory and general repair responses, helps protect the integrity of the vascular system after injury. The complex sequence of events described in detail below is activated within seconds of tissue damage. It is easiest to divide the description of normal haemostasis into a platelet component, with formation of a loose platelet plug at the site of injury, and a coagulation component, where there is generation of a more robust fibrin scaffold (thrombus) around the platelets. This approach facilitates understanding but in practice the two mechanisms are inextricably linked.

The role of platelets

Following damage to a blood vessel there is immediate vasoconstriction to slow blood flow and reduce the risk of exsanguination. The break in the endothelial cell barrier leads to the recruitment of platelets from the circulation to form an occlusive plug. Platelets interact both with the vessel subendothelial matrix (platelet 'adhesion') and with each other (platelet 'aggregation') (Fig 6.1). The first step in this process, adhesion, does not require platelet metabolic activity. It does, however, lead to the 'activation' of platelets.

Platelets are small disc-shaped particles produced in megakaryocyte cytoplasm which have a lifespan of around

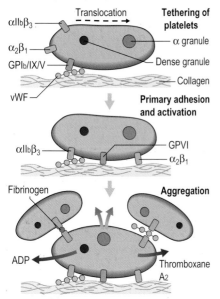

Fig 6.1 **Primary platelet adhesion, activation and aggregation.** vWF, von Willebrand factor.

10 days. They have no nucleus and no capacity for DNA biosynthesis but do have a complex infrastructure. Pores in the trilaminar platelet membrane connect with an open canalicular system allowing transport of agonists in and discharge of secretions out. The membrane receptors for agonists include:

- the glycoprotein (GP) Ia/IIa complex ($\alpha_2\beta_1$ integrin) and glycoprotein (GP) VI which are receptors for collagen
- the GPIb/IX/V complex, a receptor for vessel wall von Willebrand factor (vWF) and thrombin
- the GPIIb/IIIa complex ($\alpha_{IIb}\beta_3$ integrin), which is an agonist-induced receptor for fibrinogen and vWF (vWF is discussed in more detail on p. 74).

In the platelet cytoplasm are organelles including alpha granules (containing fibrinogen, vWF, thrombospondin and other proteins) and dense granules (containing small molecules such as ADP and calcium).

Platelet activation follows stimulation by agonists such as ADP and thromboxane A_2 interacting with surface receptors, or by direct contact with the vessel wall subendothelial matrix. Platelets convert from a compact disc to a sphere, surface receptors become activated, and cytoplasmic granules secrete their contents. The net effect is the mediation and reinforcement of aggregation and adhesion, and the promotion of further activation. Other circulating platelets adhere to the initial layer and a loose platelet plug is formed.

In addition to the formation of a physical barrier at the site of injury, platelets have a procoagulant action. The coagulation sequence described below completes much more rapidly in the presence of platelets. Following activation, platelets rearrange their membrane phospholipids and shed vesicles from their surface. The platelet surface and vesicles reveal binding sites for coagulation proteins leading to the creation of coagulation complexes (e.g. the 'prothrombinase complex') which accelerate formation of factor Xa and thrombin.

Coagulation

Although often loosely used to encompass all aspects of clot formation, the term 'coagulation' more specifically

refers to the mechanism directly leading to the conversion of the soluble plasma protein fibrinogen to the insoluble rigid polymer fibrin. The formation of the stable haemostatic plug composed of enmeshed fibrin and platelets is the culmination of a complex biochemical cascade involving circulating *coagulation factors*. This system allows extreme amplification with a robust thrombus arising from the initial stimulus of tissue injury. Most activated coagulation factors are proteolytic enzymes (serine proteases) which in the presence of cofactors cleave other factors in an ordered sequence. Thus, prothrombin (factor II), factor VII, factor IX and factor X are proenzymes which are converted to their active enzyme form (denoted by the letter 'a') by cleavage of one or two peptide bonds. Factors V and VIII are procofactors which are converted to the active cofactors (Va and VIIIa) also by cleavage of peptide bonds. The blood clotting proenzymes prothrombin and factors VII, IX and X require vitamin K for their activation (see pp. 76, 77).

The coagulation cascade, leading to the generation of thrombin and the formation of a fibrin thrombus, is classically divided into two parts: the intrinsic and extrinsic pathways (Table 6.1).

In the intrinsic pathway factor XII is activated by exposed collagen and other negatively charged components of the subendothelium. Activation of factor XII leads to the sequential activation of factors XI, IX, VIII (as cofactor), X and prothrombin. In the extrinsic pathway tissue factor complexes with factor VII with sequential activation of factors VII, X and prothrombin. Both intrinsic and extrinsic pathways terminate in the final common pathway where activated factor X, in association with the cofactor factor Va in the presence of phospholipid and calcium, converts prothrombin into thrombin. Thrombin in turn converts fibrinogen to fibrin by splitting the fibrinopeptides A and B from the centre domain to form fibrin monomers. These monomers combine spontaneously into dimers which assemble to form the fibrin polymer. Factor XIII crosslinks the fibrin polymer to consolidate the thrombus. The conventional division into two pathways is useful in the interpretation of in vitro laboratory tests of haemostasis. The prothrombin time (PT) is a simple measure of the function of the extrinsic pathway and the activated partial thrombo-plastin time (APTT) monitors the intrinsic pathway (p. 20). However, the physiological pathways at work in vivo are not so simply defined (see Fig 6.2). It seems that the intrinsic pathway is rarely relevant to coagulation in vivo – patients with hereditary deficiency of factor XII have a prolonged APTT but no bleeding disorder. The crucial protein in the initiation of blood coagulation is tissue factor, an integral membrane protein expressed on non-vascular cells. When a blood vessel is damaged, circulating factor VII comes into contact with tissue factor. The tissue factor/factor VIIa complex activates not only factor X (the extrinsic pathway) but also factor IX.

Regulation of coagulation

Blood coagulation is modulated by three major inhibitory systems:

- **Anti-thrombin.** This is the most important inhibitor of the terminal proteins of the cascade, particularly factor Xa

and thrombin. Its activity is greatly increased by interaction with heparin in the microvasculature and on the surface of endothelial cells.
- **Proteins C and S.** Protein C is a vitamin K-dependent plasma protein which inactivates the cofactors Va and VIIIa and stimulates fibrinolysis. Protein C is converted to its active enzymic form by interaction with thrombin. Protein S acts as a cofactor for protein C.
- **Tissue factor pathway inhibitor (TFPI).** TFPI inactivates factor Xa and then the TFPI/factor Xa complex inhibits factor VIIa within the VIIa/tissue factor complex.

Fibrinolysis

Once damaged endothelium is repaired the fibrin thrombus must be removed to restore normal blood flow. Thrombus removal is facilitated by a fibrin-splitting serine protease, plasmin. The fibrinolytic system is shown schematically in Figure 6.3. Release of tissue plasminogen activator (t-PA) from endothelial cells leads to conversion of the proenzyme plasminogen into plasmin. t-PA is most active when bound to fibrin, thus maximising its action at the site of the thrombus. Plasmin has the capacity to digest fibrin in addition to fibrinogen and a number of other proteins. Digestion of a cross-linked thrombus by plasmin leads to the formation of 'degradation products' which themselves act as anticoagulants. Fibrinolysis is under strict control; circulating plasmin is inactivated by the protease inhibitor α_2-antiplasmin.

Table 6.1 **The classic coagulation cascade**	
Intrinsic pathway	
Factor XIIa + Kallikrein → XIa → IXa → Xa	**Final common pathway**
Extrinsic pathway	
Factor VIIa – Tissue factor → Xa	Factor Xa → Thrombin → Fibrin

Fig 6.3 **The fibrinolytic system.** Note that, unlike the other activators listed, streptokinase is an exogenous activator derived from β-haemolytic streptococci.

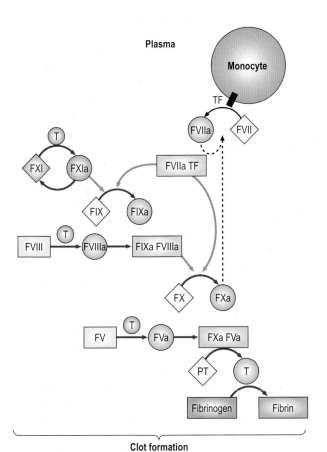

Fig 6.2 **Physiological pathways of blood coagulation.** Green arrows indicate the action of enzymes on substrates; red arrows indicate the conversion of a protein from one functional state to another after the cleavage of one or more peptide bonds. F, factor; TF, tissue factor; T, thrombin; PT, prothrombin. Reprinted with permission from Furie B, Furie BC 2004 Role of platelet P-selectin and microparticle PSGL-1 in thrombus formation. Trends in Molecular Medicine 10(4):171–178.

Haemostasis

- The clotting of blood is a critical defence mechanism protecting the integrity of the vascular system after injury.
- Platelets form an occlusive plug at the site of tissue injury. They also have procoagulant action.
- The term 'coagulation' describes the process by which fibrinogen is converted to the insoluble rigid polymer fibrin; the final thrombus is formed of enmeshed fibrin and platelets.
- The term 'coagulation cascade' describes the sequential activation of coagulation factors; in vivo the major initiator of coagulation is tissue factor.
- Fibrin generation is regulated by naturally occurring anticoagulants and fibrin is ultimately removed by the 'fibrinolytic system'.

7 History taking

Abnormalities of the blood are associated with a wide range of symptoms and these are discussed in detail under diagnostic headings in subsequent sections. The intention of this section is to give an overview of history taking in patients with blood disorders. Despite the advent of sophisticated laboratory equipment to test blood, a thorough history remains fundamental to accurate diagnosis. In practice the history may precede and then follow the knowledge of a laboratory test abnormality. Whatever the order of events, only by considering symptoms, physical signs and laboratory results in conjunction can the correct conclusion be reached and the patient be managed in the appropriate psychosocial setting (Fig 7.1).

History of the presenting complaint

Patients may be asymptomatic and have an unpredictable abnormality detected on a routine blood count. Other patients present to the doctor with complaints dependent on the nature of the change in the blood. Some will have several blood abnormalities and present with a large number of symptoms. Despite this complexity it is possible to highlight some common groups of symptoms (Table 7.1).

Symptoms attributable to anaemia (low haemoglobin concentration)

Patients with anaemia have a reduced supply of oxygen to the tissues. Symptoms include fatigue, weakness, dyspnoea, palpitations, headaches, tinnitus and chest pain (due to exacerbation of angina). The symptoms are affected not only by the severity of the anaemia but by its speed of onset. Anaemia which develops rapidly is usually less well tolerated and patients are more debilitated.

Symptoms attributable to a low white cell count (leucopenia)

It is usually a reduction in neutrophils (neutropenia) which causes clinical problems. Patients are susceptible to infections, the risk rising sharply at neutrophil counts below 0.5×10^9/L. Serious blood diseases such as acute leukaemia can present as life-threatening infections or as apparently trivial infections (e.g. a sore throat) which are unusually refractory to normal treatment. Perineal sepsis can be a particular problem.

Symptoms attributable to a low platelet count (thrombocytopenia)

Thrombocytopenia leads to a haemorrhagic tendency and common presentations include epistaxes (nose bleeds), bleeding from gums, menorrhagia (heavy periods) and excessive bleeding after trauma or surgery. Patients may also complain of easy bruising or a petechial rash. Spontaneous bleeding is usually restricted to platelet counts below 20×10^9/L. In disorders of platelet function similar symptoms may occur even when the count is normal.

Symptoms attributable to abnormal coagulation

Patients with a defect in the coagulation cascade (e.g. low factor VIII level in haemophilia A) bleed easily after surgery and trauma but the pattern of spontaneous haemorrhage is normally different to that seen in platelet disorders. The commonest complaints are of bleeding into joints (haemarthroses)

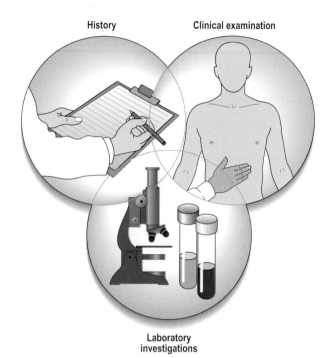

History   Clinical examination

Laboratory investigations

Fig 7.1 **The history, clinical examination and laboratory investigations are all essential in the diagnosis of a disorder of the blood.**

Table 7.1 **Common haematological abnormalities and associated symptoms**

Nature of abnormality[1]	Commonly associated symptoms
Anaemia	Fatigue, weakness, dyspnoea, palpitations, headache, dizziness, tinnitus
Leucopenia (particularly neutropenia)	Unusually severe or recurrent infections
Thrombocytopenia	Easy bruising, excessive bleeding after trauma, spontaneous bleeding from mucous membranes
Defective coagulation (e.g. key factor deficiency)	Excessive bleeding after trauma, spontaneous bleeds into joints and muscles
Infiltration by malignancy (e.g. leukaemia, lymphoma)	'Lumps' caused by lymphadenopathy, pain, neurological symptoms

[1]The haematological abnormalities have many possible causes but will always tend to lead to the symptoms shown.

and muscles. Lifelong symptoms suggest an inherited abnormality while recent onset is consistent with an acquired aetiology.

Symptoms attributable to infiltration by malignancy

Malignant disorders of the blood such as leukaemias and lymphomas have the capacity to invade tissues. Patients may complain of lumps in the neck, axillae or groin caused by lymphadenopathy or of abdominal pain or distension caused by splenomegaly. Involvement of the nervous system may manifest as headache, pain in dermatomal distribution or loss of function.

The severity, quality and temporal characteristics of pain may or may not be helpful in identifying an underlying blood disorder. The pain of the vaso-occlusive crisis of sickle cell anaemia is often distinctive whereas the chronic low back pain of myeloma is all too easily dismissed.

Systemic enquiry

A thorough systemic enquiry is essential as blood abnormalities are more often caused by a general systemic disorder than by a specific blood disease. It can be difficult to establish whether the primary problem is in the bone marrow or if the blood is 'reacting' to pathology elsewhere. One example is a high platelet count (thrombocytosis). This may be caused by the bone marrow disorder *essential thrombocythaemia* but equally can be secondary to infection, inflammation or malignancy ('reactive thrombocytosis'). Only by excluding a non-haematological aetiology can the diagnosis of essential thrombocythaemia be confidently made. On occasion the haematological diagnosis prompts a return to a particular part of the systemic enquiry. Thus the finding of unexplained iron deficiency necessitates an exhaustive enquiry for symptoms of gastrointestinal disease associated with chronic blood loss.

Past medical history

It is important to elicit a history of diseases which may have caused a haematological abnormality or which may affect the management of a primary blood disorder such as leukaemia. Where there is a known abnormality in the blood count it is helpful to establish whether previous counts have been performed. Where past results are available they will clarify whether the problem is of recent onset or longstanding. For patients presenting with easy bruising or bleeding, previous surgical exposure is of particular interest. The lack of excessive bleeding after surgery suggests that the bleeding tendency is either of limited significance or of more recent onset.

Drug history

Drugs can cause haematological problems – some commoner examples are listed in Table 7.2. A careful drug history (wherever possible verified by checking tablets) may suggest a likely offending agent. If the problem is of sufficient severity to cause concern the drug should ideally be discontinued and the blood count monitored to check resolution. It is as relevant to obtain a history of allergy in haematology as in other areas of medicine. Indeed, patients with haematological malignancies are often given an unusually large number of chemotherapeutic and antimicrobial agents and possible reactions have to be vigilantly documented to avoid repeat exposure.

Family history

As can be seen from Table 7.3, a number of blood diseases are inherited. A knowledge of the mode of inheritance is useful in diagnosis and essential in counselling the patient and family. A simple question as to the presence of 'anaemia' or a 'bleeding problem' in other family members can prevent unnecessary investigation and delay in diagnosis.

Social history

With the growing reliance on technology for diagnosis and treatment it can be surprisingly easy to forget that a blood disorder is affecting a 'real person'. An understanding of the patient's normal lifestyle is particularly important where a chronic or serious disease is diagnosed. Many people developing haematological malignancies are elderly and need support in the community, including, perhaps, visits by social workers

Table 7.2 **Possible haematological side-effects of drugs**	
Haematological abnormality	**Drugs**[1]
Marrow aplasia	Chloramphenicol (idiosyncratic) Cytotoxics (dose-related)
Haemolytic anaemia	Cephalosporins Penicillins
Leucopenia/agranulocytosis	Phenothiazines Sulphonamides
Thrombocytopenia	Quinine Thiazide diuretics

[1]Many drugs have been implicated in all these abnormalities – the examples shown are some of the more common offenders.

Table 7.3 **Some inherited blood disorders**	
Red cell disorders	
Disorders of the membrane	Hereditary spherocytosis and elliptocytosis
Disorders of haemoglobin	Thalassaemias and sickle syndromes
Disorders of metabolism	Glucose-6-phosphate dehydrogenase and pyruvate kinase deficiencies
Coagulation disorders	
Factor deficiency	Haemophilia A and B
Combined factor and platelet abnormality	von Willebrand disease
Platelet abnormality	Bernard–Soulier syndrome (rare)
White cell disorders	Rare functional disorders (e.g. chronic granulomatous disease)

The mode of inheritance of these disorders is discussed in the relevant sections.

and nurses. Often such diseases are incurable and expert management of symptoms has to be complemented by an understanding of the patient's need to sort out affairs and communicate the news to family and friends. In working adults the onset of diseases like leukaemia, with frequent clinic visits and hospitalisation, can lead to unemployment and marital and financial difficulties. In children chronic blood disorders such as haemophilia and haemoglobinopathies may cause time lost from school and create stresses for the whole family. Good practice of clinical haematology requires consideration of the far-reaching effects of the diagnosis and necessary treatment on the patient.

Miscellaneous

Alcohol misuse can cause blood changes, the most common being macrocytosis (enlarged red cells). A positive history will prevent unnecessary investigation for other causes. *Smoking* is a cause of moderate polycythaemia (elevated haematocrit/haemoglobin level) and appears to be associated with an increased incidence of acute myeloid leukaemia. *Travel* to tropical areas raises the possibility of malaria and other tropical diseases which can affect the blood.

> ### History taking
>
> - In the diagnosis of blood disorders, the history is complementary to the clinical examination and laboratory testing.
>
> - Blood abnormalities such as anaemia, leucopenia and thrombocytopenia lead to predictable groups of symptoms.
>
> - Blood abnormalities may be caused by systemic diseases, familial disorders and drugs. A thorough systemic enquiry, past medical history, drug history and family history should be elicited.
>
> - Serious and chronic blood diseases (e.g. leukaemia, haemoglobinopathies, haemophilia) have major social implications for children and adults; these should be explored not ignored.

8 Examining the patient

Abnormalities of the blood may arise as a result of a primary disorder of the bone marrow (e.g. leukaemia) or from a wide range of systemic disorders. A thorough clinical examination is vital both to confirm a likely diagnosis and to exclude coexistent problems. There is not space here to detail all the elements of clinical examination; we have concentrated on aspects of the examination most relevant to patients with a primary blood disorder.

Look at the patient!

It is easy to examine a patient carefully without properly observing them. A deliberate inspection of the patient's face while taking the history may reveal vital clues even before the formal examination is commenced. Common examples include the pallor of iron deficiency anaemia, the lemon tint of megaloblastic anaemia, the jaundice of a haemolytic anaemia, and the plethora of polycythaemia. Before laying a hand on the patient, a careful inspection of the mouth and skin may also point to particular blood abnormalities or disorders (Table 8.1). The patient's ethnic origin can be of relevance. Sickle cell anaemia is an unlikely diagnosis in a patient with white skin while pernicious anaemia is equally unlikely in a patient with black skin. Children with chronic blood disorders such as haemoglobinopathies are frequently thinner and shorter than their healthy peers.

General examination

Careful observation should be followed by a methodical examination of the major systems. The possible abnormalities in each system which may be seen in blood diseases are too numerous to detail here. They are referred to in the relevant sections describing each disease. Although examination should be ordered, in a busy clinical practice it is often necessary to prioritise. Rectal examination is not routine in all patients with blood disorders but is definitely indicated in unexplained iron deficiency to exclude an otherwise asymptomatic rectal carcinoma; it is contraindicated in patients with suspected leukaemia and neutropenia. Similarly, an exhaustive examination of the major joints is not universally performed but is crucial in a patient with haemophilia.

Examination of the lymph nodes

Lymph nodes may be enlarged in primary blood disorders and systemic diseases. Enlargement is referred to as 'lymphadenopathy' or just 'adenopathy'. The differential diagnosis differs in generalised and localised forms of lymphadenopathy (Table 8.2). In practice, palpable lymphadenopathy is usually limited to the cervical, axillary and inguinal areas.

Enlargement of the *cervical lymph nodes* is the most common cause of a swelling in the neck and, if massive, may be easily visible (Fig 8.1). Following careful inspection of the neck, it is easiest to examine the cervical nodes from behind the seated patient, methodically palpating the anatomical areas detailed in Figure 8.2. As for all lumps, it is important to document not only the size and location of enlarged nodes, but also the shape, consistency and presence of tenderness. Lymphadenopathy secondary to infection is more often tender than that due to malignancy. Nodes involved by carcinoma are characteristically stony hard while those involved by lymphoma are more 'rubbery'. The presence of cervical adenopathy should always prompt a thorough examination of the head and neck to detect a local cause (e.g. malignancy or infection); formal ear, nose and throat examination is often indicated.

The *axillary nodes* are best examined with the patient supine and the arm supported by the side, the examiner using the right hand to gently palpate the left axilla and the left hand for the right axilla. Anatomically, the nodes are divided into medial, lateral, posterior, central and apical groups. Examination of *inguinal nodes* is most easily performed while examining the abdomen. Care must be taken not to confuse inguinal adenopathy with an irreducible femoral hernia. Enlarged abdominal lymph nodes may cause an abnormal fullness of the central abdomen on palpation.

On occasion it is difficult to be certain that nodes are pathologically enlarged. Interpretation must take account of the patient's age and occupation. Large tonsillar glands are common in children, while people exposed to repeated minor injuries of the hands and feet often have

Table 8.1 **Observation of the patient with a blood disorder. Some common signs and their possible clinical relevance**	
Clinical sign	**Possible haematological abnormality**
Face	
Pallor	Any anaemia
Lemon tint	Megaloblastic anaemia
Jaundice	Haemolytic anaemia
Plethora	Polycythaemia
Mouth	
Ulcers	Neutropenia
Glossitis	Megaloblastic anaemia
	Iron deficiency anaemia
Angular stomatitis	Iron deficiency anaemia
Candida ('thrush')	Immunosuppression
Skin	
Pallor	Any anaemia
Jaundice	Haemolytic anaemia
Excessive bruising	Coagulation disorder, thrombocytopenia
Purpuric/petechial rash	Thrombocytopenia
Leg ulcers	Sickle cell anaemia

Fig 8.1 **Massive cervical lymphadenopathy.**

Table 8.2 **Common causes of lymphadenopathy**
Localised
Local bacterial or viral infection
Lymphoma
Metastatic malignancy
Generalised
Systemic infection
– bacterial (e.g. tuberculosis)
– viral (e.g. Epstein–Barr, HIV)
Lymphoma
Other haematological malignancy (e.g. leukaemia)
Inflammatory disease (e.g. connective tissue disorder, sarcoid)
Disseminated malignancy

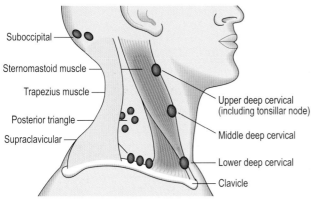

Fig 8.2 **Lymph nodes of the neck.**

Table 8.3 **Common causes of splenomegaly**		
Degree of enlargement	**Centimetres palpable below costal margin**	**Causes**
Slight	0–4	Various acute and chronic infections (e.g. septicaemia, tuberculosis)
Moderate	4–8	Haemolytic anaemia Infectious mononucleosis Portal hypertension
Massive	Greater than 8	Myelofibrosis Chronic myeloid leukaemia Polycythaemia vera Lymphoma Malaria Leishmaniasis

Note: The division by size is clinically helpful but disorders associated with massive splenomegaly may also cause lesser degrees of enlargement.

Fig 8.3 **Schematic view of splenic enlargement.** The notch is frequently not palpable. The arrow shows the normal direction of enlargement.

Fig 8.4 **Examination of the spleen.**

inspiration. If the spleen is not palpable using this technique, it is worth rolling the patient slightly onto the right side with the examiner's left hand held firmly behind the left lower ribs (Fig 8.4). This latter manoeuvre may lift forward a slightly enlarged spleen and make it palpable on deep inspiration.

The following features are typical of an enlarged spleen:

- It has a characteristic shape and sometimes a palpable notch on its upper edge.
- You cannot get above it.
- It moves with respiration.
- It is dull to percussion.
- It cannot be felt bimanually or balloted.

In practice an enlarged spleen is most likely to be misidentified as an enlarged left kidney. However, the kidney is not dull to percussion (it is covered by the colon) and it can be felt bimanually and balloted. It is worth listening with a stethoscope over an enlarged spleen as inflammation of the capsule may cause an audible 'splenic rub'. The spleen is usually uniformly enlarged and it is not generally possible to identify the underlying disorder by palpation alone. The degree of enlargement does, however, give a diagnostic clue (see Table 8.3).

some lymphadenopathy in the draining areas. A period of observation can be helpful. If serious doubt persists then a surgical biopsy is indicated.

Examination of the spleen

The spleen is enlarged in many blood disorders and in some systemic diseases (Table 8.3). The presence of a palpable spleen and its characteristics often narrows the differential diagnosis considerably. Examination of the spleen is frequently done badly. It is easy to miss a slightly enlarged spleen which is just palpable ('tippable') and it is also embarrassingly easy to miss a spleen which is massively enlarged. However, neither of these mistakes is likely if the examination is conducted as below.

The patient should be examined on a suitable examination couch or bed and should be encouraged to relax. The whole abdomen is exposed. The examiner sits or kneels to allow palpation with a (warm) hand with the forearm horizontal to the abdomen. First, the abdomen is inspected for a visible mass

and the patient is asked if they have any abdominal tenderness. It is normal to palpate the whole abdomen and then examine the major organs in turn. The spleen enlarges from below the tenth rib along a line heading for the umbilicus (Fig 8.3). Palpation for the spleen is commenced in the right lower quadrant of the abdomen, otherwise massive enlargement can be missed. The hand is moved in stages towards the tip of the left tenth rib while the patient takes deep breaths. The edge of an enlarged spleen connects with the tips of the index and middle fingers during deep

Examining the patient

- The clinical examination is an important part of the diagnosis of blood disorders.
- It is helpful to carefully observe the patient prior to the formal examination of systems.
- In routine clinical practice some aspects of examination are prioritised (e.g. rectal examination in unexplained iron deficiency).
- Proper examination of the lymph nodes requires familiarity with the normal anatomical groups and the causes of enlargement.
- Examination of the spleen is frequently badly performed; with poor technique even massive splenomegaly can be missed.

9 Laboratory haematology I – Blood and bone marrow

Diagnosis of most blood disorders is possible from a combination of clinical history, clinical examination and relatively routine laboratory tests. Haematology laboratories are heavily dependent on complex electronic machinery. The ubiquitous full blood count (FBC) is the archetypal haematological investigation and is performed by specialised automated cell counters. However, despite the accessibility of modern technology, the more simple traditional techniques of blood and bone marrow film spreading, staining, and light microscopy remain essential parts of the haematologist's repertoire.

The blood count

Many of the diseases discussed in this book are first suggested by an abnormality in the blood count (often referred to as the full blood count). The test is performed on a small specimen of anticoagulated venous blood; the normal anticoagulant is ethylene diamine tetra-acetic acid (EDTA). A typical report is illustrated in Figure 9.1. As can be seen, it contains a large amount of numerical information pertaining to the three cell lines in the peripheral blood: red cells (and haemoglobin), white cells (with a differential count of each specific cell type) and platelets.

When interpreting the report it is sensible to initially focus on the haemoglobin (Hb) concentration, total white cell count (WBC) and platelet count – most blood abnormalities of clinical significance are associated with a derangement of at least one of these values. Much of the remaining information details the nature of the red cells and their degree of haemoglobinisation, and the precise make-up of the white cell count. The former values are helpful in the diagnosis of anaemia, and the latter in the diagnosis of a variety of diseases of white cells (e.g. leukaemias) and reactions to systemic disease. To understand the role of the automated blood count in clinical practice, and particularly its limitations, it is helpful to understand how the numerical values are generated.

Automated haematology counters

The two essential functions of the automated blood cell counter are the measurement of Hb concentration in the blood and the counting and sizing of blood cells.

Most counters use a modification of the traditional *cyanmethaemoglobin method* to measure Hb concentration. In essence, blood is diluted in a solution where Hb is converted to cyanmethaemoglobin and then the Hb concentration derived from the light absorbance (optical density) of the resultant solution measured by a spectrophotometer. Automated machines have at least two channels for cell counting. In one, red cells and platelets may be counted and in the other red cells are lysed leaving white cells for analysis. Extra channels are often used for differential white cell and reticulocyte counting.

There are two basic methods for cell counting and sizing: electrical impedance and light scattering. The electrical impedance method relies on blood cells being very poor conductors of electricity. Thus, when the cells are passed in a stream through a narrow aperture across which an electrical current is maintained, the individual cells create an increase in electrical impedance of a size proportional to the cell volume. In the

Fig 9.1 **Typical blood count report.**

Fig 9.2 **Blood film.**
(a) Macroscopic;
(b) light microscopy.

light scattering method the cells deflect a beam of light (often a laser beam) and a detector converts the scatter into pulses proportional to cell size. For sophisticated measurements such as the differential white cell count the two methods can be used together with the addition of other modalities reliant on biochemical reactions and light absorbance.

Sophisticated though this technology is, automated cell counters are ultimately no substitute for the trained human eye. Results outside the machine's numerical normal range or the presence of unusual circulating cells (e.g. leukaemic cells) should be flagged as being abnormal. This alerts the operator who will return to the original blood sample to make a film.

The blood film

A blood film is simply made by smearing a drop of anticoagulated venous blood onto a glass slide with a glass spreader (Fig 9.2a). In larger laboratories film spreading can be automated. Following drying, the film is fixed with methanol and stained. Routine stains are based on *Romanowsky's method* – commonly used variants are the May–Grünwald–Giemsa (MGG) stain and Wright's stain. Constituent dyes include methylene blue, azure B and eosin. Once stained, the blood film should be systematically studied under the light

Table 9.1 **Some morphological terms used in blood film reports**

Red cells

Hypochromia	Pale staining of cells
Polychromasia	Grey-blue tint to cells (usually reticulocytes)
Anisocytosis	Variation in cell size
Poikilocytosis	Variation in cell shape
Macrocytosis/microcytosis	Increase/decrease in cell size
Spherocyte	Small spherical densely stained cell
Burr cell	Crimpled cell membrane
Target cell	Increased staining in middle of area of central pallor – suggests increased surface area
Basophilic stippling	Small basophilic inclusions in cytoplasm (RNA)
Howell–Jolly bodies	Nuclear remnants in cytoplasm
Schistocyte	Fragmented cell

White cells

Hypersegmented neutrophils	Increased nuclear segmentation
Left-shifted neutrophils	Reduced nuclear segmentation
Toxic granulation	Increased neutrophil cytoplasmic granularity
Atypical lymphocytes	Morphology variable; often seen in viral infections
Blasts	Leukaemic cells

Platelets

Clumping	Sticking together; can cause artefactually low count

Note: Causes of these morphological abnormalities are discussed in the disease sections.

microscope – the normal appearance of a film stained by the MGG method is illustrated in Figure 9.2b. Alternative stains are sometimes needed. Visualisation of reticulocytes requires the use of a dye such as methylene blue on live unfixed cells ('supravital stain'). Malarial parasites are most easily seen following staining at a specific pH.

The first step in film examination is a decision as to whether the film is of adequate quality. Either poor staining techniques or prolonged storage of the specimen may make the film worthless. Any comment on the film appearance is usually appended to the blood count report. The nomenclature used in film reporting can appear obscure; some more commonly used morphological terms are listed in Table 9.1. Microscopic images of blood cells are now routinely photographed using digital cameras. These images may increasingly be used to create 'virtual slides' or employed with cell recognition systems for automated morphological screening.

Where the film is significantly abnormal, examination of the bone marrow can give further diagnostic information.

Bone marrow examination

The clinical procedure for obtaining samples of bone marrow is described on page 106. From the favoured site, the posterior iliac crest, it is possible to obtain both a marrow *aspirate* sample and a marrow *trephine* biopsy.

Aspirate

The aspirate is simply sucked through the needle and spread onto a glass slide; the marrow particles are normally easily visible (Fig 9.3a). The marrow is fixed and stained as for a blood film and additionally stained by Perl's method to demonstrate iron. Microscopy and reporting is systematic with reference to the overall cellularity, the appearance and number of each normal cell line, possible infiltration by malignant cells, and any other pathological features. The advantage of the aspirate specimen is that individual cells are well preserved and subtle morphological changes can be detected. The major disadvantage is that the normal architecture of the marrow is lost. In the investigation of haematological malignancy (e.g. leukaemia) marrow aspirate samples are often also used for immunophenotyping and cytogenetic and molecular genetic testing.

Fig 9.3 **Bone marrow aspirate.**
(a) Macroscopic;
(b) light microscopy.

Fig 9.4 **Bone marrow trephine specimen.**
(a) Macroscopic;
(b) light microscopy.

Trephine biopsy

The trephine biopsy (Fig 9.4) is sectioned and normally stained by haematoxylin and eosin (H&E) and Giemsa methods. Silver impregnation can be used to demonstrate marrow fibrosis and Perl's stain to highlight iron. The trephine is less good than the aspirate for identifying morphological abnormalities of individual cells but it is better for detecting abnormalities of marrow architecture and infiltration by solid malignancy. The two types of bone marrow sample are thus complementary.

Laboratory haematology I – blood and bone marrow

- Many blood disorders are first suggested by an abnormality in the blood count – particularly in the haemoglobin concentration, total white cell count or the platelet count.

- Automated haematology counters measure haemoglobin concentration and count and size blood cells.

- Where the blood count is abnormal, examination of the blood film often reveals morphological abnormalities undetectable by the automated counter.

- Significant blood abnormalities can be further investigated by examination of the bone marrow – aspirate and trephine biopsy specimens provide complementary information.

10 Laboratory haematology II – Coagulation and the acute phase response

Simple tests of blood coagulation

Despite the complexity of haemostasis (p. 12), it is possible to make a general assessment of coagulation with a few relatively simple first-line tests. As an initial screen of haemostatic function the following tests should be combined with a blood count and film to determine platelet number and appearance.

The prothrombin time (PT)

The test is performed by adding thromboplastin to the patient's platelet-poor plasma, warming, and then adding calcium. The time to clot formation is recorded in seconds and the PT may be expressed as the ratio of the patient's time to a normal control time. The thromboplastin used should have been calibrated to allow this result to be converted to the international normalised ratio (INR) – the ratio which would have been obtained if the international reference preparation for thromboplastin had been used in the test (see p. 80). The PT is essentially a measure of the efficiency of the extrinsic clotting system (factor VII) in addition to the functioning of factors V and X, prothrombin and fibrinogen.

Activated partial thromboplastin time (APTT)

This test is sometimes referred to as the partial thromboplastin time with kaolin (PTTK) or the kaolin cephalin clotting time (KCCT). Patient platelet-poor plasma is combined with contact factors (kaolin, phospholipid) and calcium and the time to clot formation recorded in seconds. The test measures the overall efficiency of the intrinsic pathway (i.e. factors VIII, IX, XI, XII) as well as the function of factors V, X, prothrombin and fibrinogen.

Quantitation of plasma fibrinogen

In most laboratories this has replaced the thrombin time as a first-line test. Several accurate methods are available for the quantitative assay of plasma fibrinogen. Fibrinogen is an acute phase reactant (see below) and is frequently elevated in sick patients. Causes of low levels include disseminated intravascular coagulation (DIC) and severe liver disease.

Common clinical causes of abnormal first-line coagulation tests are shown in Table 10.1. Second-line tests may be needed for more precise diagnosis. In mixing experiments (or correction tests) patient plasma is mixed with normal or factor-deficient plasma prior to repeating first-line tests. If a particular coagulation factor is thought to be lacking, a quantitative assay can then be performed. A circulating inhibitor of coagulation is suggested by failure of the coagulation abnormality to be corrected by the addition of normal plasma. Many routine tests are now automated. Most coagulation instruments rely on measurement of changes in optical density to detect clot formation.

Measurement of the acute phase response

In assessing patients with ill-defined symptoms it can be helpful to measure activation of the acute phase response, the body's response to tissue damage. Evidence of activation of the acute phase response suggests a physical cause for symptoms. Possibilities include trauma, infections, neoplasia and autoimmune disease. Serial measurements can be useful in monitoring the effects of treatment. The most widely used measurements of the acute phase response are the erythrocyte sedimentation rate (ESR), the plasma viscosity, and C-reactive protein.

ESR

In this simple and inexpensive test venous blood (in citrate anticoagulant) is drawn up into a vertical tube (Fig 10.1) and allowed to stand for 1 hour. The red cells settle out of suspension and the length of plasma cleared after the hour is measured. The normal values are less than 5 mm/hour in men and less than 7 mm/hour in women, although values of up to 15 mm/hour are not infrequent in those over 60 years old. The test mainly reflects fibrinogen levels but is also influenced by α_2-macroglobulin, immunoglobulins and albumin. These proteins buffer the electrostatic repellent forces on the red cell membrane and allow the cells to come together and form reversible aggregates or rouleaux which fall more quickly through the plasma. The ESR result is affected by the haemoglobin concentration with high values seen in anaemia and low values in polycythaemia. A fresh sample must be processed as the result also changes over time.

Table 10.1 **Common causes of abnormal first-line clotting tests**

Test	Prolonged prothrombin time	Prolonged APTT	Low fibrinogen
Common causes	Warfarin	Heparin[1]	DIC
	Liver disease	Haemophilia	Severe liver disease
	Vitamin K deficiency	vWD	
	DIC	DIC	
		Liver disease	
		Lupus anticoagulant	

APTT, activated partial thromboplastin time; DIC, disseminated intravascular coagulation; vWD, von Willebrand disease.
[1]Unfractionated heparin.

Fig 10.1 **Measurement of the ESR.**

Table 10.2 **Clinical significance of the plasma viscosity**		
	Plasma viscosity (mPa·s) measured at:	
	25°C	37°C
Normal range[1]	1.50–1.72	1.15–1.35
Acute/chronic organic diseases (malignancy, infection, etc.)	1.75–2.55	1.36–1.99
Need to exclude paraproteinaemias/ hyperviscosity syndrome	>2.55	>2.00

[1]Slightly higher levels can be seen in normal older people.

Plasma viscosity

This test also measures the acute phase response indirectly, the result correlating with fibrinogen and immunoglobulin levels. The plasma viscosity has some advantages over the ESR. The normal range is the same in males and females and the result is independent of haemoglobin concentration. The sample can be taken from the EDTA anticoagulated blood count bottle and the test does not need to be performed immediately. The normal range, which is temperature dependent, is detailed in Table 10.2. Plasma viscosity measurement has direct pathophysiological relevance in myeloma where very high values are seen in the *hyperviscosity syndrome*.

C-reactive protein (CRP)

This easily measured protein is elevated in most types of tissue injury. The CRP is usually increased within 6–8 hours of the insult. The normal range is up to 10 mg/L with levels of 10–40 mg/L in severe viral infections, levels of 40–300 mg/L in bacterial infections and levels over 300 mg/L in severe burns. CRP results are not influenced by anaemia.

Other possible measures of the acute phase reaction include quantitation of fibrinogen, haptoglobins, alpha-1-antitrypsin and anti-chymotrypsin. These all rise following tissue damage but some acute phase reactants (notably albumin and transferrin) actually fall.

Electrophoresis

Electrophoresis has two routine applications in haematology. In the diagnosis of haemoglobinopathies (e.g. thalassaemia), cellulose acetate electrophoresis at alkaline pH is used to separate the abnormal haemoglobins. Citrate agar electrophoresis at a lower pH may be helpful in selected cases. In the investigation of myeloma, serum and urine electrophoresis is performed to detect the monoclonal immunoglobulin or light chains characteristic of the disease (Fig 10.2).

Flow cytometry

Flow cytometry is essentially the measurement of the characteristics of cells passing in a fluid stream through a detection apparatus. The automated cell counters described in the previous section are the major application of the flow cytometry principle in haematology but the technique also plays a key role in the diagnosis of haematological malignancy. Leukaemic cells often have a particular 'immunophenotype' – a characteristic pattern of detectable antigens on the cell surface and in the cell cytoplasm (see also relevant disease sections). The antigens are identified by *cluster differentiation* (CD) numbers (e.g. CD13 is a myeloid antigen; see Appendix II). Cells from peripheral blood or a bone marrow aspirate sample are incubated with specific CD monoclonal antibodies which are

Fig 10.2 **Urine electrophoresis.** The highlighted sample demonstrates proteinuria and the presence of Bence Jones (immunoglobulin light chain) protein (red arrow) in a patient with myeloma and renal failure.

Fig 10.3 **Flow cytometry.** The use of a combination of myeloid and lymphoid antibodies shows multiple different cell lines and maturation stages each in a different colour.

conjugated with a fluorochrome, a molecule which emits light at a specific wavelength when excited by a laser. The flow cytometer is then used to detect populations of cells labelled by the fluorescent marker (Fig 10.3). Flow cytometry may be used in conjunction with molecular methods for the detection of minimal residual disease in leukaemia.

> *Laboratory haematology II – coagulation and the acute phase response*
>
> ■ Despite the complexity of haemostasis the coagulation mechanism can be assessed with a few relatively simple 'first-line' tests.
>
> ■ The term 'acute phase response' describes the body's response to tissue damage; commonly used measures include the ESR, plasma viscosity and C-reactive protein.
>
> ■ Electrophoresis is routinely used in the diagnosis of haemoglobinopathies and in the investigation of myeloma.
>
> ■ Flow cytometry methodology is exploited in automated blood cell counters and plays a key role in the characterisation of leukaemia.

11 Introduction and classification

Definition

The term 'anaemia' refers to a reduction of haemoglobin or red cell concentration in the blood. With the widespread introduction of automated equipment into haematology laboratories the haemoglobin concentration has replaced the haematocrit (or 'packed cell volume') as the key measurement. Haemoglobin concentration can be determined accurately and reproducibly and is probably the laboratory value most closely correlated with the pathophysiological consequences of anaemia. Thus, anaemia is simply defined as a haemoglobin concentration below the accepted normal range.

The normal range for haemoglobin concentration varies in men and women and in different age groups (Table 11.1). The definition of normality requires accurate haemoglobin estimation in a carefully selected reference population. Subjects with iron deficiency (up to 30% in some unselected populations) and pregnant women must be excluded or the lower level of normality will be misleadingly low. Normal haemoglobin ranges may vary between ethnic groups and between populations living at different altitudes.

Prevalence

The prevalence of anaemia and the aetiologies vary in different populations. In developed countries where most studies have been performed, anaemia is more common in women than in men. Particularly susceptible groups include pregnant women, children under 5 years and the elderly. The majority of cases in younger people are caused by iron deficiency. Anaemia is surprisingly common in the elderly, affecting roughly 10% of people over 65 years. Up to a third of these cases remain unexplained (see p. 92). In developing countries, factors influencing the prevalence of anaemia include climate, socioeconomic conditions and, most importantly, the incidence of coexistent diseases.

General features

In anaemia the blood's reduced oxygen-carrying capacity can lead to tissue hypoxia. The clinical manifestations of significant anaemia (see also p. 14) are to a large extent due to the compensatory mechanisms mobilised to counteract this hypoxia. Cardiac overactivity causes palpitations, tachycardia and heart murmurs. The dyspnoea of severe anaemia may be a sign of incipient cardiorespiratory failure. Pallor is due primarily to skin vasoconstriction with redistribution of blood flow to tissues with higher oxygen dependency such as the brain and myocardium.

Anaemia is one of the most common clinical problems presenting in general practice, in hospitals and in medical examinations. Usually characteristic symptoms and signs prompt a blood count to confirm the diagnosis but on occasion an unexpectedly low haemoglobin estimation in a 'routine' blood count precedes the clinical consultation. Whatever the sequence of events, anaemia is not in itself an adequate diagnosis; further enquiry to establish the underlying cause is essential.

A logical approach to anaemia demands a clear understanding of both its possible causes and its clinical and laboratory features. There are two major classifications – both have advantages and they are best used together.

Classification

Morphological classification

As already discussed (p. 18), modern electronic laboratory equipment can provide estimations of red cell indices in addition to haemoglobin concentration. Abnormal red cell indices should be confirmed by microscopic examination of blood films. The 'morphological' classification is based on a correlation between red cell indices and the underlying cause of anaemia. The most important measurements are of red cell size (mean cell volume or MCV) and red cell haemoglobin concentration (mean cell haemoglobin (MCH) or mean cell haemoglobin concentration (MCHC)).

Anaemias with raised, normal and reduced red cell size (MCV) are termed macrocytic, normocytic and microcytic, respectively. Anaemias associated with a reduced haemoglobin concentration within red cells are termed hypochromic and those with a normal MCH are termed normochromic. Characteristic combinations are of microcytosis and hypochromia, and normocytosis and normochromia. As can be seen in Figure 11.1, this terminology is helpful in narrowing the differential diagnosis of anaemia. It is perhaps least helpful in normocytic anaemia as the possible causes are numerous and diverse.

The value of the blood film in diagnosis should not be underestimated. For instance, combined iron deficiency (a cause of microcytosis) and folate deficiency (a cause of macrocytosis) may cause an anaemia with a normal MCV. However, inspection of the film will reveal a dual population of microcytic hypochromic red cells and macrocytic red cells.

Aetiological classification

Figure 11.2 illustrates a classification of anaemia based on cause. It is less immediately helpful than the morphological classification in forming a differential diagnosis but it does illuminate the pathogenesis of anaemia. The fundamental division is between excessive loss or destruction of mature red cells, and inadequate production of red cells by the marrow.

Loss of red cells occurs in haemorrhage and excessive destruction in haemolysis. A normal bone marrow will respond by increasing red cell production with accelerated discharge of young red cells (reticulocytes) into the blood. Inadequate red cell production may result from insufficient erythropoiesis (i.e. a quantitative lack of red cell precursors) or ineffective erythropoiesis (i.e.

Table 11.1 **Normal haemoglobin concentrations at different ages**		
Age	Mean haemoglobin (g/L)	Lower limit of normal (g/L)
Birth (cord blood)	165	135
1–3 days (capillary)	185	145
1 month	140	100
2–6 months	115	95
6 months–2 years	120	105
2–6 years	125	115
6–12 years	135	115
12–18 years:		
female	140	120
male	145	130
Adult:		
female	140	115
male[1]	155	135

[1]Normal haemoglobin concentration probably slightly lower after 65 years.

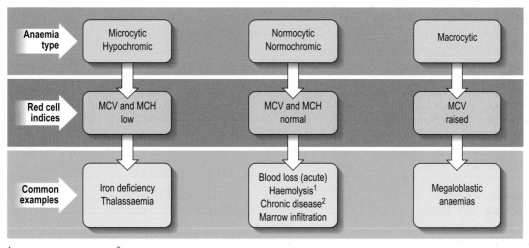

[1] Occasionally macrocytic   [2] Occasionally microcytic hypochromic

Fig 11.1 **Classification of anaemia based on red cell measurement.**

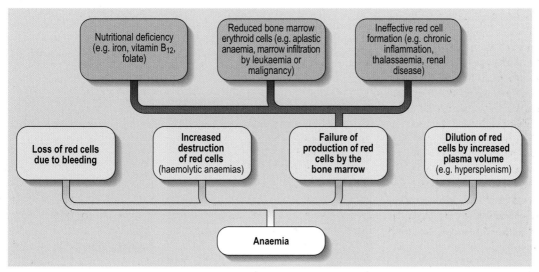

Fig 11.2 **Classification of anaemia based on cause.**

defective erythrocytes destroyed in the marrow). Examples of insufficient erythropoiesis include bone marrow hypoplasia, as in aplastic anaemia, and infiltration of the marrow by a leukaemia or other malignancy. Inefficient erythropoiesis is seen in disorders such as megaloblastic anaemia, thalassaemia and myelodysplastic syndromes.

The above provides a useful framework for thinking about anaemia. In reality different mechanisms can operate simultaneously. The anaemia of thalassaemia is caused by both ineffective erythropoiesis and haemolysis.

Management

The treatment of specific types of anaemia is discussed in subsequent sections. However, some general statements can be made. Whenever possible, the cause of anaemia should be determined before treatment is instituted.

Blood transfusion should only be used where the haemoglobin is dangerously low, where there is risk of a further dangerous fall in haemoglobin (e.g. rapid bleeding), or where no other effective treatment of anaemia is available. Prompt blood transfusion can be life-saving in a profoundly anaemic patient but it should be undertaken with great caution as heart failure can be exacerbated. Mild anaemia in the elderly should not be overlooked as it is a frequent cause of debility and has been linked with increased mortality.

Anaemia: introduction and classification

- Anaemia is defined as a haemoglobin concentration below the accepted normal range.
- The normal range for haemoglobin is affected by sex, age, ethnic group and altitude.
- The clinical features of anaemia are largely caused by compensatory measures mobilised to counteract hypoxia.
- Anaemia can be classified according to red cell morphology or aetiology.
- Red cell indices and morphology correlate with the underlying cause of anaemia.
- Wherever possible the cause of anaemia should be determined before treatment is started.
- Blood transfusion is only required in a minority of cases.

12 Iron deficiency anaemia

Iron

Iron is a constituent of haemoglobin and rate limiting for erythropoiesis. The metabolism of iron in the body is dominated by its role in haemoglobin synthesis (Fig 12.1). Normally, the total iron content of the body remains within narrow limits: absorption of iron from food (usually up to 3–4 mg/day) must replace any iron losses. Iron is not excreted as such but is lost in desquamated cells, particularly epithelial cells from the gastrointestinal tract. Menstruating women will lose an additional highly variable amount of iron, and in pregnant women the rate of iron loss is about 3.5 times greater than in normal men. The storage forms of iron, ferritin and haemosiderin, constitute about 13% of total body iron. The small peptide hepcidin plays a key role in iron metabolism and absorption (see p. 36).

Iron deficiency

Clinically significant iron deficiency is characterised by an anaemia which can usually be confidently diagnosed on the basis of the clinical history and simple laboratory tests. It cannot be over-stressed that the diagnosis of iron deficiency is not adequate in itself – a cause for the deficiency must always be sought.

Causes

The likely cause will vary with the age, sex and geographic location of the patient (Table 12.1). Iron deficiency is usually caused by long-term blood loss, most often gastrointestinal or uterine bleeding and less commonly bleeding in the urinary tract or elsewhere. Particularly in elderly patients, deficiency may be the presenting feature of gastrointestinal malignancy (Fig 12.2). Hookworm

Table 12.1 Causes of iron deficiency

Very common
- Bleeding from the gastrointestinal tract (e.g. benign ulcer, malignancy, hookworm)
- Menorrhagia

Other
- Pregnancy
- Malabsorption (e.g. coeliac disease, *Helicobacter pylori* gastritis[1])
- Malnutrition
- Bleeding from urinary tract
- Pulmonary haemosiderosis

[1]*May also cause bleeding.*

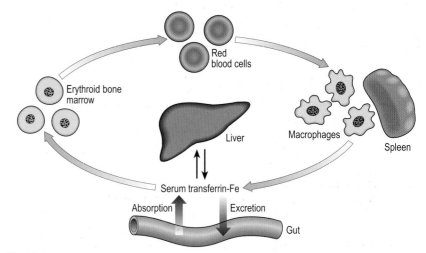

Fig 12.1 **The normal iron cycle.** Iron is absorbed from the gut into plasma where it is transported to the bone marrow for haemoglobin synthesis. Dying red cells are engulfed by macrophages in the reticuloendothelial system, and iron is recycled into the plasma for reuse. Iron is transported in the plasma bound to the glycoprotein, transferrin. Transferrin receptors exist on most cells in the body. Of the total 4–5 g of iron in the body only about 0.1% is being recycled at any given time. The rest is in tissue-specific proteins such as haemoglobin (66% of total body iron) and myoglobin, or stored in ferritin.

Fig 12.2 **Carcinoma of the colon.** A 53-year-old man presented to his doctor complaining only of tiredness. A blood count was consistent with iron deficiency (Hb 76 g/L, MCV 69 fl) and this was confirmed by a low serum ferritin level. History and examination revealed no obvious cause for his iron deficiency. Colonoscopy revealed a large bowel carcinoma which was successfully resected.

Fig 12.3 **Glossitis and angular stomatitis in iron deficiency.**

infection is the commonest cause of iron deficiency worldwide. Malabsorption and increased demand for iron, as in pregnancy, are other possible causes. Poor diet may exacerbate iron deficiency but is rarely the sole cause outside the growth spurts of infancy and teenage years.

Clinical features

These can be conveniently grouped into three categories:

- **General symptoms and signs of anaemia** (see pp. 14 and 22).

- **Symptoms and signs specific to iron deficiency.** Iron is required by many tissues in the body, shortage particularly affecting endothelial cells. Patients with long-standing deficiency may develop nail flattening and koilonychia (concave nails), sore tongues and papillary atrophy, angular stomatitis (Fig 12.3), dysphagia due to an oesophageal web (Plummer–Vinson syndrome) and gastritis. Many patients have none of these and their absence is thus of little significance. Iron deficiency in young children can contribute to psychomotor delay and behavioural problems (see also p. 91).

- **Symptoms and signs due to the underlying cause of iron deficiency.** Patients may spontaneously complain of heavy periods, indigestion or a change in bowel habit. Once the diagnosis of iron deficiency is known, it is often useful to retake the history and

Fig 12.4 **Blood film from a patient with iron deficiency.** The red cells are hypochromic (pale staining) and microcytic.

re-examine the patient with a view to detecting any clue of an underlying disorder. Rectal examination should be routine.

Diagnosis

The diagnosis may be suspected on the basis of the history and examination but laboratory investigations are required for confirmation.

The blood count

Iron deficiency causes a hypochromic microcytic anaemia. The automated red cell analyser generates a report with haemoglobin, MCV and MCH values below the normal range (see p. 22). There is a variation in red cell size (anisocytosis) reflected by a high red cell distribution width (RDW). A blood film will show characteristic features (Fig 12.4).

Confirmatory tests

Further tests are helpful in confirming the diagnosis (Table 12.2) and excluding other causes of a hypochromic microcytic anaemia (see p. 23). Measurement of serum ferritin is probably the most useful of these tests: a low level always indicates iron deficiency but a normal level does not guarantee normal stores as ferritin is increased in chronic inflammation and liver disease. In occasional difficult cases (e.g. where the patient has recently been transfused) a bone marrow aspirate is helpful in showing absence of iron stores. In practice the most likely confusion is with the anaemia of chronic disease (p. 36).

Management

This is divisible into investigations of the underlying cause and the correction of iron deficiency.

Table 12.2 Tests to confirm iron deficiency

Test	Result in iron deficiency	Comment
Ferritin	Low	Level increased in chronic inflammation/liver disease
Transferrin saturation	Low	Low levels also in elderly and chronic disease
Serum iron	Low	Levels fluctuate significantly and low in chronic disease
Transferrin concentration[1]	High	Useful test as low in anaemia of chronic disease
Zinc protoporphyrin	High	Late finding only
BM iron	Low	Informative but invasive investigation
Serum transferrin receptor level	High	Also high in haemolysis
Percentage of hypochromic red cells	High	Limited availability
Reticulocyte haemoglobin content	Low	Limited availability

BM, bone marrow.
[1]Total iron binding capacity (TIBC) may alternatively be used.

Investigation of underlying cause

Where the likely cause is apparent, further investigations can be highly selective. Thus in a young woman with severe menorrhagia and no other symptoms it can be assumed that uterine bleeding is the cause of iron deficiency, and investigation of the gastrointestinal (GI) tract is not necessary. A gynaecological referral would be adequate. Complaints of indigestion or a change in bowel habit should prompt an endoscopy or a colonoscopy or barium enema as first investigations. However, often there are no symptoms suggesting a site of blood loss. The GI tract is by far the most common site in men and post-menopausal women. Faecal occult blood testing is inadequately sensitive to exclude gastrointestinal bleeding and therefore a reasonable approach to this common problem is to commence with colonoscopy and, if normal, to proceed to upper GI endoscopy. If upper GI endoscopy is performed first in an elderly patient and shows a benign ulcerative lesion then assessment of the lower GI tract should probably still be performed as coexistent colonic neoplasms are found in a significant minority of cases. Anti-tissue transglutaminase (tTG-IgA) is a simple screening method for coeliac disease. If the GI tract is normal, rare causes of iron deficiency should be considered (see Table 12.1). In 20% of cases of iron deficiency no cause is found.

Correction of iron deficiency

Oral iron is given to correct the anaemia. The normal regimen is ferrous sulphate 200 mg three times a day (providing 195 mg elemental iron daily). Side-effects, including nausea, epigastric pain, diarrhoea and constipation, are best managed by reducing the dosage rather than changing the preparation. An adequate response to oral iron is an increase in haemoglobin of 20 g/L every 3 weeks. Iron is given for at least 6 months to ensure body stores are replete. There are several possible causes of a failure to respond to oral iron (Table 12.3). Parenteral iron (intramuscular or intravenous) can be used where oral therapy is unsuccessful because of poor tolerability or compliance or where there is continuing blood loss or malabsorption. Preparations include iron dextran, iron sucrose and ferric caboxymaltose. Anaphylactic reactions can occur and a test dose may be indicated.

Table 12.3 Failure to respond to oral iron – possible causes

- Wrong diagnosis (i.e. other cause of anaemia)
- Non-compliance
- Malabsorption
- Continued bleeding

Iron deficiency anaemia

- Iron is a constituent of haemoglobin and is essential for erythropoiesis.
- Iron deficiency is most often caused by long-term blood loss.
- Iron deficiency causes a hypochromic microcytic anaemia.
- The anaemia is usually easily corrected with oral iron supplements.
- It is important to establish the cause of iron deficiency – it may be the presenting feature of gastrointestinal malignancy.

13 Megaloblastic anaemia

The megaloblastic anaemias are characterised by delayed maturation of the nucleus of red cells in the bone marrow due to defective synthesis of DNA. Red cells either die in the marrow ('ineffective haematopoiesis') or enter the bloodstream as enlarged, misshapen cells with a reduced survival time. In clinical practice megaloblastic anaemia is almost always caused by deficiency of vitamin B_{12} (cobalamin) or folate (pteroylmonoglutamate). It is one of the most common causes of a macrocytic anaemia.

Why does deficiency of vitamin B_{12} or folate lead to megaloblastic anaemia?

Key characteristics of these essential vitamins are summarised in Table 13.1.

Both folate and vitamin B_{12} are necessary for the synthesis of DNA (Fig 13.1). Folate is needed in its tetrahydrofolate form (FH_4) as a cofactor in DNA synthesis. Deficiency of B_{12} leads to impaired conversion of homocysteine to methionine causing folate to be 'trapped' in the methyl form. The resultant deficiency in methylene FH_4 deprives the cell of the coenzyme necessary for DNA formation.

All dividing cells in the body suffer from the impaired DNA synthesis of B_{12} and folate deficiency. However, the actively proliferating cells of the bone marrow are particularly affected. As RNA synthesis progresses unhindered in the cytoplasm, the erythroid cells develop nuclear–cytoplasmic imbalance with abundant basophilic cytoplasm and enlarged nuclei. The chromatin pattern in the nucleus is characteristically abnormal; one author has described it as resembling 'fine scroll work', another as 'sliced salami' (Fig 13.2). The slowed synthesis of DNA leads to prolonged cell cycling and the cells being discharged into the blood without the normal quota of divisions. Red cells are enlarged and egg-shaped and the neutrophils hypersegmented due to retention of surplus nuclear material (Fig 13.3).

Clinical syndromes

Vitamin B_{12} deficiency
Pernicious anaemia

This classic cause of vitamin B_{12} deficiency is an autoimmune disorder. Most patients have IgG autoantibodies targeted against gastric parietal cells and the B_{12} transport protein intrinsic factor. The precise pathogenesis, and particularly the role of the autoantibodies, is incompletely understood but B_{12} deficiency ultimately arises from reduced secretion of intrinsic factor (IF) by parietal cells and, hence, reduced availability of the B_{12}–IF complex which is absorbed in the terminal ileum.

Table 13.1 **Vitamin B_{12} and folate**

Characteristic	Vitamin B_{12}	Folate
Average dietary intake/day (μg)	20	250[1]
Minimum adequate intake/day (μg)	1–2	150[1]
Major food sources	Animal produce only	Liver, vegetables
Normal body stores	Sufficient for several years	Sufficient for a few months
Mode of absorption	Combined with transport protein (IF) secreted by gastric parietal cells – then absorbed through ileum via special receptors	Dietary folate converted to methyl THF and absorbed in duodenum and jejunum

THF: tetrahydrofolate; IF: intrinsic factor.
[1]500 μg daily required in pregnancy.

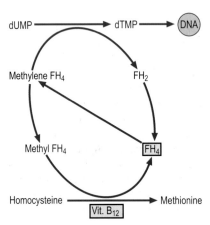

Fig 13.1 **The cause of megaloblastic anaemia.** Both vitamin B_{12} and folate (FH4) are necessary for normal synthesis of DNA (see text).

Fig 13.2 **Bone marrow aspirate in megaloblastic anaemia.** The immature red cells show nuclear–cytoplasmic imbalance with enlarged abnormal nuclei and basophilic cytoplasm.

The clinical hallmarks of pernicious anaemia are gastric parietal cell atrophy and achlorhydria, a more generalised epithelial cell atrophy and megaloblastic anaemia. The disease is most common in northern Europe in women greater than 50 years of age and is familial. Affected patients classically have premature greying of the hair and blue eyes and may develop other autoimmune disorders including vitiligo, thyroid disease and Addison's disease. Slight jaundice is caused by the haemolysis of ineffective erythropoiesis.

Patients usually have symptoms of anaemia and the generalised epithelial abnormality can manifest as glossitis (Fig 13.4) and angular stomatitis. The archetypal neurological complication – 'subacute combined degeneration' – arises from demyelination of the dorsal and lateral columns of the spinal cord. Patients most commonly complain of an unsteady gait, and if B_{12} deficiency is not corrected there can be progression to irreversible damage of the central nervous system with paralysis and dementia. There is a possible increased incidence of carcinoma of the stomach and colorectal cancer in pernicious anaemia.

Fig 13.3 **Peripheral blood film in megaloblastic anaemia.** There is a macrocytosis and the neutrophils are hypersegmented.

Fig 13.4 **Painful glossitis in pernicious anaemia.**

Diagnosis

1. *Blood count and film.* There is a macrocytic anaemia with the typical film appearance of megaloblastic anaemia. There may be leucopenia and thrombocytopenia.
2. *Bone marrow aspirate.* This is not always necessary. It will confirm megaloblastic anaemia but will not illuminate the underlying cause.
3. *Estimation of vitamin B_{12} and folate levels.* In pernicious anaemia the serum vitamin B_{12} level is normally very low but the assay is not entirely reliable and a trial of therapy may be justified where clinical and blood features strongly suggest deficiency. Serum methylmalonate and homocysteine levels are raised in B_{12} deficiency but their role in diagnosis is limited by their being often increased in normal people and a range of other disorders. Serum folate may be elevated and the red cell folate reduced (folate is trapped in its extracellular methyl FH_4 form – see Fig 13.1).

Table 13.2 **The megaloblastic anaemias**	
Vitamin B_{12} deficiency	
Deficiency of gastric intrinsic factor	Pernicious anaemia
	Gastrectomy
Intestinal malabsorption	Ileal resection/Crohn's disease
	Stagnant loop syndrome
	Tropical sprue
	Fish tapeworm
	Congenital malabsorption
Dietary deficiency (rare)	Vegans
Folate deficiency	
Dietary deficiency	
Malabsorption	Coeliac disease
	Tropical sprue
	Small bowel disease/resection
Increased requirement	Pregnancy
	Prematurity
	Haemolytic anaemia
	Myeloproliferative/malignant/ inflammatory disorders
Other causes	
Drug-induced suppression of DNA synthesis	Folate antagonists
	Metabolic inhibitors
	Nitrous oxide (prolonged use)
Inborn errors	Hereditary orotic aciduria

4. *Autoantibodies.* Parietal cell antibodies are found more commonly in the serum than IF antibodies (90% vs 50%) but whereas IF antibodies are almost diagnostic of pernicious anaemia, parietal cell antibodies occur in about 15% of healthy elderly people.
5. *Tests for vitamin B_{12} absorption.* The urinary secretion (Schilling) test was formerly much used but radioactive cyanocobalamin is not available now and the test is obsolete.

Treatment

Vitamin B_{12} levels are usually replenished by intramuscular injection of the vitamin. Several injections of 1 mg hydroxycobalamin are given over the first few weeks and then either one injection every 3 months or daily oral vitamin B_{12} 1–2 mg daily for life. The increase in reticulocytes in the blood peaks 6–7 days after the start of treatment.

In practice, ill patients with megaloblastic anaemia are often started on both B_{12} and folate supplements after a blood sample has been taken for assay of the vitamins. When the results are known the unnecessary vitamin can be stopped. Blood transfusion is best avoided as it may lead to circulatory overload – where judged necessary to correct hypoxia, it is undertaken with extreme caution. Platelet transfusion is used for bleeding caused by severe thrombocytopenia but this is unusual. Hypokalaemia occasionally requires correction.

Other causes of vitamin B_{12} deficiency

These are mostly abnormalities of the stomach and ileum (Table 13.2). As normal body stores are sufficient for 2 years, clinically apparent deficiency from any cause will develop slowly.

Folate deficiency

Folate deficiency is caused by dietary insufficiency, malabsorption, excessive utilisation or a combination of these (Table 13.2). Patients may complain of symptoms of anaemia or of an underlying disease. The increased risk of thrombosis is because of associated hyperhomocysteinaemia (see p. 79). There is a macrocytic anaemia and a megaloblastic bone marrow. In significant deficiency both serum and red cell folate are usually low but the latter is the better measure of tissue stores. In addition to a thorough dietary history patients may need investigations for malabsorption (e.g. jejunal biopsy).

Folate deficiency is treated with oral folic acid 5 mg once daily. This is given for several months at least, the precise duration of therapy depending on the underlying cause. Folate is prescribed prophylactically in pregnancy (400 µg daily) with a reduction in neural tube defects in the fetus and also in groups of patients at high risk of deficiency (Table 13.2). Before folate is prescribed, vitamin B_{12} deficiency must be excluded (or corrected) as subacute combined degeneration of the cord can be precipitated.

> ### *Megaloblastic anaemia*
>
> - Megaloblastic anaemia is a common cause of a macrocytic anaemia.
> - In clinical practice it is almost always caused by deficiency of vitamin B_{12} or folate.
> - Vitamin B_{12} deficiency normally arises from malabsorption – the classic clinical syndrome is the autoimmune disorder pernicious anaemia.
> - Folate deficiency is more often due to frank dietary deficiency or increased dietary requirements as in pregnancy.
> - Vitamin B_{12} deficiency should be excluded or corrected before folate is administered as subacute combined degeneration of the cord can be precipitated.

14 Haemolytic anaemia I – General features and inherited disorders

General features of haemolysis

The term 'haemolytic anaemia' describes a group of anaemias of differing aetiology that are all characterised by abnormal destruction of red cells. The hallmark of these disorders is reduced lifespan of the red cells rather than underproduction by the bone marrow.

In classification of the haemolytic anaemias there are three main considerations:

- The mode of acquisition of the disease: is it an inherited disorder or a disorder acquired in later life?
- The location of the abnormality: is the abnormality within the red cell (intrinsic) or outside it (extrinsic)?
- The site of red cell destruction: red cells may be prematurely destroyed in the bloodstream (intravascular haemolysis) or outside it in the spleen and liver (extravascular haemolysis).

The simple classification in Table 14.1 relies upon division of the main clinical disorders into inherited and acquired types. In general, it can be seen that inherited disorders are intrinsic to the red cell and acquired disorders extrinsic. The inherited disorders can be subdivided depending on the site of the defect within the cell – in the membrane, in haemoglobin, or in metabolic pathways. Acquired disorders (discussed in the next section) are broadly divided depending on whether the aetiology has an immune basis.

Diagnosis of a haemolytic anaemia

Recognition of the general clinical and laboratory features of haemolysis usually precedes diagnosis of a particular clinical syndrome. Where haemolysis leads to significant anaemia the resultant symptoms are as for other causes of anaemia. However, the increased red cell breakdown of the haemolytic anaemias causes an additional set of problems. Accelerated catabolism of haemoglobin releases increased amounts of bilirubin into the plasma such that patients may present with jaundice (Fig 14.1). Where the spleen is a major site of red cell destruction there may be palpable splenomegaly. Severe prolonged haemolytic anaemia in childhood can lead to expansion of the marrow cavity and associated skeletal

Table 14.1 Classification of the haemolytic anaemias

Inherited disorders	
Red cell membrane	Hereditary spherocytosis and hereditary elliptocytosis
Haemoglobin	Thalassaemia syndromes and sickling disorders
Metabolic pathways	Glucose-6-phosphate dehydrogenase and pyruvate kinase deficiency
Acquired disorders	
Immune	Warm and cold autoimmune haemolytic anaemia
Isoimmune	Rhesus or ABO incompatibility (e.g. haemolytic disease of newborn, haemolytic transfusion reaction)
Non-immune and trauma	Valve prostheses, microangiopathy, infection, drugs or chemicals, hypersplenism

Fig 14.1 **Mild jaundice in a patient with hereditary spherocytosis.**

abnormalities including frontal bossing of the skull.

Initial laboratory investigations of haemolysis will include an automated blood count, a blood film and a reticulocyte count. The blood count will show low haemoglobin. Many cases of haemolysis have 'normochromic normocytic' red cell indices although some are moderately macrocytic. The latter observation is caused by the increased number of large immature red cells (reticulocytes) in the peripheral blood following a compensatory increase in red cell production by the bone marrow. Reticulocytes have a characteristic blue tinge with Romanowsky stains and their presence in the film causes 'polychromasia'. A reticulocyte count is performed either manually on a blood film stained with a supravital stain or by the automated cell counter.

Simple laboratory tests to detect increased breakdown of red cells are also useful indicators of haemolysis. In addition to moderately raised serum bilirubin (often 30–50 mol/L), there may be raised levels of urine urobilinogen and faecal stercobilinogen. Bilirubin itself is unconjugated and therefore does not appear in the urine. Haptoglobin, a glycoprotein bound to free haemoglobin in the plasma, is depleted in haemolysis. In intravascular haemolysis, haemoglobin and haemosiderin can be detected in the urine.

Fig 14.2 **Hereditary spherocytosis.** Spherocytes in a blood film.

Fig 14.3 **Increased osmotic fragility in hereditary spherocytosis.** Spherocytes are more fragile than normal red cells and lyse at higher saline concentrations. The sensitivity of the test is increased by incubating the cells at 37°C.

Haemosiderin is present for several weeks after a haemolytic episode and is simply demonstrated by staining urine sediment for iron.

Examination of the bone marrow is not usually necessary in the work-up of haemolysis but, where performed, will show an increased number of immature erythroid cells. Formal demonstration of reduced red cell survival by tagging of cells with radioactive chromium (^{51}Cr) and in vivo surface counting of radioactivity to identify the site of red cell destruction are other possible investigations infrequently performed in practice.

Inherited disorders

Disorders of the red cell membrane
Hereditary spherocytosis
This is the most common cause of inherited haemolytic disease in northern Europeans. The disease is heterogeneous with a variable mode of inheritance. There are many possible gene mutations with alterations in spectrin, ankyrin and other membrane proteins. In a blood film the red cells are spheroidal ('spherocytes') with a reduced diameter and more intense staining than normal red cells (Fig 14.2). These abnormal red cells are prone to premature destruction in the microvasculature of the spleen.

The severity of haemolysis is variable and the disease may present at any age. Fluctuating levels of jaundice and palpable splenomegaly are common features. Occasionally, patients develop severe anaemia associated with the transient marrow suppression of a viral infection; this so-called 'aplastic crisis', which may intervene in any form of chronic haemolysis, is often caused by parvovirus B19. Prolonged haemolysis may lead to bilirubin gallstones.

Diagnosis is facilitated by the presence of a family history. The combination of general features of haemolysis and spherocytes in the blood is suggestive of hereditary spherocytosis but not diagnostic as spherocytes may also be seen in autoimmune haemolysis. The two haemolytic disorders are distinguished by the direct antiglobulin test, which is negative in hereditary spherocytosis and nearly always positive in immune haemolysis. Useful screening tests for hereditary spherocytosis include measurement of osmotic fragility (Fig 14.3) and flow cytometric analysis of eosin-5-maleimide binding. In difficult cases, gel electrophoretic analysis of red cell membranes is helpful.

In patients with milder disease folate supplements are considered but no other treatment is required. In more serious cases the spleen is removed. This should ideally be performed after 6 years of age with counselling regarding the infection risk.

Hereditary elliptocytosis
This is generally a mild disorder with similarities to hereditary spherocytosis. There is a variable deficiency of spectrin tetramers. Red cells are elliptical except in the rare subtype *hereditary pyropoikilocytosis* when they are more distorted and heat labile. Splenectomy may be indicated for severe haemolysis.

Abnormalities of haemoglobin
These disorders are referred to collectively as the 'haemoglobinopathies'. Thalassaemia and sickle cell syndromes are discussed in later sections.

Abnormalities of red cell metabolism
The red cell has metabolic pathways to generate energy and also to protect it from oxidant stress (Fig 14.4). Loss of activity of key enzymes may lead to premature destruction; there are two common examples.

Glucose-6-phosphate dehydrogenase (G6PD) deficiency
G6PD is a necessary enzyme in the generation of reduced glutathione which protects the red cell from oxidant stress. Deficiency is X-linked, affecting males; female carriers show half normal G6PD levels. The disorder is most common in West Africa, southern Europe, the Middle East and South-East Asia. Patients are usually asymptomatic until increased oxidant stress leads to a severe haemolytic anaemia, often with intravascular destruction of red cells. Common triggers include fava beans, drugs (many, including antimalarials and analgesics) and infections. The disease can alternatively present as jaundice in the neonate. Diagnosis requires demonstration of the enzyme deficiency by direct assay – this should not be done during acute haemolysis as reticulocytes have higher enzyme levels than mature red cells and a 'false normal' level may result. Treatment is to stop any offending drug and to support the patient. Blood transfusion may be necessary.

Pyruvate kinase (PK) deficiency
In this autosomal recessive disorder patients lack an enzyme in the Embden–Meyerhof pathway. Red cells are unable to generate adequate ATP and become rigid. All general features of haemolysis can be present, but clinical symptoms are often surprisingly mild for the degree of anaemia as the block in metabolism leads to increased intracellular 2,3-DPG levels facilitating release of oxygen by haemoglobin. Splenectomy may help in reducing transfusion requirements.

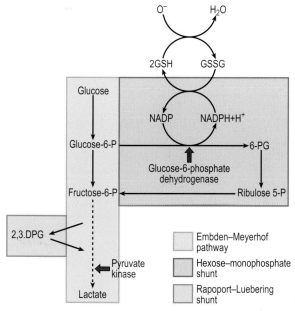

Fig 14.4 **Schematic diagram of red cell metabolism.** This shows the key roles of pyruvate kinase in the Embden–Meyerhof pathway (the cell's source of ATP) and glucose-6-phosphate dehydrogenase in the hexose-monophosphate shunt (the cell's protection from oxidant stress). The broken line represents several intermediate steps.

> ### Haemolytic anaemia I – general features and inherited disorders
>
> - 'Haemolytic anaemias' are caused by abnormal destruction of red cells.
>
> - Most inherited haemolytic disorders have a defect within the red cell while most acquired disorders have the defect outside the cell.
>
> - Haemolysis causes characteristic clinical features and laboratory abnormalities. It may be intra- or extravascular.
>
> - Hereditary spherocytosis and hereditary elliptocytosis are haemolytic disorders caused by a deficiency in the red cell membrane.
>
> - Glucose-6-phosphate dehydrogenase and pyruvate kinase are key enzymes in red cell metabolism; inherited deficiency leads to haemolysis.

15 Haemolytic anaemia II – Acquired disorders

Autoimmune haemolytic anaemia

Autoimmune haemolytic anaemia (AIHA) is an example of an acquired form of haemolysis with a defect arising outside the red cell. The bone marrow produces structurally normal red cells and premature destruction is caused by the production of an aberrant autoantibody targeted against one or more antigens on the cell membrane. Once an antibody has attached itself to the red cell, the exact nature of the haemolysis is determined by the class of antibody and the density and distribution of surface antigens. IgM autoantibodies cause destruction by agglutination or by direct activation of serum complement. IgG class antibodies generally mediate destruction by binding of the Fc portion of the cell-bound immunoglobulin molecule by macrophages in the spleen and liver. The disparate behaviour of different types of autoantibody provides the explanation for a number of different clinical syndromes.

Classification

Table 15.1 shows a simple approach to the classification of autoimmune haemolytic anaemia. The disease can be divided into 'warm' and 'cold' types depending on whether the antibody reacts better with red cells at 37°C or 0–5°C. For each of these two basic types of autoimmune haemolysis there are a number of possible causes and these can be incorporated into the classification. A diagnosis of autoimmune haemolysis may precede diagnosis of the causative underlying disease.

Clinical presentation and management
Warm autoimmune haemolytic anaemia

Warm AIHA (Figs 15.1 and 15.2) is the most common form of the disease. The red cells are coated with either IgG alone, IgG and complement, or complement alone. Premature destruction of these cells usually takes place in the reticuloendothelial system. Approximately half of all cases are idiopathic but in the other half there is an apparent underlying cause (Table 15.1). The autoantibody is produced by polyclonal B-cells and is usually nonspecific with reactivity against basic membrane constituents present on virtually all red cells. Patients present with the clinical and laboratory features of haemolysis discussed in the last section. Splenomegaly is

Table 15.1 **Classification of the autoimmune haemolytic anaemias**	
Warm AIHA (usually IgG)	
Primary (idiopathic)	
Secondary	Lymphoproliferative disorders
	Other neoplasms
	Connective tissue disorders
	Drugs
	Infections
Cold AIHA (usually IgM)	
Primary (cold haemagglutinin disease)	
Secondary	Lymphoproliferative disorders
	Infections (e.g. mycoplasma)
	Paroxysmal cold haemoglobinuria[1]

[1]Caused by a biphasic polyclonal IgG antibody (Donath–Landsteiner).

Fig 15.1 **Blood film in warm AIHA.** Spherocytes and polychromasia are present.

Fig 15.2 **Increased reticulocytes in warm AIHA.** The reticulocyte ribosomal RNA is stained supravitally by brilliant cresyl blue.

a frequent examination finding in severe cases. The most characteristic laboratory abnormality in warm AIHA is a positive direct antiglobulin test (DAT) sometimes known as the Coombs' test (p. 83). A major priority in management is the identification and treatment of any causative

disorder. It is particularly important to stop an offending drug – cephalosporin antibiotics are most commonly implicated. Where the haemolysis itself requires treatment, steroids are normally used (e.g. prednisolone 1–2 mg/kg daily). In idiopathic AIHA most patients will respond to steroids with a significant rise in haemoglobin and diminished clinical symptoms. However, the disease is usually controlled rather than cured and relapses often occur when steroids are reduced or stopped. Where refractoriness to steroids develops, splenectomy is usually indicated. Other immunosuppressive drugs (e.g. azathioprine, ciclosporin), intravenous immunoglobulin, cytotoxic agents and the monoclonal antibody rituximab may all be helpful in difficult cases.

Cold autoimmune haemolytic anaemia

In cold AIHA the antibody is generally of IgM type with specificity for the I red cell antigen. It attaches best to red cells in the peripheral circulation where the blood temperature is lower. As is seen in Table 15.1, this kind of haemolysis can occur in the context of a monoclonal (i.e. malignant) proliferation of B-lymphocytes in the so-called 'idiopathic cold haemagglutinin syndrome' or in a variety of lymphomas. The other major cause is infection.

The severity of haemolysis varies and agglutination (clumping) of red cells (Fig 15.3) may cause circulatory problems such as acrocyanosis, Raynaud's phenomenon and ulceration. The haemolysis, where longstanding, is often worse in the winter. On occasion red cell destruction is intravascular due to direct lysis by activated complement. Where this occurs free haemoglobin is released into the plasma (haemoglobinaemia) and may appear in the urine (haemoglobinuria), giving it a dark colour. Cold AIHA arising from infection is usually self-limiting. Where it is chronic the mainstay of treatment is keeping the patient warm, particularly in the extremities. In forms associated with lymphoproliferative disorders, cytotoxic drugs (e.g. chlorambucil) or rituximab may be helpful. Steroids are generally ineffective.

Isoimmune haemolytic anaemia

Here alloantibodies (isoantibodies) cause haemolysis as a result of transfusion or

Fig 15.3 **Cold agglutination in the blood film of a patient with cold autoimmune haemolytic anaemia.**

transfer across the placenta. These antibodies are conventional antibodies specific for foreign antigens on incompatible red cells. Haemolytic blood transfusion reactions are discussed on page 84 and haemolytic disease of the newborn on page 90.

Microangiopathic haemolytic anaemia

Collectively, microangiopathic haemolytic anaemia (MAHA) is one of the most frequent causes of haemolysis. The term describes intravascular destruction of red cells in the presence of an abnormal microcirculation. There are many causes of MAHA (Table 15.2) but common triggers are the presence of disseminated intravascular coagulation (DIC), abnormal platelet aggregation and vasculitis. Characteristic laboratory findings include red cell fragmentation in the blood film (Fig 15.4) and the coagulation changes seen in DIC (see p. 79). Two specific syndromes merit brief description.

Haemolytic uraemic syndrome (HUS)

HUS mainly affects infants and children. The three main features are MAHA, renal failure and thrombocytopenia. The disease can occur as seasonal epidemics caused by *Escherichia coli* producing verotoxin; it is then preceded by bloody diarrhoea. Treatment is essentially supportive with dialysis for renal failure. Mortality ranges from 5 to 15%.

Thrombotic thrombocytopenic purpura (TTP)

This rare congenital or acquired disorder has many similarities to HUS. It is characterised by MAHA, thrombocytopenia (often severe), fluctuating neurological symptoms, fever and renal failure. Platelet microvascular thrombi are mediated by ultra-large von Willebrand factor

Table 15.2 **Causes of microangiopathic haemolytic anaemia**
Haemolytic uraemic syndrome (HUS)[1]
Thrombotic thrombocytopenic purpura (TTP)[1]
Carcinomatosis
Vasculitis
Severe infections
Pre-eclampsia
Glomerulonephritis
Malignant hypertension

[1]*Some authorities believe that HUS and TTP are effectively a single disorder TTP-HUS.*

multimers which accumulate due to deficiency of a protease (ADAMTS 13). Daily plasma exchange is the mainstay of treatment; mortality rates are 10–20%.

Other acquired haemolytic anaemias

Haemolysis associated with red cell fragmentation may also occur due to the mechanical effects of defective heart valves or in long distance runners who effectively stamp repeatedly on a hard surface ('march haemoglobinuria'). Certain drugs (e.g. dapsone and sulfasalazine) can cause oxidative intravascular haemolysis in normal people if taken in sufficient dosage. Many infections can cause haemolysis, either by direct invasion of red cells or via the circulatory changes already discussed. The anaemia of malaria often has a haemolytic component (pp. 98–99).

Paroxysmal nocturnal haemoglobinuria (PNH) (Fig 15.5) is a rare example of acquired haemolysis caused by an intrinsic red cell defect. In this clonal disorder arising from a somatic mutation in the *PIG-A* gene in a stem cell, the mature blood cells have faulty anchoring of several proteins to membrane glycophospholipids containing phosphatidylinositol. Clinical features are highly variable and include intravascular haemolysis, pancytopenia and recurrent thrombotic episodes, including portal vein thrombosis. There is coexistent marrow damage and PNH is often associated with aplastic anaemia and may even terminate in acute

Fig 15.4 **Blood film in microangiopathic haemolytic anaemia.** Fragmented red cells and thrombocytopenia.

Fig 15.5 **Haemosiderinuria caused by chronic intravascular haemolysis in PNH (Perls' reaction).**

leukaemia. The traditional diagnostic test exploited the cell's unusual sensitivity to complement lysis (Ham test). Flow cytometry is now used to show the cells' characteristic lack of certain surface proteins (CD55, CD59) and to quantitate the PNH clone. Management is largely supportive with blood transfusion and anticoagulation. More recently, eculizumab, a monoclonal antibody blocking activation of terminal complement, has been given to reduce haemolysis and the risk of thrombosis. Allogeneic stem cell transplantation is the only curative option but is used very selectively (e.g. in severe marrow failure).

> ## *Haemolytic anaemia II – acquired disorders*
>
> - Autoimmune haemolytic anaemia (AIHA) can be divided into 'warm' and 'cold' types dependent on the temperature at which the antibody reacts optimally with red cells.
>
> - For each type of AIHA there are possible underlying causes which must be identified and treated.
>
> - The term 'microangiopathic haemolytic anaemia' (MAHA) describes the intravascular destruction of red cells in the presence of an abnormal microenvironment. Clinical syndromes associated with MAHA include haemolytic uraemic syndrome and thrombotic thrombocytopenic purpura.
>
> - Paroxysmal nocturnal haemoglobinuria (PNH) is a rare example of acquired haemolysis caused by an intrinsic red cell defect.

16 The thalassaemias

The thalassaemias are a heterogeneous group of inherited disorders of haemoglobin synthesis. They are characterised by a reduction in the rate of synthesis of either alpha or beta chains and are classified accordingly (i.e. α-thalassaemia, β-thalassaemia). The basic haematological abnormality in the thalassaemias is a hypochromic microcytic anaemia of variable severity. Unbalanced synthesis of α- and β-globin chains can damage red cells in two ways. Firstly, failure of α and β chains to combine leads to diminished haemoglobinisation of red cells to levels incompatible with survival. Even those hypochromic cells released into the circulation transport oxygen poorly. The second mechanism for red cell damage is the aggregation of unmatched globin chains – the inclusion bodies lead to accelerated apoptosis of erythroid precursors in the bone marrow (ineffective erythropoiesis) and destruction of more mature red cells in the spleen (haemolysis). In general, the clinical severity of any case of thalassaemia is proportionate to the degree of imbalance of α- and β-globin chain synthesis.

Thalassaemias are among the most common inherited disorders. Gene carriers have some protection from falciparum malaria. Cases occur sporadically in most populations but the highest thalassaemia gene frequency is in a broad geographical region extending from the Mediterranean through the Middle East and India to South-East Asia.

Classification

The classification illustrated in Table 16.1 is based on the mode of inheritance of thalassaemia.

As the α-globin chain gene is duplicated on each chromosome there may be total loss of α-globin chain production (termed α^0 or $-/$haplotype) or partial loss of α-chain production resulting from loss of only one gene (termed α^+ or $-\alpha/$haplotype).

The most important clinical syndromes are *haemoglobin (Hb)-Barts hydrops syndrome* ($--/--$), which is incompatible with life, and *Hb H disease* ($-\alpha/--$). At the molecular level the α-thalassaemias result from loss of α-gene function due to gene deletion or non-deletional mutations; different types of mutations may be co-inherited.

Table 16.1 **Classification of thalassaemia**

Type of thalassaemia	Heterozygote	Homozygote
α-Thalassaemia[1]		
α^0 ($--/$)	Thal. minor	Hydrops fetalis
α^+ ($-\alpha/$)	Thal. minor	Thal. minor
β-Thalassaemia		
β^0	Thal. minor	Thal. major
β^+	Thal. minor	Thal. major or intermedia

[1]*Compound heterozygosity ($--/-\alpha$) leads to HbH disease.*

β-Thalassaemias are autosomal recessive disorders characterised by reduced (β^+) or absent (β^0) production of β chains. The heterozygous ('trait' or 'minor') form of the disease is usually symptomless while homozygosity is associated with the clinical disease β-thalassaemia 'major'. Homozygous mild (β^+) thalassaemia may, however, lead to a less severe clinical syndrome termed 'thalassaemia intermedia'. The β-thalassaemias are very heterogeneous at the molecular level – the large majority of mutations are single base substitutions (point mutations) and insertions or deletions of one to two bases.

Although molecular analysis may be needed, diagnosis of the major syndromes is normally possible from consideration of the clinical features and simple laboratory tests. The latter must include a blood count and blood film, and haemoglobin electrophoresis with quantification of the different types of haemoglobin (i.e. HbA, HbA_2, HbF).

Other structural Hb variants may coexist with thalassaemias giving rise to a wide range of clinical disorders. Only the more common thalassaemia syndromes are discussed here.

Clinical syndromes

α-Thalassaemias

Hb-Barts hydrops syndrome ($--/--$)
Here deletion of all four genes leads to complete absence of α-chain synthesis. As the α-globin chain is needed for fetal haemoglobin (HbF) as well as adult haemoglobin (HbA) (see p. 5) the disorder is incompatible with life and death occurs in utero (hydrops fetalis).

HbH disease ($-\alpha/--$)
This disorder arises from deletion of three of the four α-globin genes and is found most commonly in South-East Asia. The clinical features are variable but there is often a moderate chronic haemolytic anaemia (Hb 70–110 g/L) with splenomegaly and sometimes hepatomegaly. Severe bone changes and growth retardation are unusual. The blood film shows hypochromic microcytic red cells with poikilocytosis, polychromasia and target cells. The HbH molecule is formed of unstable *tetramers* of unpaired β chains (β_4). It is best detected by electrophoresis but may be demonstrated as red cell inclusion bodies in reticulocyte preparations.

α-Thalassaemia traits
Deletion of a single α-globin chain leads only to a slight lowering of red cell mean corpuscular volume (MCV) and mean corpuscular haemoglobin (MCH) and even deletion of two genes usually only minimally lowers the haemoglobin with a raised red cell count and hypochromia and microcytosis. These carrier states can be difficult to identify in the routine laboratory as haemoglobin electrophoresis is normal. Occasional HbH bodies may be detected in reticulocyte preparations. Definitive diagnosis requires DNA analysis.

β-Thalassaemias
β-Thalassaemia major
The characteristic severe anaemia (Hb less than 70 g/L) is caused by α-chain excess leading to ineffective erythropoiesis and haemolysis. Anaemia first becomes apparent at 3–6 months when production of HbF declines. The child fails to thrive and develops hepatosplenomegaly. Compensatory expansion of the marrow space causes the typical facies with skull bossing and maxillary enlargement (Fig 16.1a). The 'hair-on-end' radiological appearance of the skull (Fig 16.1b) is due to expansion of bone marrow into cortical bone. If left untreated further complications can include repeated infections, bone fractures and leg ulcers. Red cell membrane abnormalities contribute to hypercoagulability.

Laboratory testing should precede blood transfusion. There is a severe hypochromic microcytic anaemia with a characteristic blood film (Fig 16.2) and Hb electrophoresis demonstrates absence or near absence of HbA with small amounts of HbA_2 and the remainder HbF (Fig 16.3).

With intense supportive therapy, increasing numbers of patients in the

Fig 16.1 **β-Thalassaemia major. (a)** Typical facies; **(b)** skull X-ray showing 'hair-on-end' appearance.

Fig 16.2 **Blood film in β-thalassaemia major.**

Fig 16.3 **Haemoglobin electrophoresis (cellulose acetate, pH 8.5).** The patterns obtained in normality and some common thalassaemia syndromes are shown. Other screening methods include high-performance liquid chromatography and isoelectric focusing.

Table 16.2 **Possible causes of thalassaemia intermedia**
■ Mild defects of β-globin chain production, e.g. homozygous mild β⁺-thalassaemia
■ Homozygosity or compound heterozygosity for severe β-thalassaemia with co-inheritance of α-thalassaemia or genetic factors enhancing γ-chain production
■ Heterozygous β-thalassaemia with co-inheritance of additional α-globin gene
■ δβ-thalassaemia and hereditary persistence of fetal haemoglobin
■ HbH disease

developed world survive into adulthood. Blood transfusion remains the mainstay of management. Raising the haemoglobin concentration both reduces tissue hypoxia and suppresses endogenous haematopoiesis which is largely ineffective. There is improved growth and development and reduced hepatosplenomegaly. Transfusion is generally given to maintain a haemoglobin level of at least 90–100 g/L. Splenectomy can reduce the transfusion frequency. With such regular transfusion iron chelation is necessary to minimise iron overload. Without chelation, accumulation of iron damages the liver, endocrine organs and heart with death in the second or third decades. The most commonly used regimen is subcutaneous desferrioxamine given for 5–7 days per week. Compliance may be problematic (especially in teenagers) but where good there is a considerably improved life expectancy. Oral iron chelators (e.g. deferiprone, deferasirox) are emerging as an acceptable alternative. Endocrine disturbances related to iron overload will require appropriate therapy.

Allogeneic stem cell transplantation is a serious option. In 'best risk' patients the probability of survival exceeds 90%. Experimental therapies include drugs designed to stimulate fetal haemoglobin production (e.g. erythropoietin, hydroxycarbamide) and gene therapy (see p. 103).

Thalassaemia intermedia

Thalassaemia intermedia is a clinical syndrome which may result from a variety of genetic abnormalities (Table 16.2). The clinical features are less severe than in β-thalassaemia major as the α/β-globin chain imbalance is less pronounced. Patients usually present later than is the case for β-thalassaemia major (often at 2–4 years), and have relatively high haemoglobin levels (80–100 g/L), moderate bone changes and normal growth. Transfusion may be required but requirements are less than in β-thalassaemia major.

β-Thalassaemia trait (minor)

Heterozygotes for β⁰ or β⁺ are usually asymptomatic with hypochromic microcytic red cells and slightly reduced haemoglobin levels. The red cell count is elevated. The key diagnostic feature is a raised HbA₂ level (4–7%). The disorder may be confused with iron deficiency leading to unnecessary investigations. If both parents have β-thalassaemia trait there is a 25% chance of a child having β-thalassaemia major.

Prenatal diagnosis

This depends on early identification of couples at risk and sensitive counselling. Adequate amounts of fetal DNA can be obtained around the 10th week of gestation by chorionic villus sampling. Current technologies allow reliable identification of single point mutations from very small DNA samples. Techniques are being developed to analyse fetal DNA obtained from maternal plasma or peripheral blood.

The thalassaemias

- The thalassaemias are a heterogeneous group of inherited disorders where there is a reduction in the rate of synthesis of haemoglobin α chains (α-thalassaemia) or β chains (β-thalassaemia).

- There may be both ineffective erythropoiesis and haemolysis. The basic haematological abnormality is a hypochromic microcytic anaemia.

- There are several clinical syndromes. In general the severity is proportionate to the degree of imbalance of α- and β-globin chains.

- β-Thalassaemia major leads to severe anaemia requiring regular blood transfusion and iron chelation.

- Thalassaemia trait is a symptomless clinical disorder which should not be confused with iron deficiency. Genetic counselling is required in selected cases.

17 Sickle cell syndromes

The sickle cell syndromes are a group of haemoglobinopathies which primarily affect the Afro-Caribbean population. The common feature of these diseases is inheritance of an abnormal haemoglobin β-chain gene – the gene is designated β^S. Inheritance of two β^S genes leads to a serious disorder termed sickle cell anaemia. A similar syndrome can result from inheritance of the β^S gene with another abnormal β gene such as the haemoglobin C gene or β-thalassaemia gene. Inheritance of the β^S gene with a normal β-chain gene (β^A) causes the innocuous sickle cell trait (Fig 17.1).

Pathophysiology

The abnormal β^S gene has a high incidence in tropical and subtropical regions as the abnormal haemoglobin produced (HbS) gives some protection against falciparum malaria. HbS differs from normal haemoglobin (HbA) in that glutamic acid has been replaced by valine at the sixth amino acid from the N-terminus of the β-globin chain. The clinical features of sickle cell anaemia arise from the propensity of red cells containing haemoglobin S to undergo 'sickling'. In the deoxygenated state HbS undergoes a conformational change leading to the creation of haemoglobin tetramers which aggregate to produce large polymers. The red cell loses its normal deformability and becomes characteristically sickle-shaped (Fig 17.2). Damage to the membrane leads to increased rigidity and the ultimate sequestration of the red cell in the reticuloendothelial system causing haemolytic anaemia. The inflexible sickle cells also become lodged in the microcirculation causing stasis and obstruction.

Clinical syndromes

Sickle cell anaemia (HbSS)
This classic form of sickle cell syndrome is enormously variable in severity.

Haemolytic anaemia
The haemoglobin is generally in the range 60–100 g/L. Because HbS releases oxygen more readily than HbA, the symptoms of anaemia are often surprisingly mild. Intercurrent infection with parvovirus or folate deficiency can block erythropoiesis and cause a sudden fall in haemoglobin – the 'aplastic crisis'.

Fig 17.1 **Inheritance of sickle cell syndromes.** Two pedigrees showing inheritance of sickle cell syndromes. In the first family one child is unaffected, one has sickle cell trait and one has sickle cell anaemia. In the second family one child has inherited the abnormal sickle gene and the HbC gene; this double heterozygosity leads to haemoglobin SC disease.

Fig 17.2 **Blood film in sickle cell anaemia.**

Fig 17.3 **Dactylitis in sickle cell anaemia.** (Reproduced with permission from Linch D C, Yates A P 1996 *Colour Guide Haematology* Churchill Livingstone, Edinburgh.)

Vascular-occlusive crises
Acute, episodic, painful crises are a potentially disabling feature of sickle cell anaemia. They may be triggered by infection or cold. Patients complain of musculoskeletal pain which may be severe and require hospital admission. Hips, shoulders and vertebrae are most affected. Attacks are generally self-limiting but infarction of bone can occur and must be distinguished from salmonella osteomyelitis. Avascular necrosis of the femoral head is a crippling complication. Other organs are vulnerable to infarction; most serious is neurological damage which may manifest as seizures, transient ischaemic attacks (TIAs) and strokes. Vaso-occlusion in infancy is responsible for the 'hand–foot syndrome', a type of dactylitis damaging the small bones of hands and feet (Fig 17.3).

Sequestration crises
These arise from sickling and infarction within particular organs. Specific syndromes include 'acute chest syndrome' with occlusion of the pulmonary vasculature, 'girdle sequestration' caused by occlusion of the mesenteric blood supply, and hepatic and splenic sequestration.

Other complications
These are multiple, usually caused by vascular stasis and local ischaemia.

- *Genitourinary.* Papillary necrosis with haematuria; loss of ability to concentrate urine; nephrotic syndrome; priapism.
- *Skin.* Lower limb ulceration.
- *Eyes.* Proliferative retinopathy; glaucoma.
- *Hepatobiliary.* Liver damage; pigment gallstones.

Diagnosis
Diagnosis depends on the following:

- Blood film appearance (see Fig 17.2).
- *Screening tests for sickling.* The blood sample is deoxygenated (e.g. with sodium metabisulphate) to induce sickling.
- *Haemoglobin electrophoresis.* In sickle cell anaemia (HbSS) there is no HbA detectable (Fig 17.4).

Management

General. Patients need support in the community and easy access to centres experienced in the management of sickle cell anaemia. Prophylaxis is important. Patients should avoid factors known to precipitate crises, take folate supplements (because of chronic haemolysis) and be prescribed penicillin and pneumococcal vaccine (because of hyposplenism caused by infarction). Infections require prompt treatment. Transcranial Doppler ultrasonography can identify children at high risk of stroke. Annual retinal screening is recommended.

Painful vascular-occlusive crises. First-line treatment is rest, increased fluids and adequate oral analgesia. Constitutional upset or pain not relieved by oral analgesia necessitates hospital admission with continued rest, warmth, intravenous fluids and opiate analgesia. Psychological support is vital.

Blood transfusion. Acute or chronic simple red cell transfusion may be given to relieve severe anaemia and to reduce the amount of circulating sickle haemoglobin. Chronic transfusions are the most effective intervention to prevent recurrent cerebrovascular events. Other indications for transfusion include complications such as chest syndrome and priapism. Blood transfusion is not usually required for episodes of pain. Exchange transfusion is preferred to simple transfusion for rapid reduction of HbS levels or where simple transfusion would cause hyperviscosity or circulatory overload. Blood is phenotypically matched to reduce the chance of alloimmunisation. Iron chelation may be required.

Pregnancy and surgery. Transfusion is not routinely indicated in an uncomplicated pregnancy but may be needed for severe anaemia or other sickle-cell-related complications. During surgery it is important to avoid hypoxia and dehydration. Preoperative simple transfusion or even exchange transfusion may be appropriate for high-risk procedures.

Hydroxycarbamide. Increasing the level of fetal haemoglobin in red cells with the antimetabolite hydroxycarbamide can reduce the severity of the disease. Clinical trials have been encouraging with significant reductions in painful crises, major complications, blood transfusion, hospital admissions and mortality rates. It is important to ensure compliance as clinical benefit may not be immediate. There are concerns regarding the leukaemogenic and teratogenic effects of hydroxycarbamide but with cautious use and patient education (e.g. appropriate contraception) the risks appear to be low.

Stem cell transplantation. Allogeneic stem cell transplantation offers the possibility of a cure in selected high risk patients but it will not be more widely applicable until the toxicity is reduced (see p. 56).

Gene therapy. Gene therapy has the potential to provide a cure without the risks of allogeneic stem cell transplantation (see p. 103).

Prognosis

The risk of early death is inversely related to fetal haemoglobin levels. The most common causes of death are infection in infancy, cerebrovascular accidents in childhood and adolescence and respiratory complications in adult life.

Doubly heterozygous sickling disorders

Here patients inherit the β^S gene and another abnormal β gene – usually HbC or β-thalassaemia. HbSC disease is similar to HbSS but there is a tendency for fewer painful crises and a higher incidence of proliferative retinopathy and avascular necrosis. The severity of sickle cell/β-thalassaemia depends on whether patients have the β^+ or β^0 genotype. The less common HbS/β^0 form has a similar clinical picture to HbSS.

Sickle cell trait (HbAS)

Sickle cell trait normally causes no clinical problems as there is enough HbA in red cells (approximately 60%) to prevent sickling. However, haematuria occasionally occurs as a result of renal papillary necrosis and additional care is required during pregnancy and anaesthesia. Diagnosis is by a sickling test and Hb electrophoresis (see Fig 17.4). Life expectancy is normal although there may be a slightly increased risk of sudden death during intense exercise in young adults.

Counselling and prenatal diagnosis

Genetic counselling is needed by those affected with either the homozygous disease, compound heterozygosity or the trait. Prenatal diagnosis is possible using mutation analysis on PCR-amplified DNA from chorionic villi (see p. 100).

Screening strategies

Screening of all newborn babies for sickle cell syndromes is recommended to reduce the risk of early death from infection. Preconception testing and antenatal testing of pregnant women is performed depending on individual risk and the local prevalence of sickle cell disease. A similar approach is adopted prior to surgery.

Fig 17.4 **Cellulose acetate electrophoresis to separate haemoglobins A, F, S and C.** Lane 4, control sample; Lanes 2, 3, 6, 7, normal; Lane 1, sickle cell anaemia; Lane 5, sickle cell trait.

Sickle cell syndromes

- The sickle cell syndromes are a group of haemoglobinopathies which primarily affect people of African origin.

- Inheritance of two β^S genes leads to the serious clinical disorder sickle cell anaemia (HbSS).

- Clinical problems in sickle cell anaemia include chronic haemolytic anaemia, vascular-occlusive crises, sequestration crises and susceptibility to infection.

- Routine management of sickle cell anaemia entails prophylactic measures, supportive care during vascular-occlusive crises and the selective use of blood transfusion and hydroxycarbamide.

- Sickle cell trait (HbAS) is an innocuous clinical disorder but genetic counselling is often needed.

18 Anaemia of chronic disease

Anaemia of chronic disease (ACD) is a term used to describe a type of anaemia seen in a wide range of chronic inflammatory, infective and malignant diseases (Table 18.1). The anaemia often becomes apparent during the first few months of illness and then remains fairly constant (Fig 18.1). It is rarely severe (haemoglobin ≥90 g/L; packed cell volume (PCV) ≥0.30) but there is some correlation with the intensity of the underlying illness. For instance, in infection the anaemia is often more marked where there is a persistent fever and in malignancy where there is widespread dissemination. Patients may suffer no symptoms from their anaemia or have only slight fatigue. The importance of this type of anaemia arises not from its severity but from its ubiquity. It is widely misunderstood (for such a common disorder) and ill patients are frequently subjected to excessive haematological investigation and unnecessary treatment with haematinics. The term ACD should not be used to describe other causes of anaemia such as haemolysis or bleeding which may also complicate chronic disorders. It has been argued that the designation ACD is inappropriate but other suggested terms (e.g. anaemia of inflammation) appear even less satisfactory. The anaemia of chronic renal failure is variously referred to as ACD although it has its own specific features (see p. 96).

Incidence

Because its causes are common, ACD is probably only second to iron deficiency as a cause of anaemia. It has been estimated to account for approximately half of all hospital cases of anaemia not explained by blood loss.

Pathophysiology

The causation of the anaemia of chronic disease has been extensively studied but questions remain. Key factors in aetiology are summarised in Figure 18.2. Inflammatory cytokines such as tissue necrosis factor (TNF) and interleukin-1 and -6 are implicated in all of these processes.

There is a modest shortening of red cell lifespan which leads to an increased demand for bone marrow production. The marrow struggles to respond adequately as there is blunting of the expected increase in erythropoietin secretion and also diminished responsiveness of erythroid precursor cells to erythropoietin. Hepcidin, a peptide hormone, appears to be an important mediator of ACD. This acute phase reactant protein is released from the liver following stimulation by interleukin-6. Actions of hepcidin include inhibition of microbial infection, macrophage iron recycling and intestinal iron absorption. Its role in iron balance and transport is mediated via binding to ferroportin, the major cellular iron efflux protein. Patients with inflammation and anaemia have elevated serum and urine levels of hepcidin. Abnormalities of iron metabolism are well documented in ACD. These include:

- reduced iron absorption from the gastrointestinal tract
- decreased plasma iron concentration
- excessive retention of iron in reticuloendothelial cells (macrophages) with diminished release to erythroid cells.

The high prevalence of ACD has led to the suggestion that it may have some benefits for those with chronic inflammation. Perhaps withdrawal of iron by increased storage in the reticuloendothelial system limits its availability to microorganisms or tumour cells. Decreased haemoglobin levels reduce the oxygen-carrying capacity of the blood and might reduce the oxygen supply to unwelcome microorganisms and cells. Cell-mediated immunity is probably strengthened by reduced levels of metabolically active iron in the circulation as iron inhibits the activity of IFN-γ.

Diagnosis

Most patients will have a documented chronic disorder and a moderate anaemia. On occasion the anaemia is a more dominant feature and the underlying cause is not immediately apparent. The anaemia is usually of normochromic normocytic type although it can be slightly hypochromic microcytic. The blood film appearance is often unremarkable but there may be changes 'reactive' to the underlying disorder such as a neutrophil leucocytosis, thrombocytosis and rouleaux formation. There is a reticulocytopenia. Inflammatory markers such as C-reactive protein (CRP) and erythrocyte sedimentation rate (ESR) are often raised. Serum iron concentration and transferrin concentration are usually reduced. The serum ferritin level is normal or high (as an acute phase reactant). In practice, ACD is most commonly confused with mild iron deficiency anaemia, particularly if the MCV and MCH are reduced. However, the two forms of anaemia should be distinguishable as in uncomplicated iron deficiency the transferrin concentration is elevated and the ferritin level is low. In difficult cases the serum

---

Table 18.1 **Common causes of the anaemia of chronic disease**

- Malignancy
- Rheumatoid arthritis
- Various connective tissue disorders
- Chronic infection
- Extensive trauma
- Chronic renal failure[1]
- Chronic heart failure

[1]See also page 96.

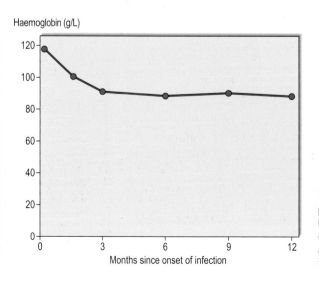

Haemoglobin (g/L)

Months since onset of infection

Fig 18.1 **ACD in a patient with chronic infection.** The rate of development of anaemia and its final severity are typical of ACD.

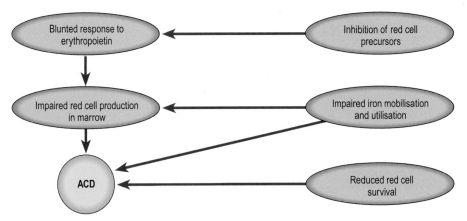

Fig 18.2 **Overview of the aetiology of ACD.** Cytokines such as TNF, interleukin-1 and interleukin-6 and the peptide hepcidin play key roles (see text).

Table 18.2 **Comparison of clinical and laboratory findings in ACD and iron deficiency anaemia**

Characteristic	ACD	Iron deficiency
Severity of anaemia	Hb usually ≥90 g/L	Very variable
Symptoms of anaemia	Usually mild	May be severe
Coexistent chronic disease	Yes	Variable
Red cell indices (MCV, MCH)	Normochromic Normocytic[1]	Hypochromic Microcytic
Blood film appearance	Often normal or reactive[2]	Hypochromia Microcytosis Poikilocytosis Target cells
Serum iron	Reduced	Reduced
Transferrin concentration	Reduced or normal	Increased
Ferritin	Normal or increased	Reduced[3]
Serum transferrin receptor	Normal	Increased
Serum transferrin receptor-ferritin index[4]	Low	High
Marrow iron stores	Normal or increased	Reduced

[1]May be slightly hypochromic microcytic.
[2]'Reactive' changes in a blood film may accompany the underlying disorder; possible abnormalities include rouleaux formation, a neutrophil leucocytosis and thrombocytosis.
[3]Unless there is a coexistent acute phase response when the ferritin level may be normal.
[4]Transferrin receptor concentration divided by serum ferritin concentration (or log of plasma ferritin concentration).

transferrin receptor concentration and the serum transferrin receptor-ferritin index may be useful (Table 18.2). Measurement of the percentage of hypochromic red cells or reticulocyte haemoglobin content can be helpful in detecting coexistent iron-restricted red cell production in a patient with ACD. Reliable hepcidin assays are under development and are likely to enter routine clinical practice. Bone marrow examination is not routinely required but where performed will show normal or increased marrow iron stores with decreased marrow sideroblasts (Fig 18.3).

It should be remembered that anaemia in a patient with a chronic medical disorder may be of multifactorial origin. It is important not to misdiagnose ACD as something else but equally it cannot be assumed that every patient with long-standing disease and a low haemoglobin has only ACD.

Management

As the anaemia is usually non-severe and not progressive, the management is primarily that of the underlying disorder. The rationale for treating the anaemia itself is to avoid immediate deleterious effects (e.g. on the cardiovascular system), to improve quality of life, and possibly to improve the prognosis of the underlying condition.

Fig 18.3 **Bone marrow aspirate stained with Perls stain showing increased reticuloendothelial iron stores in ACD.**

Occasionally, patients cannot adequately compensate for the anaemia and require blood transfusion. Recombinant human erythropoietin and its derivatives can be effective in relieving anaemia, particularly in rheumatoid arthritis and malignancy. Their use is restricted by concerns of increased risk of thromboembolic events and higher rates of tumour recurrence; they should only be used selectively and in the lowest effective dose. In the absence of coexistent iron deficiency, oral iron supplements are rarely helpful. Intravenous iron may be beneficial, especially if combined with erythropoietin, but there is limited experience outside the field of renal medicine. Further studies are needed to evaluate the effect of amelioration of the anaemia on the course of the underlying disease. Possible future therapies for ACD include alternative stimulators of erythropoiesis, hepcidin antagonists and novel anti-inflammatory agents.

Anaemia of chronic disease (ACD)

- ACD is seen in a wide range of chronic malignant, inflammatory and infective disorders.

- The pathogenesis of ACD is complex. There is a reduction in both red cell production and survival. Hepcidin is likely to be a key mediator.

- The anaemia is usually of normochromic, normocytic type, non-progressive and is rarely severe.

- Treatment is primarily that of the underlying disorder. Blood transfusion and erythropoietin may help in selected cases. Iron supplementation has a limited role.

19 Introduction

The leukaemias are a heterogeneous group of malignant blood disorders. In this introductory section, general characteristics such as definitions, aetiology and classification are discussed. Each of the more common types of leukaemia is subsequently described in more detail.

Definition

Leukaemia is a type of cancer caused by the unregulated proliferation of a clone of immature blood cells derived from mutant haematopoietic stem cells. The disease is the result of multiple acquired genetic and epigenetic events which can vary widely between patients. Leukaemic transformation is assumed to occur at or near the level of the leukaemic stem cell prior to definite lineage commitment. The leukaemic cells do not differentiate normally. They may avoid standard mechanisms of cell death (apoptosis) and they may also retain the stem cell signature of self-renewal. This relentless proliferating clone of aberrant cells eventually squeezes out normal cells from the bone marrow causing marrow failure and death.

Incidence

Leukaemia is not a common disorder but it is a significant cause of death from cancer (Fig 19.1). There is a male preponderance in most types of leukaemia. Geographic variations exist; for instance, chronic lymphocytic leukaemia is the predominant form of leukaemia in the Western world but is much less frequent in Japan, South America and Africa.

Aetiology

As for other malignancies, the evolution of leukaemia is likely to be a multistep process. Thus, accumulated genetic mutations corrupt normal cellular pathways controlling proliferation and differentiation and lead to the production of an autonomous proliferating stem cell clone ('clonal evolution'). It is easiest to think about the aetiology in terms of these acquired genetic abnormalities and other more general predisposing factors.

Genetic abnormalities

Cytogenetic analysis and particularly molecular genetic techniques have revealed various acquired non-random chromosomal derangements which play a fundamental role in leukaemogenesis (Fig 19.2). There are a number of different types of possible chromosomal change.

Chromosomal translocations

One chromosome breaks and donates a fragment to another chromosome which reciprocates by returning a fragment of its own. Such translocations can result in the movement of proto-oncogenes to new sites where they have the capacity to cause leukaemic transformations. The classical example of a balanced translocation is the 'Philadelphia chromosome', found in 95% of cases of chronic myeloid leukaemia (CML), where breakages in chromosomes 9 and 22 result in the creation of a new fusion gene (*BCR-ABL*) which encodes a novel protein with intense tyrosine kinase activity. In a manner incompletely understood, this protein causes deregulated myeloid cell growth.

Chromosome deletions and additions

A chromosome may be completely or partly deleted, for example monosomy 7 in acute myeloid leukaemia (AML). Here a normal gene may be lost, allowing expression of a recessive cancer gene. Conversely, an additional chromosome may be gained.

Submicroscopic mutations

A change in the base sequence of certain oncogenes may predispose to leukaemia. The *RAS* oncogene which encodes a protein vital in signal transduction is mutated in 50% of cases of AML.

Epigenetic mechanisms

Epigenetic changes, where there is a change in gene function (e.g. altered DNA methylation) but not structure, may play a role in leukaemia.

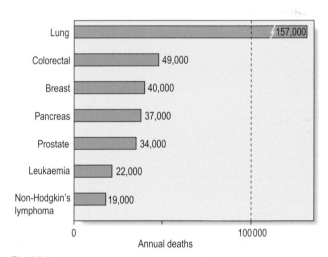

Fig 19.1 **Annual causes of death from malignancy in the year 2011** (estimated data from United States).

Fig 19.2 **Fluorescence in situ hybridisation (FISH) study of a complex karyotype (including t(8;16)) in a patient with acute myeloid leukaemia.**

Table 19.1 **Factors predisposing to leukaemia**
Radiation exposure
Previous chemotherapy (particularly alkylating agents)
Occupational chemical exposure (e.g. benzene)
Some genetically determined disorders (e.g. Down syndrome)
Viral infection (only HTLV-1 proven as a causative factor)
Myelodysplastic and myeloproliferative disorders
Other possible (e.g. cigarette smoking)

Particular chromosome changes are often associated with specific types of leukaemia (e.g. the Philadelphia chromosome in CML). However, few abnormalities are entirely specific – the Philadelphia chromosome can be found in cases of acute leukaemia. It should also be noted that not all cases of leukaemia have a detectable cytogenetic abnormality. The incidence of abnormality is partly dependent on the laboratory expertise available.

Predisposing factors

In a small subpopulation of leukaemic patients there is another obvious predisposing factor – the more common of these are listed in Table 19.1.

The incidence of acute leukaemia and chronic myeloid leukaemia increases with radiation dose exposure in all age groups. Classic studies have included people exposed to the atomic bombs in Japan and patients receiving radiotherapy for ankylosing spondylitis in the middle years of the 20th century. Results from studies of diagnostic radiation and adult leukaemia are inconsistent and in appropriate radiological procedures the benefit is likely to outweigh what appears to be at most a very small risk. Paternal preconception exposure to ionising radiation has been associated with an increased incidence of acute leukaemia in offspring.

Cytotoxic chemotherapy, particularly with alkylating agents, leads to an increased risk of leukaemia (Fig 19.3). The risk appears to be greatest in older

Fig 19.3 **Peripheral blood film in a young woman with acute myeloid leukaemia.** She had received chemotherapy for choriocarcinoma several years previously.

patients also treated with radiotherapy. The best established occupational leukaemogenic exposure is undoubtedly to benzene. A number of genetically determined diseases also predispose to leukaemia. Here the liability to leukaemia is probably caused by factors such as increased chromosomal breakage (e.g. Fanconi's anaemia) and immunosuppression (e.g. ataxia telangiectasia).

Viruses are known to be the main cause of leukaemia in many animals but in humans the only well-proven association is of the HTLV-1 virus with the rare disorder T-cell leukaemia lymphoma (Fig 19.4). Myelodysplastic syndromes (pp. 50–51) and myeloproliferative disorders (pp. 64–67) may transform to acute myeloid leukaemia.

Classification

In such a potentially complex group of disorders it is helpful to use a relatively simple classification. The leukaemias can most broadly be divided into acute and chronic types depending on their clinical course. The classification illustrated here (Table 19.2) further divides

Fig 19.4 **Bone marrow trephine appearance in human T-cell leukaemia lymphoma.** The only human leukaemia with a known viral causation.

leukaemias into their cell of origin (i.e. myeloid or lymphoid) and refers to the microscopic appearance (morphology) of the leukaemic cells. The traditional classification of the acute leukaemias is that of the FAB group – the abbreviation being for the French, American and British nationalities of the terminologists – but this has been overtaken by the World Health Organization (WHO) system. Basic morphological techniques (e.g. microscopic inspection of a blood film and bone marrow sample) remain important in the initial diagnosis but cytogenetic and molecular genetic techniques are becoming increasingly important in classification as acquired genetic changes frequently have prognostic significance and can guide treatment.

In the following pages are discussed acute myeloid leukaemia, acute lymphoblastic leukaemia, chronic myeloid leukaemia and chronic lymphocytic leukaemia. Together these four diseases constitute the overwhelming majority of leukaemias in clinical practice. A few rarer types of leukaemia are discussed separately.

Table 19.2 **Classification of leukaemia**[1]	
Acute leukaemia	Acute myeloid leukaemia
	Acute lymphoblastic leukaemia
Chronic leukaemia	Chronic myeloid leukaemia
	Chronic lymphocytic leukaemia
Other types	Hairy cell leukaemia
	Prolymphocytic leukaemia
	T-cell leukaemia lymphoma

[1] See specific disease sections for more detail.

Leukaemia: introduction

■ Leukaemia is a type of cancer caused by the unregulated proliferation of a clone of immature blood cells.

■ Leukaemia is a heterogeneous group of clinical disorders classified on the basis of their clinical course (acute or chronic) and their cell of origin (myeloid or lymphoid).

■ The aetiology of leukaemia is likely to be multifactorial with known predisposing factors such as radiation exposure present in only a minority of cases. Acquired genetic and epigenetic abnormalities play a fundamental role in leukaemogenesis with certain changes associated with particular types of leukaemia.

20 Acute myeloid leukaemia

Introduction

Acute myeloid leukaemia (AML) is a malignant clonal disorder of haematopoietic progenitor cells. Leukaemic transformation usually occurs at a very early stage of myeloid development, probably at or near the haematopoietic stem cell, but it may develop in a more mature cell. The disease is heterogeneous. The malignant cells acquire genetic alterations which upset their normal mechanisms of self-renewal, proliferation and differentiation. Ultimately the malignant clone causes marrow failure. AML is rare in childhood and the incidence increases with age; two-thirds of cases occur in people aged over 60 years.

Classification

The WHO system has now largely superseded the French-American-British (FAB) classification. The newer classification reduces the bone marrow leukaemic blast cell percentage differentiating AML from myelodysplastic syndrome (see p. 50) from 30% to 20%. Other key changes include the creation of specific subtypes with non-random cytogenetic or equivalent molecular abnormalities, and the distinction of patients with multilineage dysplasia and also previous chemotherapy. The major FAB subtypes are included in the 'other' category with the exception of acute promyelocytic leukaemia (previously FAB M3) which is now in the 'recurrent translocations' group due to the inevitable presence of t(15;17). It can be seen (Table 20.1) that occasional cases of AML show megakaryocytic or erythroid differentiation. Gene mutations are likely to become increasingly important in classification.

Clinical features

In practice there is little uniformity in presentation. Some patients are remarkably asymptomatic while others are seriously ill. Bone marrow infiltration by leukaemic blast cells usually leads to anaemia, neutropenia and thrombocytopenia. Thus, patients often have symptoms of anaemia, infection and haemorrhage.

One subtype of AML deserves special consideration as it must be treated as a medical emergency:

Table 20.1 WHO classification of acute myeloid leukaemia

AML with recurrent genetic abnormalities[1]
AML with t(18;21)(q22;q22)
AML with inv (16)(p13;q22) or t(16;16) (p13.1;q22) (M4 Eo)
AML with t(15;17)(q22;q12) (M3:M3V)
AML with t(9;11) (p22;q23)
AML with t(6;9) (p23;q34)
AML with inv(3) (q21;q26.2) or t(3;3) (q21;q26.2)
AML (megakaryoblastic) with t(1;22) (p13;q13)
AML with myelodysplasia-related changes
Therapy related myeloid neoplasms
AML not otherwise specified[2]
AML with minimal differentiation (M0)
AML without maturation (M1)
AML with maturation (M2)
Acute myelomonocytic leukaemia (M4)
Acute monoblastic/ monocytic leukaemia(M4/5)
Acute erythroid leukaemia (M6)
Acute megakaryoblastic leukaemia (M7)
Acute basophilic leukaemia
Acute panmyelosis with myelofibrosis
Myeloid sarcoma
Myeloid proliferation related to Down syndrome
Blastic plasmacytoid dendritic cell neoplasm

[1]See also Table 2 for genetic changes.
[2]FAB equivalent is shown in parentheses.

- **AML with t(15;17)(q22;q12) (M3, M3V).** More traditionally referred to as *acute promyelocytic leukaemia*, this disease is associated with a high incidence of disseminated intravascular coagulation (DIC) and a high risk of spontaneous bleeding into vital organs.

Tissue infiltration is more common in subtypes with monocytic morphology and immunophenotypic features (i.e. FAB M5) – patients often present with gum infiltration (Fig 20.1), lymphadenopathy, skin deposits and hepatosplenomegaly. Central nervous system (CNS) disease is rare in AML but most frequent in monocytic/monoblastic leukaemia.

Diagnosis

Diagnosis depends on a logical sequence of tests.

1. **Blood count and film.** The white cell count (WCC) is usually elevated (up to 200×10^9/L) but may be normal or low. There is often anaemia and thrombocytopenia. Usually there are leukaemic blast cells although occasionally these are absent. There may be dysplastic changes in other cells.

2. **Bone marrow aspirate and trephine.** The bone marrow is

Fig 20.1 **Gum infiltration in acute monocytic (M5) leukaemia.**

Fig 20.2 **Bone marrow appearance in different FAB subtypes of AML. (a)** AML M2: the leukaemic blast cells show some granulocytic differentiation. **(b)** AML M3 (promyelocytic): the leukaemic cells show marked cytoplasmic granularity. **(c)** AML M4 (myelomonocytic): some of the leukaemic cells have monocytic features.

infiltrated by leukaemic blast cells (Fig 20.2). In more immature forms of AML morphological differentiation from acute lymphoblastic leukaemia (ALL) can be difficult.

3. **Cytochemistry.** Special stains are used on bone marrow and blood smears to help differentiate myeloid and lymphoid blast cells. In AML there is positivity with Sudan black and myeloperoxidase – these stains are negative in ALL. AML with

monocytic features will stain positively with a non-specific esterase stain.

4. **Immunophenotyping.** Both surface and intracellular antigens are analysed. Characteristic 'myeloid' antigens include CD13 and CD33 while CD34 positivity indicates a particularly immature cell of origin. Modern multicolour flow cytometry techniques allow quantitation of blast cells and correlate with both morphology features and the common balanced translocations.

5. **Cytogenetics.** A bone marrow sample is sent for analysis. Chromosome abnormalities are associated with particular AML subtypes and also give vital prognostic information (see Tables 20.1 and 20.2).

6. **Molecular biology.** Molecular techniques are increasingly important in classification, determining prognosis, and in monitoring response of disease to treatment (see p. 100). Sequential RT-PCR monitoring (e.g. in patients with the t(15;17) subtype in clinical remission) can predict the likelihood of relapse. Numerous genetic abnormalities are being identified – mutation of the tyrosine kinase receptor gene *FLT3* is the commonest finding in patients with normal cytogenetics and carries a poorer prognosis. Other genetic mutations (e.g. nucleophosmin 1 (NPM1), two mutations of CEPPA gene) can favourably influence prognosis.

Management

Supportive care

This includes red cell transfusion for anaemia, platelet concentrates for thrombocytopenia and broad-spectrum intravenous antibiotics for infection. An indwelling central venous catheter facilitates support during and after chemotherapy.

Chemotherapy and stem cell transplantation

The first objective of treatment with cytotoxic drugs is to achieve a 'complete remission' (CR) – defined as less than 5% blast cells in a normocellular bone marrow. Initial cytotoxic drug treatment is termed 'induction'. A CR is followed by a second sequence of drugs termed 'consolidation'. Induction and consolidation take at least several months, but

Table 20.2 **Common genetic abnormalities in AML**

Abnormality	Genes involved	Associated subtype	Prognosis[1]
t(8;21)	AML1-ETO (RUNX1 -RUNX1-T1)	M2	Good
t(15;17)	PML-RARα	M3	Good
inv 16	CBFB-MYH11	M4	Good
t(9;11)	MLL	M4/5	Poor
5 and 7 (various)	Unknown	Secondary AML[2]	Poor

[1]Compared with AML with no detectable genetic abnormality.
[2]Antecedent events include chemotherapy, myelodysplastic syndrome and myeloproliferative disorders.

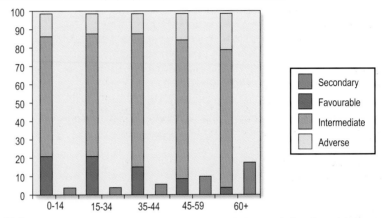

Fig 20.3 **Relationship between age of presentation and characteristics of AML.** Older patients have a higher incidence of 'poor risk' disease. (Reprinted with permission from Smith ML, Hills RK, Grimwade D 2011 Independent prognostic variables in AML. Blood Reviews 25: 40.)

longer-term 'maintenance' treatment is rarely given. The well tested combination of an anthracycline (e.g. daunorubicin) and cytosine arabinoside is standard induction therapy. Higher doses of cytosine are often used as consolidation therapy. Acute promyelocytic leukaemia (t(15;17)) is additionally treated with the differentiating agent all-*trans*-retinoic acid (ATRA), which reduces the risk of early death from bleeding and improves long-term survival compared with chemotherapy alone.

Autologous stem cell transplantation (SCT) can be used to intensify chemotherapy but the benefit has proved difficult to quantify. Surprisingly, the precise role of allogeneic SCT is also not clear-cut – most clinicians would consider a transplant from an available HLA-matched sibling in a younger patient with high-risk (see below) or relapsed disease. Novel molecular targeted therapies under exploration include anti-CD33 antibodies, *FLT3* inhibitors and demethylating agents.

Prognosis

The major factors determining outcome are age, initial response to treatment and genetic abnormalities. Approximately 80–90% of younger patients will achieve a CR with conventional chemotherapy. Younger patients with 'standard risk' disease have 5-year survivals of 40–45% with optimal therapy; this compares with around 70% for 'good risk' and 20% for 'poor risk' groups. Older patients have a greater incidence of adverse cytogenetics (Fig 20.3) and tolerate chemotherapy less well, and CR and cure rates are much lower (see p. 93). Indeed, it may be kinder not to use chemotherapy in some elderly patients. In children, intensive chemotherapy gives 5-year survival rates of around 50%.

Acute myeloid leukaemia

- AML arises out of the malignant transformation of a myeloid precursor cell.
- The WHO classification emphasises the prognostic significance of non-random chromosome abnormalities.
- Symptoms mainly result from anaemia, neutropenia and thrombocytopenia.
- Prognosis largely depends on age, initial response to treatment, and genetic abnormalities.
- Chemotherapy leads to CR rates of 80–90% in younger patients but cure rates are lower, around 45%. Allogeneic stem cell transplantation is considered in younger patients at high risk of relapse.
- Older patients tolerate chemotherapy less well and cure is rarely achievable.

21 Acute lymphoblastic leukaemia

Acute lymphoblastic leukaemia (ALL) is a clonal malignancy of lymphoid precursor cells. In over 80% of cases the malignant cells are primitive precursors of B-lymphocytes and the remainder are T-cell leukaemias. The abnormal cell may arise at various stages of early lymphocyte differentiation (see p. 8).

ALL has a peak incidence in childhood with a gradual rise in incidence in later years (Fig 21.1). The disease has distinct characteristics in children and adults. Childhood ALL is often curable by chemotherapy whereas cure is elusive in adult ALL. Poorer outcome in adult ALL is due to a combination of a greater frequency of high-risk leukaemia with more drug resistance, and less effective treatment regimens.

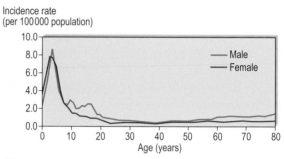

Fig 21.1 **Incidence of ALL at different ages.**

Classification

The French-American-British (FAB) morphological classification is based on characteristics of the blast cells, including cell size, nuclear–cytoplasmic ratio, number and size of nucleoli and the degree of cytoplasmic basophilia (Fig 21.2). Morphological classification is now less important than that based on immunophenotyping, cytogenetics and molecular analysis (Table 21.1).

Definition of the immunological subtypes of ALL depends on the presence or absence of various cell surface and cytoplasmic antigens. A commonly used classification divides ALL into early pre-B, pre-B, B-cell and T-cell subtypes. Mature B-cell ALL typically has L3 morphology. The current WHO classification divides most ALL subtypes into B- or T-lymphoblastic leukaemia/lymphoma under the heading 'precursor lymphoid neoplasms'. Mature B-ALL is included as Burkitt lymphoma.

In the selection of treatment it is important to differentiate between three broad groups; T-cell ALL, mature B-ALL and all other types of B-lineage ALL. Genetic abnormalities are becoming increasingly important in classification of ALL as they give vital prognostic information (Table 21.2).

Clinical features

These can be very variable. Accumulation of malignant lymphoblasts in the marrow leads to a scarcity of normal cells in the peripheral blood and symptoms may include those associated with anaemia, infection and haemorrhage. Other common complaints are anorexia and back or joint pain. T-cell ALL is associated with a large mediastinal nodal mass and pleural effusions which result in dyspnoea. Central nervous system (CNS) involvement is more often seen

Table 21.1 **Classification of ALL**

Morphological classification[1]	
L1	Small uniform blast cells with scanty cytoplasm
L2	Large heterogeneous blast cells with nucleoli and low nuclear–cytoplasmic ratio
L3	Basophilic vacuolated blast cells
Immunological classification	
B-lineage ALL	
Early pre-B	
Pre-B ALL	
B-cell	
T-lineage ALL	
Early	
Cortical	
Mature	

[1]See also Figure 21.2.

in ALL than in AML and patients can present with symptoms of raised intracranial pressure (headache, vomiting) or cranial nerve palsies (particularly VI and VII). Examination findings may include pallor, haemorrhage into the skin and mucosae, lymphadenopathy and moderate hepatosplenomegaly. In males the testes can be involved and should be routinely examined.

Diagnosis

1. Blood count and film

The white cell count may be raised, normal or low. Only 20% have white cell counts greater than 50×10^9/L. Anaemia and thrombocytopenia are common. The proportion of blast cells in the white cell count varies from 0% to 100%.

2. Bone marrow aspirate and trephine

This is essential to confirm the diagnosis and for classification.

3. Cytochemistry

Stains which classically show positivity in AML – Sudan black and myeloperoxidase – are negative in ALL.

Fig 21.2 **Morphology of ALL blast cells.** **(a)** L1 type; **(b)** L2 type; **(c)** L3 type. Note that the L2 cells have more cytoplasm and more prominent nucleoli than L1 cells. L3 type cells have cytoplasmic vacuolation.

Cytochemistry is useful in distinguishing precursor B and B-ALL from T-ALL. Reactivity with the acid phosphatase stain is seen in malignant T-lymphocytes but not in B-cells which may show periodic acid Schiff (PAS) block positivity.

4. Immunophenotyping

Useful reagents for establishing the diagnosis and identifying the immunological subtype include antibodies to CD19, CD79A and CD22 (found in most B-lineage ALLs), CD10 (the 'common ALL antigen'), CD3 and CD7 (found in T-lineage ALLs).

Table 21.2 **Chromosomal abnormalities in ALL**		
Abnormality		**Prognostic significance**
Numerical change		
High hyperdiploidy (over 50 chromosomes)		Favourable
Hyperdiploidy (47–50)		Intermediate
Pseudodiploidy (46 with structural/numerical change)		Intermediate
Hypodiploidy (less than 46)		Poor
Structural abnormality	**Genes involved**	
Philadelphia chromosome, t(9;22)[1]	BCR-ABL	Poor
t(12;21)[2]	TEL-AML1 (ETV6-RUNX1)	Good
t(1;19)	E₂A-PBX1	Good
t(v;11q23)	MLL-AF4, ENL-MLL	Poor
t(8;14)[3]	MYC	Good

[1]Must be distinguished from the lymphoid blast crisis of chronic myeloid leukaemia.
[2]Occurs in 20% cases of childhood ALL. Not detectable by standard cytogenetics.
[3]Seen in B-ALL with L3 morphology.

Table 21.3 **Factors predicting poor prognosis in ALL**
■ Increasing age[1]
■ High white cell count at presentation
■ Certain cytogenetic abnormalities (see Table 21.2)
■ Poor response to treatment[2]

[1]With the exception of children under 1 year who have a worse prognosis than older children.
[2]Assessed from the bone marrow appearance after 14 days of chemotherapy.

5. Cytogenetics

Cytogenetic analysis is doubly useful as structural abnormalities correlate with particular subtypes of ALL and both structural and numerical abnormalities give prognostic information (see Table 21.2). Varying patterns of cytogenetic abnormality may partly explain the different prognosis in children and adults. The Philadelphia chromosome, regarded as a marker of 'incurability' by chemotherapy, is found in 20–30% of adult cases but in only 2% of children.

6. Molecular techniques

Molecular analysis yields complementary and additional information to conventional cytogenetics (see Table 21.2). The cryptic t(12;21) creates a *TEL-AML1* (ETV6-RUNX1) fusion gene – this is the commonest genetic rearrangement in childhood ALL and it can only be detected by molecular techniques. Although not yet routinely available in most laboratories, global gene expression profiling reveals distinct patterns in specific subtypes of ALL (see p. 100).

Management and outcome

General principles

Patients with ALL require supportive care. Chemotherapy is the mainstay of treatment. Drug schedules vary but remission induction classically relies on three agents: vincristine, a glucocorticoid (e.g. prednisolone) and asparaginase. The anthracycline daunorubicin may be included in the induction regimen and other drugs, notably methotrexate, cyclophosphamide and cytosine arabinoside, then added in 'intensification' ('consolidation') (see p. 54 for more detail of individual drugs). The rationale for early intensification of treatment is to reduce the leukaemic cell population quickly and reduce the likelihood of drug resistance. Therapy is usually completed with a period of 'maintenance' using methotrexate and mercaptopurine. The greater chance of CNS disease in ALL (than in AML) necessitates prophylactic treatment to prevent CNS relapse. The usual method is intrathecal and systemic chemotherapy with the possible addition of cranial irradiation in those at highest risk.

The ultimate choice of management is influenced by a number of prognostic factors which have changed with improving treatment (Table 21.3). Where clinical and laboratory features predict a poor response to chemotherapy alone, more intensive treatments such as allogeneic stem cell transplantation (SCT) are considered. Of all the prognostic indices the most influential is age.

ALL in children

The majority of children are curable with current chemotherapy regimens. The standard strategy is intensive induction therapy, CNS prophylaxis, and maintenance treatment for 2–2.5 years. In children receiving the most intensive protocols, 5-year disease-free survivals of nearly 90% are now achievable. Autologous and allogeneic SCT is best reserved for relapse after chemotherapy or for patients with poor prognostic features. New methods for detecting minimal residual disease during treatment (e.g. after induction) allow early identification of patients at high risk of relapse. Mature B-ALL is a special case best treated with short-term fractionated intensive chemotherapy. With improved cure rates the long-term side-effects of the drugs, including endocrine problems, secondary leukaemia and cardiotoxicity, are becoming increasingly relevant. Wherever feasible, the use of agents with the safest profiles is desirable.

ALL in adults

The majority of adult patients enter remission but are not curable with chemotherapy alone and less than 40% will become long-term survivors. Most chemocurable patients are aged between 16 and 25 years with other good prognostic features. This 'good risk' subgroup resembles childhood ALL and chemotherapy alone is a reasonable initial policy with cure rates of around 75%. For adults with higher-risk disease the hope of cure is likely to depend on even more intensive therapy with either autologous or allogeneic SCT. Allogeneic SCT from an HLA-matched family donor performed in first remission gives long-term survival of around 50%. SCT using an unrelated HLA-'matched' donor is more risky but can be successful. In Philadelphia chromosome positive ALL the tyrosine kinase inhibitor imatinib is useful adjunctive therapy (see p. 45). Optimum management of adult ALL has yet to be defined and there is a need for careful consideration of all the known prognostic factors in each case. More elderly patients (over 60 years) tolerate chemotherapy less well and cure rates are very low. In these cases it is often kinder to concentrate on palliation of symptoms and provision of a short period of good quality life rather than undertaking aggressive chemotherapy with a negligible chance of success.

Acute lymphoblastic leukaemia

- ALL is a clonal malignancy of lymphoid precursor cells.
- There is a peak incidence in childhood and a gradual rise in later years.
- Accumulation of lymphoblasts in the bone marrow often leads to anaemia, infection and haemorrhage. CNS involvement is more common than in acute myeloid leukaemia.
- The majority of children are curable with standard chemotherapy regimens and CNS prophylaxis.
- In adults, cure by chemotherapy alone is much less frequent. Autologous or allogeneic stem cell transplantation may be considered in 'high-risk' cases.

22 Chronic myeloid leukaemia

Chronic myeloid leukaemia (CML) is a clonal myeloproliferative disorder which results from an acquired genetic change in a pluripotential stem cell. The disease is characterised by a gross over-production of neutrophils and their precursors (Fig 22.1). It is unusual in having three clinical phases: a relatively benign 'chronic phase' is followed by an ominous 'accelerated phase' and, finally, an almost invariably fatal acute leukaemic phase termed 'blast crisis'.

The annual incidence of CML is around one per 100 000 with presentation most common in the fifth and sixth decades of life. The diagnosis is increasingly made in asymptomatic patients having routine blood tests.

Pathogenesis

The hallmark of CML cells is the presence of a Philadelphia (Ph) chromosome – the t(9;22)(q34;q11) chromosomal translocation. Over 95% of classical CML cases are Ph positive. The Ph translocation causes the fusion of the *ABL* proto-oncogene from chromosome 9 to the interrupted end of the breakpoint cluster region (*BCR*) of chromosome 22 (Fig 22.2). The chimeric *BCR-ABL* gene created on the Ph chromosome (22q–) encodes a protein with considerably greater tyrosine kinase activity than the normal counterpart. In chronic phase CML, cells in the progenitor pool have increased proliferation due to over-expression of *BCR-ABL*. The mechanism by which the BCR-ABL oncogene affects stem cell kinetics is not well understood. It presumably deregulates signalling pathways involved in proliferation, apoptosis, cellular adhesion and genomic stability. Progression to blast crisis with production of leukaemic stem cells requires complex additional events including increased proliferation and self-renewal capacity avoidance of cell death, a block in differentiation and bypassing of normal immune responses.

Clinical features

Patients usually present in chronic phase. Typical symptoms are of anaemia, anorexia and weight loss. Splenomegaly is the most common physical finding and is often marked, causing pain, bloating and satiety. The occasional patient presents with gout or hyperviscosity associated with a very high white cell count. Neutropenia and thrombocytopenia are not normally features of chronic phase and infection and haemorrhage are rare.

After a period of stability in chronic phase, patients develop blast crisis with symptoms typical of acute leukaemia. Between chronic phase (CP) and blast crisis is an intervening period of 'acceleration'. The accelerated phase is poorly defined but

Fig 22.1 **Blood sample (right) from a patient with CML.** Note the greatly increased white cell component ('buffy coat') compared with the normal sample.

is usually associated with an insidious deterioration in the patient's health and the need for more intense treatment to control splenic size and white cell count.

Diagnosis and monitoring

The major laboratory abnormality in CP-CML is an elevated white cell count; this often exceeds 100×10^9/L. The blood film shows an increase in morphologically normal myeloid cells at all stages of differentiation but with greatest numbers of myelocytes and neutrophils (Fig 22.3). There is usually an absolute basophilia. Thrombocytosis and nucleated red cells may be present.

The bone marrow appearance is less informative than the blood film; pronounced hypercellularity and abnormal myelopoiesis is characteristic but not specific for CML. The key diagnostic abnormality is the presence of the Ph chromosome. Patients with apparent CML with Ph chromosome negativity need careful review as they may represent an atypical myeloproliferative or myelodysplastic disorder.

The accelerated phase is characterised by an increase in the number of immature cells in the peripheral blood and in blast crisis the blood appearance is dominated by the presence of myeloblasts

Fig 22.2 **The Philadelphia chromosome.** Chromosomal and molecular abnormalities in chronic myeloid leukaemia. In a translocation between chromosomes 9 and 22 (t(9;22)) the oncogene *ABL* on chromosome 9 is moved to the breakpoint cluster region (*BCR*) of chromosome 22. The resulting *BCR-ABL* hybrid gene encodes a protein with high tyrosine kinase activity.

Fig 22.3 Blood film in CML showing myeloid cells of varying maturity.

Table 22.1 Evaluation of response to imatinib in chronic phase CML

Time after start of treatment	Response		
	Optimal	Suboptimal	Failure
3 months	CHR and at least minor CyR	No CyR	No CHR
6 months	At least partial CyR	Less than partial CyR	No CyR
12 months	CCyR	Partial CyR	Less than partial CyR
18 months	MMR	Less than MMR	Less than CCyR
Any time	Stable or improving MMR	Loss of MMR. Presence of BCR-ABL mutations	Loss of CHR. Loss of CCyR. Clonal evolution[1]

CHR: complete haematological remission; CyR: cytogenetic response; CCyR: complete cytogenetic response; MMR: major molecular response.
[1]Additional chromosome abnormalities in Ph+ cells.

(65% of cases) or lymphoblasts (35%). The most widely used staging system, devised by Sokal, is based on patient age, spleen size, blood blast cell count and platelet count. Monitoring of the response to treatment is now central to management. This involves examination of the peripheral blood, bone marrow metaphase cytogenetics and measurement of BCR-ABL transcripts using real-time quantitative polymerase chain reaction (RQ-PCR). The results allow the patient's response to be defined at key time points (see Table 22.1). Where there is failure or a suboptimal response, alternative therapy is considered.

Treatment

Recent advances have revolutionised the management of chronic phase CML. It has been transformed from a disease with a very poor prognosis to a chronic subclinical disorder controlled with oral medication.

Chronic phase

Patients presenting with a very high white cell count may have symptoms of hyperviscosity and can benefit from leucapheresis.

Drug therapy. Hydroxycarbamide can also be used to rapidly reduce an initial high white cell count. Tyrosine kinase inhibitors (TKIs) are the treatment of choice. Imatinib at a dose of 400 mg daily orally is normally used as first-line. Patients achieving the milestones shown in Table 22.1 have an excellent prognosis, with long-term survival rates exceeding 90% and a very low risk of transformation to accelerated phase or blast crisis. For patients who are unable to tolerate imatinib or who become resistant, so-called second generation TKIs such as dasatinib and nilotinib can be effective. Both these drugs are more potent than imatinib and are likely to be increasingly used as initial treatment. Third generation agents (e.g. bosutinib) are under investigation.

Stem cell transplantation (SCT). Allogeneic SCT is at present the only proven curative treatment for CML. Patients have survived for more than 10 years after SCT with no detectable BCR-ABL transcripts in blood or bone marrow. The 5-year leukaemia-free survival after HLA- identical sibling SCT is around 60%. Results have been best when SCT has been performed in chronic phase within 1 year of diagnosis. The use of low intensity conditioning prior to allogeneic transplantation (see p. 57) potentially allows the procedure in older patients. In younger patients the use of an unrelated HLA-matched donor is possible but results are poorer than for sibling donor SCT.

Autologous stem cell transplantation can induce Ph-negative haematopoiesis but the therapeutic value is unproven.

Choice of treatment in chronic phase. The number of allogeneic SCTs performed for CP-CML has fallen sharply in the imatinib era. TKI therapy is now unquestionably the treatment of choice in the vast majority of patients. Allogeneic SCT still has a role in patients who fail TKI therapy although it is not currently clear how this failure should be defined. Patients who do not respond to two TKIs should probably receive allogeneic SCT if feasible.

Advanced disease

In the accelerated phase and blast crisis, options remain limited. Patients may be helped by allogeneic SCT but results are much inferior to those achieved in CP. Blast crisis can be treated with the combination chemotherapy regimens used in acute leukaemia, and some patients (particularly those with lymphoblastic transformation) will initially respond and return to chronic phase. Unfortunately, such 'remissions' are usually short-lived. Imatinib can also give good responses but these are rarely sustained.

Chronic myeloid leukaemia

- CML is a clonal myeloproliferative disorder arising from an acquired genetic change in a pluripotential stem cell.
- The hallmark of CML cells is the Philadelphia chromosome (t(9;22)) and the resultant chimeric BCR-ABL gene.
- There is gross overproduction of neutrophils and their precursors.
- CML has an indolent chronic phase followed by a period of acceleration and a final, generally fatal, acute leukaemic phase.
- Tyrosine kinase inhibitors (e.g. imatinib) have much improved the prognosis of CP-CML.
- Allogeneic stem cell transplantation is the only well proven curative treatment but is associated with significant mortality.

23 Chronic lymphocytic leukaemia

Chronic lymphocytic leukaemia (CLL) is a disease characterised by a clonal proliferation of antigen-stimulated mature B-lymphocytes. It is the most frequent form of leukaemia in the Western world and is a disease of the elderly; almost all patients are over 50 years old at diagnosis. Recent research has highlighted the biological diversity of CLL. The disease can be most broadly divided into two types dependent on whether the leukaemic cells have a mutation of the immunoglobulin heavy chain variable region (IgV_H) gene. Patients with cells lacking this mutation tend to have more aggressive disease with shortened survival.

Clinical features

Many patients survive long periods with minimal symptoms, while others have a rapid demise with bone marrow failure, bulky lymphadenopathy and hepatosplenomegaly. Fortunately, the former group is in the majority. Indeed, the diagnosis is increasingly made by chance on a routine blood count. Elderly patients with early CLL are very likely to die from other causes.

Where problems do arise, patients commonly complain of symptoms of anaemia, lymphadenopathy, unusually persistent or severe infections and weight loss. The most frequent findings on examination are lymphadenopathy and splenomegaly. In more advanced cases other tissues such as skin, the gastrointestinal tract, the central nervous system, lungs, kidneys and bone may be infiltrated by leukaemic cells. Occasionally there is transformation into a poorly differentiated large cell lymphoma which carries a poor prognosis (*Richter syndrome*). The immunodeficiency in CLL is caused mainly by hypogammaglobulinaemia, which predisposes to infections (Fig 23.1) and also accounts for an increased incidence of other malignancies.

Diagnosis

The diagnosis is suggested by a high lymphocyte count confirmed by the blood film appearance. Lymphocyte counts in CLL exceed $5 \times 10^9/L$ and may reach levels of $500 \times 10^9/L$ or more. The cells resemble normal mature lymphocytes but are often slightly larger with a tendency to burst during preparation of blood films, resulting in 'smear

(a)

(b)

Fig 23.1 **CLL is a cause of acquired immunosuppression. (a)** Oral candidiasis; **(b)** severe chickenpox.

cells' (Fig 23.2). Unexplained persisting lymphocytosis in an elderly person should always suggest CLL. The diagnosis is made by proving that the lymphocytosis is a proliferation of clonal B-cells; this is most simply demonstrated by using in situ or flow cytometry techniques (see p. 21) to show that the cells have characteristic B-lymphocyte antigens and that a single immunoglobulin light chain (kappa or lambda) exists on the cell surface (i.e. it is a monoclonal population). The bone marrow aspirate shows increased numbers of small lymphocytes and a trephine biopsy is worthwhile as the pattern of lymphocyte infiltration gives prognostic information. The blood film appearance may suggest autoimmune haemolysis or autoimmune thrombocytopenia, both of which can complicate CLL.

The term *monoclonal B-cell lymphocytosis* is used where there are fewer than $5 \times 10^9/L$ monoclonal B-lymphocytes in the blood in the absence of other disease features such as lymphadenopathy. In the majority of cases the

Fig 23.2 **Blood film in CLL.** The malignant cells resemble mature lymphocytes but are prone to burst during film preparation leading to the formation of smear cells.

Table 23.1 **Binet staging system for CLL**	
Stage A	No anaemia or thrombocytopenia Fewer than three lymphoid areas[1] enlarged
Stage B	No anaemia or thrombocytopenia Three or more lymphoid areas enlarged
Stage C	Anaemia (Hb less than 100 g/L) and/or platelets less than $100 \times 10^9/L$

[1]*Lymphoid areas are cervical, axillary and inguinal lymphadenopathy (uni- or bilateral), spleen and liver.*

immunophenotye is identical to CLL and some of these patients will progress to CLL over time.

Staging

Staging is important in CLL as it helps in making a rational decision as to whether to commence treatment, and it also gives useful prognostic information. The easiest method is the Binet adaptation of the previous Rai system (Table 23.1); this is simple to apply and correlates closely with survival.

Other variables are increasingly important in predicting prognosis. As gene sequencing is expensive and time-consuming, expression of the signalling molecule ZAP-70 can be used as a surrogate marker for unmutated IgV_H genes and a poor prognosis (Table 23.2).

Management

When to start treatment

There has to be a reason to start treatment in CLL – many patients with early stage disease are completely well and need reassurance as to its relatively benign nature. Early treatment may slow progress but does not improve survival and can lead to significant side-effects including other neoplasms, and the emergence of resistant disease.

Choice of treatment

Treatment should be commenced when the patient develops significant symptoms, when the disease is progressing rapidly or when it is already at an advanced clinical stage. For many years, oral chlorambucil (usually given intermittently) has been the traditional first-line agent for treatment. Chlorambucil is still useful in older patients and where there is significant comorbidity but it has now been mostly replaced in first-line treatment by the more effective purine analogue fludarabine. The combination of fludarabine with other agents has brought benefits with higher levels of complete remission (Fig 23.3) translating into a survival advantage; the current favoured regimen is a combination of fludarabine, cyclophosphamide and the monoclonal antibody rituximab (anti-CD20). The alkylating agent bendamustine is a promising new approach to first-line treatment. Steroids (e.g. prednisolone) are best reserved for patients with pancytopenia or autoimmune complications such as haemolysis or immune thrombocytopenia. Treatment decisions are increasingly influenced by risk factors (see Table 23.2) in addition to stage – for instance, patients with 17p deletions are known to respond poorly to fludarabine and may be considered for more novel therapies such as alemtuzumab (anti-CD52) and ibrutinib.

Radiotherapy can be used as palliation, particularly where enlarged lymph nodes or spleen cause compressive problems. Splenectomy can be beneficial for painful splenomegaly or autoimmune cytopenia. In hypogammaglobulinaemia and recurrent infection, regular intravenous immunoglobulin has been shown to be well tolerated and quality of life is often improved.

None of the above drug regimens or other treatment modalities will cure CLL; the emphasis is on control of symptoms and prolongation of life. In the rare younger patient with CLL a more aggressive approach to treatment may be justified to try and eradicate disease. Allogeneic stem cell transplantation should be considered in younger fit patients with refractory CLL or with very poor prognostic features (e.g. 17p deletion).

Table 23.2 Other prognostic factors in CLL[1]

Factor	Prognosis	
	Good	Poor
Age	Younger	Older
Response to therapy (e.g. CR[2])	Yes	No
Lymphocyte morphology	Typical	Atypical
Histopathology of marrow trephine	Non-diffuse infiltration	Diffuse infiltration
No. of lymphocytes in blood	Low (e.g. $<50\times10^9$/L)	High (e.g. $>50\times10^9$/L)
Lymphocyte doubling time	Long (e.g. >12 months)	Short (e.g. <12 months)
Immunophenotype	FMC7− CD38−	FMC7+ CD38+
β_2-microglobulin	Low	High
Cytogenetics	del 13q14	del 11q22, trisomy 12, del 17p13[3]
Mutation IgV$_H$ genes	Yes	No
ZAP-70 expression	No	Yes

[1]Factors not included in Binet staging system.
[2]Complete remission.
[3]p53 mutation/deletion.

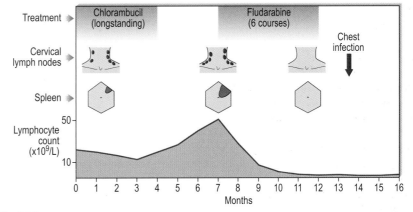

Fig 23.3 **Efficacy of fludarabine in CLL.** Fludarabine, usually in combination with other agents, is now the favoured first-line treatment. Its general superiority over chlorambucil is demonstrated in this patient – the chest infection is a reminder that fludarabine is, however, more immunosuppressive than chlorambucil.

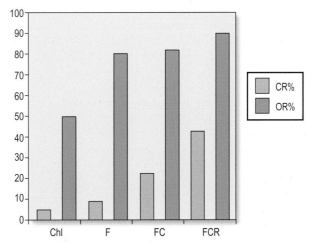

Fig 23.4 **The combination of different agents as first-line treatment for CLL leads to improved response rates.** (Reproduced from Hallek M 2009 State-of-the-art treatment of chronic lymphocytic leukaemia. American Society of Haematology Educational Book). CR, complete remission; OR, overall response; Chl, chlorambucil; F, fludarabine; C, cyclophosphamide; R, rituximab.

Chronic lymphocytic leukaemia

- CLL is the commonest form of leukaemia in the Western world. It is a disease of the elderly.
- There is a clonal proliferation of B-lymphocytes.
- Symptoms/signs include anaemia, recurrent infections, weight loss, lymphadenopathy and hepatosplenomegaly.
- The clinical course is often indolent but it can be more aggressive in advanced stages.
- Chemotherapy is often not immediately needed in early CLL.
- The combination of fludarabine, cyclophosphamide and rituximab (FCR) is the initial treatment of choice in most cases.

24 Other leukaemias

Hairy cell leukaemia

Hairy cell leukaemia (HCL) is a rare chronic B-cell leukaemia characterised by distinctive biological features and unusual sensitivity to treatment. The name of the disease is a reference to the distinctive appearance of the malignant cell (Figs 24.1 and 24.2).

Clinical features

Patients often have non-specific symptoms including fatigue and weight loss. Infection, the main cause of morbidity and mortality, and bleeding are other possible presentations. The spleen is the probable site of origin of the malignant clone and splenomegaly is found in over 80% of cases. This may be massive and is usually not accompanied by lymphadenopathy. The liver is enlarged in 50% of patients.

Diagnosis

Most cases of HCL have a pancytopenia and there may be circulating hairy cells in the blood film. Neutropenia and monocytopenia are often particularly marked, accounting for the frequency of infection. Hairy cells strongly express the markers of mature activated B-cells: CD19, CD11c, CD20, CD22 and CD25 and CD103. The bone marrow is normally difficult to aspirate because of increased fibrosis; the trephine will show a variable number of infiltrating hairy cells. Where splenectomy is performed, the sinuses and cords are seen to be infiltrated by a uniform population of lymphoid cells with blood-filled spaces lined by hairy cells (the pathognomonic 'pseudosinuses' of HCL). There is no specific karyotypic abnormality.

Management

A minority of patients (perhaps 10%) are asymptomatic and in the first instance may require no intervention. Treatment options are as follows.

Nucleoside analogues

Purine analogues are highly effective treatment, producing a more complete and durable response than other therapies (Fig 24.3). Both cladribine and pentostatin give excellent long-term survivals (90–95% at 10 years) and death from HCL is rare.

Interferon alfa

Although less effective than nucleosides, interferon alfa may still be used in patients with severe cytopenia or where the myelosuppressive effects of nucleosides are unacceptable. In the latter patients, G-CSF may also be helpful.

Major side-effects of interferon alfa include systemic symptoms such as pyrexia, lethargy and depression. Following cessation, the disease normally slowly relapses but it will often respond to reintroduction of the drug.

Splenectomy

This produces improvement in symptoms and cytopenia but responses are not particularly durable and it is now less used than previously.

Prolymphocytic leukaemia

Prolymphocytic leukaemia (PLL) may be connected with chronic lymphocytic leukaemia (p. 46), but it more often presents de novo and is best regarded as a distinct disease. The malignant cell is usually of B-lineage and is more mature than the B-CLL cell. Thus, in addition to characteristic B-cell antigens, the cells show a high density of surface immunoglobulin and clonal rearrangements of both heavy and light chain immunoglobulin genes. *TP53* mutations are commonly found. Approximately 20% of cases are of T-cell lineage.

Clinical features and diagnosis

PLL is very much a disease of the elderly with a maximum incidence in the eighth decade of life. The most common clinical presentation of B-PLL is massive splenomegaly. Lymphadenopathy is usually not conspicuous. In T-PLL, involvement of lymph nodes and other tissues including liver and skin is more common. The characteristic PLL blood abnormality is a marked lymphocytosis (normally greater than 100×10^9/L). Anaemia is normal but platelet numbers are often well preserved. Prolymphocytes are large cells recognised by their condensed nucleus with a single prominent nucleolus surrounded by abundant cytoplasm. B- and T-cell types are not distinguishable by routine microscopy.

Management

PLL has a poorer prognosis than chronic lymphocytic leukaemia. The disease is usually aggressive and the median survival is 3 years with an even bleaker outlook in the T-cell variant. Most patients are elderly and the disease is frequently refractory to conventional chemotherapy. Palliative options include splenic irradiation, splenectomy and leucapheresis to control the high white cell count. Survival in B-PLL may be improved by use of fludarabine and rituximab while alemtuzumab (anti-CD52 monoclonal antibody) is emerging as first-line treatment for T-PLL.

T-cell large granular lymphocyte leukaemia

T-cell large granular lymphocyte leukaemia (T-LGL) is a clonal disorder

Fig 24.1 **Normal lymphocyte and hairy cell.**

Fig 24.2 **Hairy cells seen with electron microscopy.**

Fig 24.3 **Response of hairy cell leukaemia to treatment with cladribine (2-CDA).** Bone marrow examinations 1 and 2 showed numerous hairy cells, and bone marrow 3 a remission.

Table 24.1 **Common clinical and laboratory features in ATLL**
Clinical
Lymphadenopathy
Skin lesions
Splenomegaly
Hepatomegaly
Pulmonary lesions
Laboratory
High white cell count
Anaemia
Thrombocytopenia
Hypercalcaemia

of cytotoxic T-lymphocytes. It is often associated with autoimmune disorders such as rheumatoid arthritis. The most common blood manifestation is severe chronic neutropenia although anaemia and thrombocytopenia may also occur. Patients can suffer from recurrent infections, 'B symptoms' such as fever and weight loss, and hepatosplenomegaly. Although the disorder is unequivocally a leukaemia rather than a reactive process, it is generally indolent with responses to immunosuppressive treatment.

Adult T-cell leukaemia lymphoma

Adult T-cell leukaemia lymphoma (ATLL) is a malignant disorder of relatively mature T-lymphocytes. It is rare but of great interest as it is conclusively caused by a virus. The majority of patients with ATLL have antibodies to HTLV-1 and definitive evidence for the aetiological role of this retrovirus has come from studies showing monoclonal integration of proviral DNA in the leukaemic cells.

The disease is mostly seen in areas endemic for HTLV-1, notably in parts of Japan and in the islands of the Caribbean. There is a long latent period from infection to overt disease and less than 5% of infected people actually develop ATLL. Patients most commonly present in the fifth decade and, as its name suggests, ATLL may behave as a leukaemia

or a lymphoma. In the most acute form presentation is with a frank leukaemia. The malignant cells in the blood are pleomorphic but often have very irregular polylobulated nuclei. Even within the leukaemic group there is great heterogeneity with chronic and smouldering forms. In 25% of cases the disease is better described as a lymphoma as there is no demonstrable blood involvement. Despite the variability of the pathology there are well-defined clinical and laboratory features which should prompt consideration of the diagnosis, particularly in a person from an HTLV-1 endemic area (Table 24.1). In practice, lymphoma-type ATLL may be confused with other forms of T-non-Hodgkin's lymphoma. Leukaemic ATLL must be distinguished from *Sezary syndrome*, a lymphoproliferative disorder with circulating T-cells and skin changes including erythroderma and exfoliative dermatitis.

Diagnosis

This requires morphological examination and immunophenotyping of blood lymphocytes or a lymph node biopsy. HTLV-1 positivity is established by serological testing and by DNA analysis of affected tissue where available. Chromosome abnormalities are found in up to 90% of cases but are not specific for ATLL.

Management

Therapy is offered to patients with acute, lymphomatous or unfavourable prognosis chronic type ATLL while patients with typical chronic or smouldering disease are normally first observed. Treatment is unsatisfactory and the median survival in aggressive disease is less than 1 year. The lymphoma type of ATLL has a slightly better outlook than the leukaemia type. Acute forms are frequently resistant to conventional lymphoma chemotherapy protocols (e.g. CHOP) and more intensive regimens with central nervous system prophylaxis are generally recommended. The combination of interferon alfa and the antiviral agent zidovudine may give responses where chemotherapy has failed. Allogeneic stem cell transplantation can be considered in younger patients with a suitable donor.

The chronic and smouldering leukaemia forms can run a protracted course but eventually transform to an acute phase. Skin lesions may be helped by extracorporeal photochemotherapy.

Other leukaemias

■ Hairy cell leukaemia (HCL) is a malignant proliferation of B-cells with a characteristic hairy appearance. Pancytopenia and splenomegaly are common. Nucleoside analogue drugs are usual first-line treatment and the prognosis is good.

■ Prolymphocytic leukaemia is a B-cell (or less often a T-cell) malignancy typified by presentation in the elderly, a high white cell count, splenomegaly and a poor prognosis.

■ T-cell LGL leukaemia most commonly manifests as chronic severe neutropenia.

■ Adult T-cell leukaemia lymphoma is a malignant disorder of T-lymphocytes associated with infection by the HTLV-1 virus. It may present as leukaemia or lymphoma.

25 The myelodysplastic syndromes

The myelodysplastic syndromes (MDS) are a group of clonal disorders of the bone marrow. Their common feature is bone marrow failure as a result of ineffective haematopoiesis rather than reduced haematopoietic activity. A hypercellular marrow and peripheral blood cytopenia with characteristic dysplastic morphological abnormalities form the basis for diagnosis. In early disease there is increased apoptosis of marrow progenitors causing peripheral blood cytopenia but in later MDS there is actually decreased apoptosis with characteristic gene mutations, enhanced survival of myeloblasts and potential expansion of a leukaemic clone. Patients may develop frank acute myeloid leukaemia (AML; see p. 40). Increased marrow angiogenesis and autoimmunity also occur.

MDS is predominantly a disease of the elderly, although it may affect all ages. It can arise de novo or follow previous chemotherapy or radiotherapy for another malignancy. It seems to be increasing in incidence.

Classification

This is not straightforward. The French-American-British (FAB) classification divides MDS into five subtypes depending on morphological features and particularly the number of blood and marrow leukaemic blast cells. The more recent WHO system (Table 25.1) divides MDS into unilineage or multilineage dysplasia, refractory anaemia with ring sideroblasts and dysplasia with excess blasts. The FAB entity chronic myelomonocytic leukaemia (CMML) is now included in the overlap 'MDS with myeloproliferative disorder' category. It is likely that cytogenetic and molecular abnormalities will be increasingly incorporated into the classification; a current example is 5q– syndrome, a distinct subtype of MDS associated with a response to novel therapy and a good prognosis.

Clinical features

The diagnosis may follow a routine blood count in an asymptomatic patient. Where symptoms do occur they range from a mild anaemia to the consequences of severe marrow failure with profound anaemia, leucopenia and thrombocytopenia (Fig 25.1). Abnormal haematopoiesis can cause functional abnormalities of cells, and infection and haemorrhage may be more severe than would be predicted from the degree of cytopenia. Pronounced symptoms are predictably more common in the subtypes with increased blast cells. CMML, like the acute monocytic leukaemias, has specific features including splenomegaly (rare in other forms of MDS), skin infiltration and serous effusions.

Diagnosis

Morphology

The diagnosis of MDS depends on careful morphological examination of the blood film and bone marrow aspirate and trephine specimens (Fig 25.2). Common abnormalities include:

- *Peripheral blood.* Red cells – anisopoikilocytosis, macrocytosis. Neutrophils – hypogranulation, pseudo-Pelger forms. Platelets – giant forms.
- *Bone marrow.* Erythroid cells – multinuclearity, nuclear budding, ring sideroblasts. Myeloid cells – hypogranularity, increased blast cells. Megakaryocytes – giant forms or micromegakaryocytes.

Where there are changes in all three lines the term 'trilineage dysplasia' is used. The bone marrow trephine biopsy usually confirms marrow hypercellularity, although fibrosis and even hypocellularity may occur.

Genetics

Around 50% of cases of MDS show cytogenetic abnormalities. Common changes include monosomy 7 or 7q–, trisomy 8, monosomy 5 or 5q–, and loss of the Y chromosome. The incidence of chromosome abnormalities increases with the severity of the disease and risk of leukaemic transformation.

Work is ongoing to better characterise the complex molecular basis of MDS. Mutations of genes encoding cell surface receptors (e.g. *KIT*), signal transduction proteins (e.g. *RAS*), transcription factors (e.g. *AML1*), epigenetic modifiers (e.g. *MLL*) and protein degradation pathways (e.g. *CBL*) have been identified.

Prognostic factors

The outcome is closely linked to the classification and the risk of transformation to leukaemia. The International Prognostic Scoring System (IPSS) – based on the number of blood cytopenias, percentage of bone marrow blasts and karyotype – is a simple prognostic tool which can be used to direct

Table 25.1 **WHO classification of myelodysplastic syndrome**
Refractory anaemia with unilineage dysplasia
Refractory anaemia (RA)
Refractory neutropenia (RN)
Refractory thrombocytopenia (RT)
Refractory anaemia with ring sideroblasts (RARS)
Refractory cytopenia with multilineage dysplasia (RCMD)
Refractory anaemia with excess blasts (RAEB)[1]
MDS with isolated del (5q)
MDS, unclassifiable
Myelodysplastic/myeloproliferative neoplasms (MDS/MPN)
Chronic myelomonocytic leukaemia (CMML)
Atypical chronic myeloid leukaemia
Refractory anaemia with ring sideroblasts and thrombocytosis (RARST)

[1]Defined as 5–10% blasts in bone marrow.

Fig 25.1 **Purpuric rash in myelodysplastic syndrome.** The patient was thrombocytopenic.

Fig 25.2 **Myelodysplastic syndromes.** Morphological changes in the blood film and bone marrow aspirate. **(a)** Pseudo-Pelger neutrophil with bilobed nucleus. **(b)** Dysplastic megakaryocyte in the bone marrow. **(c)** Iron stain of the bone marrow showing 'ring sideroblasts'.

treatment (Table 25.2). Median survivals vary from 6 years in the low risk group to less than a year in patients at higher risk. Patients with low risk disease have an average period of 10 years before the onset of AML whereas for high risk patients this is only a few months.

Treatment

Supportive care

In patients with significant marrow failure, supportive care is crucial to ameliorate symptoms and prolong life. Regular blood transfusion is often necessary to control symptoms of anaemia, and haemorrhage is managed with platelet transfusions. Patients receiving multiple blood transfusions can benefit from iron chelation therapy. This may reduce not just iron overload but also transfusion dependency. Infections require swift intervention with broad-spectrum antibiotics.

Specific treatments

Treatment needs to be individualised according to the type of disease and age of the patient.

Low-risk MDS

In patients with low-risk MDS, the main goal of treatment is to improve cytopenias. Anaemia may respond to erythropoietin alone or combined with G-CSF. Immunosuppression with anti-thymocyte globulin (ALG) can give good results in younger patients with marrow hypocellularity. The immunomodulatory agent lenalidomide is

particularly effective in patients with del (5q), often leading to resolution of anaemia and transfusion independence. After a long period when low-risk MDS patients received only supportive care, it is likely that many will now receive at least a trial of growth factors or a novel agent.

High-risk MDS

In high-risk MDS (e.g. RAEB; see Table 25.1), the primary aim is to prolong survival and delay transformation to AML. In younger patients, AML-type chemotherapy and allogeneic stem cell transplantation, the only potentially curative treatment, are possible options. The hypomethylating agent azacitidine has shown efficacy in higher risk subgroups with significantly prolonged survivals and delay of onset of AML. It is given subcutaneously as outpatient therapy and is generally well tolerated.

Table 25.2 **The International Prognostic Scoring System for Primary MDS**

Prognostic variable	0	0.5	1	1.5	2	Risk group	Score
Bone marrow blasts (%)	<5	5–10	–	11–20	21–30	Low	0
						Int-1	0.5–1
Karyotype	Good[1]	Intermediate	Poor[2]	–	–	Int-2	1.5–2
Cytopenias	0/1	2/3	–	–	–	High	≥2

Int: Intermediate
[1]*E.g. normal, del (5q).*
[2]*E.g. complex or chromosome 7 abnormalities.*

The myelodysplastic syndromes

- MDS is a heterogeneous group of clonal disorders of the bone marrow; the abnormal clone differentiates ineffectively, leading to a hypercellular marrow and blood cytopenia.
- MDS may affect all ages but is predominantly a disease of the elderly.
- Diagnosis depends on the presence of characteristic morphological changes in the blood and marrow.
- Classification into subtypes relies on bone marrow morphology and cytogenetics.
- Prognosis is highly variable.
- Supportive care remains crucial but growth factors and other specific therapeutic agents (e.g. lenalidomide, azacitidine) are increasingly used. Chemotherapy and stem cell transplantation may be considered in younger patients with high-risk disease

26 Aplastic anaemia

The term aplastic anaemia is a misnomer in that the disorder so described is characterised by a pancytopenia arising from failure of production of all the normal cells of peripheral blood. The underlying cause is a reduction in the number of pluripotential stem cells. This deficit may be exacerbated by an abnormality in the marrow microenvironment or an autoimmune reaction against the abnormal haematopoietic tissue.

Aplastic anaemia is rare (approximately 2–5 cases/million/year worldwide) and affects all ages. It must be emphasised that it is not a subtype of leukaemia. However, the disease's presenting clinical characteristics, the management problems of marrow failure (including fulminating septicaemia and haemorrhage) and the possible evolution to a clonal marrow disorder dictate its inclusion in this section.

Classification and aetiology

Aplastic anaemia (AA) may be part of a congenital syndrome, be secondary to well-defined insults to the bone marrow, or arise apparently spontaneously with no identifiable cause. A simple classification is shown in Table 26.1. The most common congenital disorder is *Fanconi's anaemia*. Affected children suffer from defective DNA repair and the aplasia often coexists with skeletal deformities, skin pigmentation (Fig 26.1) and renal abnormalities. To date, fifteen genes (termed FANC) have been identified. *Dyskeratosis congenita*, another form of constitutional aplasia, is distinguished by a later onset, nail dystrophy, leukoplakia of mucosal surfaces and a high incidence of epithelial tumours. There is defective telomere maintenance and patients usually have

very short telomeres. This is also observed in 10–15% of patients with acquired AA.

Infections known to predispose to AA include viral hepatitis and parvovirus infection. Exposure to chemicals, drugs and radiation can damage stem cells. Drugs may depress haematopoiesis idiosyncratically or predictably (Table 26.2). In roughly two-thirds of patients, no cause is apparent and AA is termed 'idiopathic'. Improved haematopoiesis following immunosuppression (see below) suggests that in at least some cases the abnormal stem cell compartment is further compromised by poorly defined immune phenomena.

Clinical features

Patients with marrow failure predictably present with anaemia, unusually frequent or severe infections (caused by neutropenia) and a haemorrhagic

Table 26.1 Classification of aplastic anaemia

1. Idiopathic AA	
2. Congenital AA	Fanconi's anaemia
	Dyskeratosis congenita
3. Secondary AA	Drugs – idiosyncratic or dose-related
	Chemicals
	Ionising radiation
	Infection

Table 26.2 Drugs associated with aplastic anaemia[1]

Predictable	Cytotoxic agents
Idiosyncratic	Chloramphenicol
	Sulfonamides
	Phenylbutazone
	Indometacin
	Gold salts
	Penicillamine
	Carbamazepine
	Phenytoin
	Carbimazole

[1]This is a selective list of more commonly implicated agents.

tendency (caused by thrombocytopenia). The onset may be gradual or fulminant. Symptoms or signs of an underlying systemic disorder (e.g. Fanconi's) or possible trigger (e.g. hepatitis) may be present. An exhaustive history, including drug and occupational exposure, and a thorough examination are mandatory.

Diagnosis

There are really two questions. Is the pancytopenia due to aplastic anaemia? Is this idiopathic AA or aplasia secondary to an identifiable cause (Table 26.3)?

A reasonable sequence of investigations is as follows:

1. Blood count and film
There is a pancytopenia and reticulocytopenia. To define AA there must be at least two of the following: (1) haemoglobin less than 100 g/L; (2) neutrophils less than 1.5×10^9/L; (3) platelets less than 50×10^9/L. There are no abnormal cells in the blood film.

2. Bone marrow aspirate and trephine
This is the key diagnostic test. The marrow aspirate can be highly suggestive of aplasia with grossly hypocellular

Table 26.3 Causes of pancytopenia

Marrow failure or infiltration
- Aplastic anaemia
- Myelodysplastic syndrome
- Leukaemia
- Myelofibrosis
- Infiltration by other malignancy (e.g. lymphoma, carcinoma)
- Infection (e.g. tuberculosis)
- Megaloblastic anaemia
- Prolonged starvation

Hypersplenism
- Portal hypertension
- Felty syndrome (rheumatoid arthritis)
- Storage disorders

Fig 26.1 **Fanconi's anaemia. (a)** Digital abnormalities in brothers with the syndrome. **(b)** Skin pigmentation.

particles but a trephine biopsy is necessary to confirm the diagnosis and quantify the degree of hypocellularity (Fig 26.2). Aplasia may be patchy and if the trephine is surprisingly cellular in the context of the blood count, then further samples should be obtained. In practice the only likely confusion is with hypocellular myelodysplastic syndrome (see p. 50) or an atypical presentation of acute leukaemia, the latter particularly in childhood.

3. Tests for an underlying cause
These include liver function tests, viral titres, vitamin B_{12} and folate levels and tests for paroxysmal nocturnal haemoglobinuria (see p. 31) and the inherited bone marrow failure syndromes. Cytogenetic analysis of the hypocellular bone marrow is often problematic but will reveal abnormal cytogenetic clones in some patients.

Measurement of severity

This is crucial as the severity defined from peripheral blood and bone marrow measurements predicts the response to treatment and survival (Table 26.4). The median survival of untreated severe AA is 3–6 months with only 20% of patients surviving longer than 1 year.

Management

Removal of cause
Where an agent such as a drug or a chemical is implicated this should be removed.

Supportive care
Blood and platelet transfusion may be life-saving but should be used judiciously as patients with AA have intact cellular and humoral immunity and can become sensitised to histocompatibility antigens. Iron chelation therapy may be required. Infection in neutropenic patients requires prompt expert management (see p. 87).

Restoring normal haematopoiesis
There are two major options: immunosuppression and stem cell transplantation.

Immunosuppression
AA is thought to be at least in part an autoimmune disease and immunosuppressive agents provide worthwhile responses and prolonged survival in 60–80% of patients with 5-year survival

Fig 26.2 Bone marrow trephine in severe aplastic anaemia. The cellularity is markedly reduced. (Compare with normal bone marrow appearance, p. 2.)

Table 26.4 **Severity of aplastic anaemia**
AA is defined as **non-severe (NSAA)** unless it is:
1. **Severe (SAA)**. Requires two of three peripheral blood criteria: <ul><li>Neutrophils less than 0.5×10^9/L</li><li>Platelets less than 20×10^9/L</li><li>Reticulocytes less than 20×10^9/L</li></ul> Within the bone marrow: <ul><li>Less than 25% haematopoietic cells, or 25–50% haematopoietic cells and less than 30% cellularity</li></ul>
2. **Very severe (VSAA)**. Requires a neutrophil count less than 0.2×10^9/L in the presence of at least one other peripheral blood criterion and the bone marrow features given for SAA

around 75%. Responses are poorer in younger patients and in severe aplastic anaemia (SAA). The best regimen is a combination of antithymocyte globulin (ATG) and ciclosporin. Both drugs are potentially toxic – ATG can produce pyrexia, rashes and hypotension while ciclosporin may cause nephrotoxicity and hypertension. Complete or partial responses to immunosuppressive treatment can take several months. Other immunosuppressive drugs which may be considered include cyclophosphamide and the anti-CD52 monoclonal antibody alemtuzumab. As further discussed below, there is concern that immunosuppression may stimulate haematopoiesis but not necessarily cure the disease.

Stem cell transplantation (SCT)
The object of allogeneic SCT is to repopulate the patient's marrow with normal stem cells from a healthy compatible donor. Transplantation from an HLA-identical sibling donor in younger patients (less than 45 years) produces long-term survival (possibly cure) in about 75–90% of cases. It is important to transplant early in the course of the disease as multiple transfusions lead to sensitisation and an increased chance of graft rejection. Minimal-intensity conditioning regimens (see p. 57) are being explored.

Immunosuppression or SCT?
Younger patients (less than 30 years) with SAA and a matched sibling donor should be transplanted. In VSAA (see Table 26.4) in this age group, the lack of a family donor should prompt a search for an HLA-matched unrelated donor. In patients 30–40 years with SAA, sibling SCT and immunosuppression produce similar survivals over 2–5 years. However, a significant proportion of patients receiving immunosuppression alone, approximately 25% at 10 years, evolve to clonal marrow diseases such as paroxysmal nocturnal haemoglobinuria, myelodysplastic syndrome and acute myeloid leukaemia. Thus in this group matched sibling SCT probably gives a better long-term prognosis. In older patients with SAA, and patients with non-severe AA, immunosuppression is generally the treatment of choice.

Growth factors
Growth factors cannot rectify the stem cell defect and are therefore not routinely used in AA. G-CSF may be useful in severe infection.

> ### *Aplastic anaemia*
> - AA is characterised by a pancytopenia arising from the failure of production of normal cells by the bone marrow.
> - There is a reduction in the number of pluripotential stem cells; there may also be an abnormal marrow microenvironment and ill-defined autoimmunity.
> - AA can be congenital, secondary to well-defined insults (e.g. drugs) or idiopathic.
> - Prognosis relates to severity, which is defined from blood and bone marrow indices. Evolution to a clonal marrow disorder such as leukaemia may occur.
> - Good supportive care is vital.
> - Major treatment modalities are immunosuppression and SCT – the choice of treatment is based on patient age, disease severity and availability of a stem cell donor.

27 Chemotherapy and related treatments

General principles

The life cycle of the normal cell is shown schematically in Figure 27.1. Conventional anti-leukaemic and lymphoma cytotoxic drugs can be broadly divided into those agents active during only one phase of the cell cycle ('phase-specific') and those acting at all stages ('phase non-specific'). In practice, most anti-leukaemic drugs act predominantly against proliferating cells and therefore affect a fraction of the malignant cell population. Thus, if in advanced acute leukaemia the total number of malignant cells is 10^{10}, a single course of chemotherapy could be expected to kill between 2 and 5 log of cells, leaving between 10^5 and 10^8 residual leukaemic cells. It can be seen that the chance of eradication of the disease by chemotherapy is favoured by early treatment when the leukaemic mass is small and by repeated courses of cytotoxic drugs. It is also logical to combine different agents to maximise the anti-leukaemic activity and exploit different toxicities ('combination chemotherapy').

Major classes of conventional cytotoxic drugs

Alkylating agents

Despite their variable structure, all alkylating agents appear to have a common mechanism with cross-linking of DNA the principal cytotoxic action. Agents commonly used in haematological practice include melphalan, chlorambucil, cyclophosphamide, busulfan and bendamustine. These are toxic to rapidly proliferating cells and the dose-limiting toxicity is myelosuppression. Other side-effects include infertility, haemorrhagic cystitis (cyclophosphamide) and an increased risk of secondary malignancy.

Antimetabolites

These drugs are compounds which interfere with the utilisation of a natural metabolite by virtue of the similarity of their chemical structure. Most are analogues of nucleic acid precursors. Commonly used examples are the folinic acid analogue methotrexate, the purine analogues 6-mercaptopurine and fludarabine, and the pyrimidine analogue cytosine arabinoside. The alkylating agent bendamustine also has some antimetabolic activity. The main toxic effect of the group is myelosuppression. Fludarabine is significantly immunosuppressive.

Topoisomerase poisons and inhibitors

This broad class of drugs includes the anthracyclines (doxorubicin, daunorubicin, mitoxantrone, idarubicin) and the epipodophyllotoxins (etoposide). The anthracyclines are cell cycle non-specific drugs. The acute dose-limiting toxicity is bone marrow suppression but the cumulative dosage is limited by cardiotoxicity. Etoposide is a phase-specific drug (active in G_2) with myelosuppression the major toxicity.

Spindle poisons

Key agents in this group are the two vinca alkaloids, vincristine and vinblastine. They are cell-cycle phase-specific, exerting a cytotoxic effect by binding to cellular microtubular protein and inhibiting mitosis. Vincristine's major adverse effects are mixed motor-sensory and autonomic neuropathies (patients usually initially complain of 'pins and needles' in the fingers or toes and constipation); vinblastine is less neurotoxic but causes more bone marrow suppression.

Side-effects of conventional cytotoxic drugs

Some toxic effects are common to many cytotoxic drugs and must be discussed with all patients receiving a relevant single agent or combination chemotherapy (Table 27.1). Myelosuppression and alopecia are often unavoidable. However, nausea and vomiting can usually be minimised or even completely avoided by modern antiemetic protocols. The probability of infertility is influenced by the agents used, the total dosage, the duration of administration and the age and sex of the patient. Strategies to minimise infertility include prechemotherapy storage of germ cells (unfortunately, fertility is often abnormal at presentation) or choice of regimens which are relatively non-sterilising. Gonadal failure occurs more commonly in women and may be managed by hormone replacement therapy; androgens are used in men. Chemotherapy is associated with an increased risk of secondary

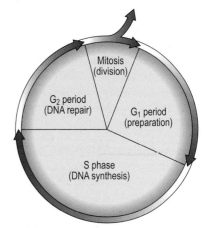

Fig 27.1 **The cell cycle.**

Table 27.1 **Common adverse effects of cytotoxic drugs**	
Short-term effects	**Long-term effects**
Myelosuppression	Infertility
Nausea and vomiting	Secondary malignancy
Alopecia	
Mucositis	

Note: If extravasated from the vein some drugs can cause severe tissue injury.

malignancy including leukaemia and solid tumours. Alkylating agents are particularly leukaemogenic.

Multi-drug resistance

The major problem in the treatment of leukaemia and other haematological malignancies is the emergence of cells resistant to chemotherapy. Genes capable of conferring resistance to cytotoxic drugs have been characterised. Of particular note is the P-glycoprotein or multi-drug resistance gene (MDR1), as its over-expression can lead to resistance to many of the agents used in the treatment of leukaemia. The MDR1 gene encodes a membrane protein which acts as an ATP-dependent efflux pump transporting organic compounds out of the cell. Elevated MDR1 levels appear to predict a poor prognosis in acute myeloid leukaemia. A number of MDR-reversing agents (e.g. ciclosporin, PSC-833, zosuquidar) have been given in conjunction with normal chemotherapy in AML but so far with little benefit.

Other treatments for haematological malignancy

Conventional chemotherapy currently plays the major role in the treatment of most haematological malignancies but, as these selected examples demonstrate, there is increasing emphasis on more targeted therapies which exploit particular characteristics of tumour cells and cause fewer systemic side-effects.

Differentiating agents

In most cases, attempts to induce maturation of malignant cells have been disappointing. One notable exception is the drug all-*trans*-retinoic acid (ATRA) in acute promyelocytic leukaemia (associated with t(15;17)). At pharmacological concentrations ATRA overcomes the suppressive effect of the PML-RARα fusion protein, allowing leukaemic promyelocytes to differentiate into neutrophils. Addition of ATRA to normal chemotherapy reduces the severity of APL-related coagulopathy and gives a significantly better survival than chemotherapy alone. The major side-effect is 'ATRA syndrome' where a rising white blood cell count accompanies systemic upset with cardiopulmonary and renal problems.

Monoclonal antibodies

Monoclonal antibodies (MoAbs) promise tumour-targeted therapy with minimal toxicity. They may be unconjugated or conjugated to a toxin or radioisotope. One potential target is the CD20 antigen which is present in over 90% of B-cell lymphomas. An unconjugated chimeric human-mouse anti-CD20 MoAb (rituximab) is widely used in association with chemotherapy in follicular and diffuse large B-cell non-Hodgkin's lymphomas. Newer anti-CD20 agents (e.g. ofatumumab) are being investigated. The linking of a radionucleotide to anti-CD20 may improve efficacy. Other MoAbs in clinical practice include anti-CD52 (alemtuzumab) in chronic lymphocytic leukaemia, anti-CD33 (Mylotarg) in acute myeloid leukaemia and anti-CD30 (brentuximab) in Hodgkin's lymphoma.

Tyrosine kinase inhibitors (TKIs)

Imatinib mesilate (Glivec), a specific small molecule inhibitor of BCR-ABL, is very effective drug therapy for chronic myeloid leukaemia (CML) (see also p. 45). In patients who develop resistance to imatinib more potent BCR-ABL inhibitors (e.g. dasatinib, nilotinib) can give good responses. Other TKIs entering clinical practice include JAK2 inhibitors (e.g. ruxolitinib) in myelo-

proliferative neoplasms and FLT3 inhibitors in acute myeloid leukaemia.

Proteosome inhibitors

The proteosome is an enzyme complex that plays a crucial part in cell-cycle control and gene expression by regulating cellular protein degradation. Inhibition of the proteosome ultimately results in cell death. Bortezomib (Velcade) is a proteosome inhibitor that is able to kill tumour cells selectively. It is effective in myeloma and it also has activity in non-Hodgkin's lymphomas. The most troublesome side-effect is peripheral neuropathy.

Epigenetic therapies

The term 'epigenetics' refers to heritable changes in gene expression which are not coded in the DNA sequence. Epigenetic mechanisms, including DNA and histone modifications, are potentially reversible. The hypomethylating agents azacitidine and decitabine have activity in myelodysplastic syndrome and acute myeloid leukaemia.

Anti-angiogenic agents

Myeloma is known to be associated with increased angiogenesis in the bone marrow. The anti-angiogenic agents thalidomide and lenalidomide now play key roles in the treatment of this malignancy. Both drugs have other mechanisms of action including alteration of tumour cell cycle progression and immunomodulation.

Interferon alfa

Interferon alfa is an antiviral protein with immunomodulatory and

anti-cancer activities. It has been extensively used in CML and hairy cell leukaemia but is now being largely supplanted by more effective and better tolerated agents.

Haematopoietic growth factor therapy

Several haematopoietic growth factors are routinely used in clinical haematology. Their main use is in haematological malignancy.

Supportive care in patients with blood cytopenia

G-CSF (see p. 2) is most commonly used to accelerate the production of neutrophils following chemotherapy or stem cell transplantation. The shortened period of neutropenia reduces the incidence of infections and the length of stay in hospital. It can also help maintain the dose intensity of chemotherapy. Erythropoietin is mainly used to treat the anaemia of renal failure but may ameliorate anaemia in selected patients with myelodysplastic syndrome and myeloma. Early trials of thrombopoietin-like agents to treat thrombocytopenia were unsuccessful due to the development of neutralising antibodies. Thrombopoietin receptor agonists are used in immune thrombocytopenia (see p. 69) but they have no definite role in thrombocytopenia due to marrow failure.

Stem cell mobilisation

G-CSF is used in conjunction with chemotherapy to 'mobilise' stem cells from the bone marrow to the blood prior to harvesting (see also p. 56).

Chemotherapy and related treatments

- There are several classes of conventional cytotoxic drugs with different mechanisms of action.
- In leukaemia and lymphoma it is usual to combine cytotoxic drugs in repeated courses to maximise anti-tumour activity and exploit different toxicities.
- Cytotoxic drugs have predictable short-term and long-term side-effects.
- Conventional chemotherapy is increasingly being supplemented, or even replaced, by therapies targeting particular characteristics of tumour cells (e.g. tyrosine kinase inhibitors in CML).
- Erythropoietin may be used to treat anaemia in selected patients with haematological malignancy.
- G-CSF is used to shorten the duration of neutropenia after intensive chemotherapy and to mobilise stem cells for harvesting.

28 Stem cell transplantation

The term 'stem cell transplantation' (SCT) is used to describe a number of different procedures. In allogeneic SCT the haematopoietic stem cells are provided by another individual, either a family member or an unrelated donor. In autologous SCT the patient's own stem cells are used to re-establish haematopoiesis. For many years bone marrow (BM) harvested from the pelvis was the only source of stem cells but now they are more commonly harvested from the peripheral blood (PB) by leucapheresis.

Allogeneic and syngeneic (twin) SCT

The allogeneic procedure is outlined in Figure 28.1. The patient's own haematopoietic stem cells, immune system and residual tumour cells are conventionally destroyed by conditioning treatment with high-dose chemotherapy and (usually) radiotherapy prior to intravenous infusion of stem cells harvested from the healthy donor. The ideal patient has a disease curable by allogeneic SCT but not by less toxic treatment and is young (less than 40 years old). The ideal donor, excepting the rare presence of a twin, is a sibling genotypically matched with the recipient for HLA-A, B and DR. The genes for HLA are found on chromosome 6 and so inheritance follows the rules of simple Mendelian inheritance; two siblings have a one in four chance of sharing the same two HLA haplotypes. With relatively small family size in the Western world, only around 30% of patients will have an HLA-identical sibling. Transplants from HLA-haploidentical relatives have been associated with a high rate of morbidity and mortality. An alternative strategy is to search for an unrelated volunteer donor who is a phenotypic HLA match. From the worldwide databases of 18 million HLA-typed volunteers, around 50% of Caucasian patients can be found a suitable donor. Success rates are lower in other ethnic groups. Use of a HLA-mismatched donor leads to an increase in the incidence and severity of the adverse effects of SCT. Weaker transplant reactions result from mismatch for minor histocompatibility antigens, single peptides derived from polymorphic proteins which may differ between donor and recipient.

After conditioning treatment there is a period of about 3 weeks before 'engraftment' during which the patient is severely pancytopenic and immunosuppressed and requires intensive supportive care with blood products and aggressive treatment of any infection. Major adverse events include graft failure with rejection arising from a failure to immunosuppress the patient adequately, and graft-versus-host disease (GVHD). GVHD is a potentially life-threatening disorder predominantly affecting the skin (Fig 28.2), gastrointestinal tract and liver which may occur early after transplantation (acute GVHD) or after a few months (chronic GVHD). GVHD results from donor immunocompetent cells attacking antigens in the recipient and can be abrogated by removal of T-lymphocytes from the donor stem cells. Such 'lymphocyte depletion' may lead to an increased risk of relapse of the underlying malignancy, confirming that much of the curative potential of allogeneic SCT is due to the presence of immunologically active donor cells rather than the preparative regimen (see also non-myeloablative SCT). The profound and prolonged immunosuppression of allogeneic SCT renders the patient vulnerable to life-threatening fungal and viral (e.g. cytomegalovirus) infections. Causes of late death include relapse of disease, chronic GVHD and secondary cancers related to previous chemotherapy and SCT conditioning. Peripheral blood stem cells are now used more often than bone marrow for allogeneic procedures. For related donors, PBSC give quicker engraftment and probably reduced disease relapse and improved survival although there is some increase in GVHD. Common indications for allogeneic SCT include acute leukaemia and chronic myeloid leukaemia.

Autologous SCT

The procedure is outlined in Figure 28.1. High-dose chemotherapy, and sometimes radiotherapy, is followed by reinfusion of previously stored patient stem cells. Autologous SCT has less toxicity than allogeneic SCT and therefore can be performed in older patients. It also has the advantage that the patient is the

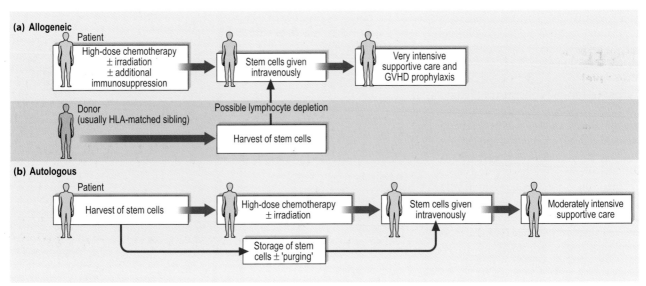

Fig 28.1 **Stem cell transplantation.**

Fig 28.2 **Acute GVHD of the skin after allogeneic SCT.**

Fig 28.3 **Peripheral blood stem cells being harvested by leucapheresis.**

donor and therefore donor unavailability and GVHD are not issues. The main disadvantage of autologous SCT compared with allogeneic SCT is an increased incidence of relapse of malignant disease. It is not clear whether this arises from resistance to the conditioning treatment or infusion of residual tumour cells in the graft. The 'purging' of tumour cells from grafts does not appear to alter survival. Peripheral blood stem cells (PBSC) have now largely replaced the use of bone marrow in autologous procedures. PBSC can be harvested from the patient's blood by leucapheresis during the recovery phase from moderate doses of chemotherapy (Fig 28.3). The growth factor G-CSF is often used to facilitate the 'mobilisation' of stem cells. Compared with the traditional bone marrow autologous transplant, PBSCT gives more rapid recovery of a normal blood count with fewer infections, less intensive supportive care and shortened hospital stay. PBSCT is currently widely used as a convenient and relatively safe method of escalating the dose of chemotherapy in patients with acute leukaemia, lymphoma and myeloma. Its role in the treatment of non-haematopoietic solid tumours and autoimmune disorders is less established.

Recent developments

Non-myeloablative allogeneic SCT ('reduced intensity')

As allogeneic SCT has evolved it has become increasingly apparent that its curative potential is not simply due to the killing of tumour cells by intensive conditioning regimens. The major therapeutic component of allogeneic SCT is thought to be donor T-lymphocytes mediating 'graft versus tumour (GVT)' or 'graft versus leukaemia (GVL)' effects.

The rationale of reduced intensity SCT is to avoid potentially harmful intensive pre-transplant conditioning and to instead harness the anti-leukaemic (or other tumour) effects of the donor allo-reactive T-lymphocytes. These cells are capable of killing leukaemic stem cells and other tumour cells resistant to conventional chemotherapy. Patients are given moderate doses of chemotherapy and immunosuppressive drugs to engender a state of host versus graft tolerance before the infusion of allogeneic donor stem cells. As the procedure is of relatively low toxicity it allows allogeneic SCT in older patients. There is, however, still a significant risk of acute and chronic GVHD. Reduced intensity conditioning regimens are being developed to try and minimise the toxicity and to maximise GVT activity. Donor lymphocyte infusions (DLIs) are another form of allogeneic cell therapy. In patients with leukaemia relapsed after allogeneic SCT, a simple infusion of lymphocytes from the original donor may induce a further remission.

Umbilical cord blood transplantation

Umbilical cord blood (UCB) is an important source of haematopoietic stem cells now being used for transplantation. UCB is readily available and large banks of stored frozen UCB are significantly extending the application of SCT. Immunocompetent cells in CB are less mature than the T- and B-lymphocytes in an adult and there is a lower risk of inducing GVHD, allowing the possibility of HLA-mismatched UCB transplantation. A cord blood unit provides a relatively low stem cell dose leading to slower haematopoietic and immune recovery. Results are better where higher cell doses are available. Emerging strategies include the use of double cord blood transplants and in vitro techniques to increase the number of haematopoietic stem cells. UCB transplantation has been mainly used in children. In adults it is considered when other donor cells are unavailable or not quickly accessible.

Stem cell transplantation

- Stem cell transplantation (SCT) procedures may be undertaken using an HLA-matched family donor or unrelated donor (allogeneic SCT), an identical twin donor (syngeneic SCT) or the patient's own stored stem cells (autologous SCT).

- Stem cells may be sourced from the bone marrow but are now more commonly derived from peripheral blood (PBSC).

- Allogeneic SCT is a more effective anti-leukaemic treatment than autologous SCT but is associated with greater toxicity including graft rejection and graft versus host disease.

- The greater curative potential of allogeneic SCT in leukaemia is largely due to a 'graft versus leukaemia (GVL)' effect mediated by donor T-lymphocytes.

- More recent developments include reduced intensity conditioning regimens exploiting GVL effects and alternative sources of stem cells (e.g. umbilical cord blood).

29 Hodgkin's lymphoma

The lymphomas are malignant disorders of lymphoid tissue subdivided into two broad groups – Hodgkin's lymphoma (HL) and non-Hodgkin's lymphoma (NHL).

Hodgkin's disease was first described by Thomas Hodgkin in 1832. In developed countries there is a bimodal age distribution with peak incidences in young adults (15–35 years) and the more elderly (over 50 years). The disease is commoner in men.

Aetiology

Hodgkin's lymphoma is an unusual malignancy in that the malignant cells, termed Reed–Sternberg cells (Fig 29.1), and mononuclear Hodgkin's cells form only a minority of the tumour. The remainder is composed of very variable numbers of other cells including lymphocytes, granulocytes, fibroblasts and plasma cells. This inflammatory cell infiltrate presumably reflects an immune response by the host against the malignant cells. Reed–Sternberg (RS) cells appear to originate from germinal-centre B-lymphocytes. In classical HL the RS cells are 'crippled' germinal-centre B-cells incapable of secreting immunoglobulins, while in lymphocyte predominant nodular HL RS cells the coding regions of the immunoglobulin genes are intact and potentially functional.

Epstein–Barr virus (EBV) may play a role in classical Hodgkin's lymphoma, particularly the mixed cellularity subtype. When the disease occurs in patients with HIV infection and after solid organ transplantation it is often EBV-associated. There is no specific chromosomal translocation associated with Hodgkin's lymphoma.

Classification

It is acknowledged in the World Health Organization (WHO) classification (see also p. 60) that 'Hodgkin's disease' comprises two distinct 'Hodgkin's lymphomas' with different clinical features: classical HL and lymphocyte predominant nodular HL (Table 29.1).

Clinical presentation

Classical Hodgkin's lymphoma
Asymmetrical and painless lymphadenopathy, most often in the cervical region, is the most common presentation. The

Fig 29.1 **Reed–Sternberg cells in a lymph node biopsy.** This giant cell is binucleated or multinucleated with large inclusion-like nucleoli and abundant cytoplasm.

Table 29.1 **WHO classification of Hodgkin's lymphoma**

Histological subtype	Histological pattern	Immunophenotype
Lymphocyte predominant nodular	Polylobulated Reed–Sternberg (RS) cells Nodular growth pattern	CD30– CD20+ CD45+
Classical Lymphocyte-rich Nodular sclerosis Mixed cellularity Lymphocyte depletion	Classical or lacunar type. RS cells in inflammatory cell background. In nodular sclerosis type are often fibrous bands	CD15+ CD30+ CD45–

nodes usually gradually enlarge but may fluctuate in size. Patterns of disease suggest contiguous spread via the lymphatic chain. Mediastinal involvement is a particular feature of the nodular sclerosing histological subtype (Fig 29.2). Splenomegaly and hepatomegaly occur but massive enlargement is rare.

Significant systemic upset affects a minority of patients (20–30%) at presentation. This includes fever, sweating (often at night), weight loss, pruritus and fatigue.

Lymphocyte predominant nodular Hodgkin's lymphoma
Most cases present with cervical adenopathy and early stage disease. The disease is more indolent than classical HL with long survivals common. However, late relapse and transformation to diffuse large B-cell NHL can occur. Treatment of advanced disease is similar to that used for classical HL (see below).

Diagnosis and staging

Diagnosis
The key investigation is biopsy of a lymph node for histological

Fig 29.2 **Chest X-ray showing mediastinal lymphadenopathy in nodular sclerosing Hodgkin's lymphoma.**

examination. This is needed to distinguish Hodgkin's lymphoma from other causes of lymphadenopathy.

Staging
Optimal treatment is determined by the stage of disease (Fig 29.3), which is derived from the following investigations:

1. *Blood count and bone marrow investigation.* A mild normochromic

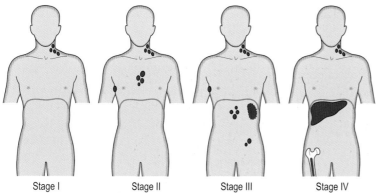

Fig 29.3 **Staging of Hodgkin's lymphoma.** Stage I, node involvement in single lymph node area (e.g. cervical); II, two or more lymph node areas on one side of diaphragm; III, nodal involvement above and below diaphragm; IV, involvement outside node areas (e.g. liver, bone marrow). The stage is followed by the letter A (absence) or B (presence) pertaining to significant systemic symptoms (one or more of: unexplained fever above 38°C, night sweats, loss of more than 10% body weight in 6 months). A single extranodal site is designated E.

Fig 29.4 **PET scan appearance in Hodgkin's lymphoma.**

or microcytic anaemia and blood eosinophilia may be present. Bone marrow aspiration and trephine biopsy to detect infiltration by disease is necessary in more advanced cases.

2. *Imaging.* A whole body computed tomography (CT) scan is the central staging procedure. In difficult cases this may be supplemented by magnetic resonance imaging (MRI). Positron emission topography (PET) scanning is increasingly used in staging and also to assess response during and after treatment (Fig 29.4). Clinical trials are needed to better define its role.

Management of classical Hodgkin's lymphoma

The challenge is to improve current high cure rates while reducing the incidence of the serious late complications of radiotherapy and chemotherapy.

Early stage disease

Patients with stage I or II disease who lack adverse features (Table 29.2) have been traditionally treated with radiotherapy alone. This is given over an extended field using a linear accelerator. Nodes above the diaphragm are treated using the 'mantle' field (like the mantle on a suit of armour) while the 'inverted Y' field includes all nodes below the diaphragm.

Radiotherapy alone fails to cure disease in 20–30% of patients and there is now more widespread use of chemotherapy in early stage disease – either alone or in combination with radiotherapy. Chemotherapy may be used in shorter courses (than for advanced disease) and the radiation field may be more restricted when combined with chemotherapy. There are various chemotherapy protocols but most common is ABVD (doxorubicin, bleomycin, vinblastine, dacarbazine), which is given intravenously as 4-weekly cycles.

Advanced stage disease

All patients with stage III or IV disease require chemotherapy with possible addition of radiotherapy for bulky disease or palliation of symptoms. ABVD is the regimen of choice for most patients. This is being compared in clinical trials with 'alternating' or 'hybrid' regimens containing a larger number of drugs. Autologous stem cell transplantation is the best choice for younger patients who fail induction chemotherapy or who have early relapse. Novel targeted therapies under investigation include the anti-CD30 monoclonal antibody-drug conjugate brentuximab vedotin.

Prognosis and late effects of treatment

Survival rates are closely linked to stage although within each stage other

Table 29.2 **Factors predicting a poor prognosis**
■ Advanced stage (most important)
■ B symptoms
■ Increased tumour bulk
■ Increased sites of disease
■ Advanced age
■ Extranodal disease
■ Poor response to chemotherapy (e.g. after two cycles)
■ Early relapse
■ Elevated erythrocyte sedimentation rate (ESR)
■ Lymphopenia
■ Anaemia

prognostic factors influence outcome (see Table 29.2). Cure rates for early stage disease are around 90% while even more advanced disease is curable in up to 80% of patients with optimal management. As in other haematological malignancies, elderly patients tolerate chemotherapy less well and cure rates are more modest. In long-term survivors there is a risk of secondary malignancy. Young women receiving mediastinal irradiation are at particularly high risk of breast cancer. Other possible late effects of treatment include cardiac disease, lung damage, sterility and endocrine dysfunction.

Hodgkin's lymphoma

- The term Hodgkin's lymphoma describes a group of lymphomas distinct from the 'non-Hodgkin's' lymphomas.

- The presumed malignant cells, Reed–Sternberg and mononuclear Hodgkin's cells, compose a minority of tumour cells.

- Common clinical presentations are palpable lymphadenopathy and constitutional symptoms.

- Prognosis is largely determined by the stage of the disease.

- Chemotherapy leads to high cure rates even in advanced disease. The late side-effects of such treatment (e.g. secondary malignancy) are significant.

30 Non-Hodgkin's lymphoma

Malignant solid tumours of lymphoid tissue which are not Hodgkin's lymphoma are termed non-Hodgkin's lymphomas (NHL). This group of lymphomas is even more heterogeneous than Hodgkin's lymphoma. The disease is the most common haematological malignancy and is currently the fifth most common cancer in the Western world. It appears to be increasing in incidence. NHL may occur at any age but the median age of presentation is 55–60 years.

Aetiology

The cause of the majority of cases of NHL is obscure. However, specific chromosomal translocations are closely associated with particular histological types. Thus, the majority of Burkitt's lymphoma cases demonstrate the t(8;14) abnormality in which the *MYC* oncogene on chromosome 8 is moved next to the immunoglobulin heavy chain region on chromosome 14. Almost 90% of follicular low-grade lymphomas are characterised by t(14;18) where the *BCL2* gene on chromosome 18 is moved to the immunoglobulin heavy chain region. This leads to excessive expression of *BCL2*, an oncogene known to inhibit apoptosis (programmed cell death). It is likely that such chromosome rearrangements require further events – perhaps co-expression of a second proto-oncogene or antigenic stimulus – to produce the clonal malignant cell. Possible triggering antigens include *Helicobacter pylori* in gastric MALT lymphoma and hepatitis C in marginal zone lymphoma. The aggressive extranodal lymphomas seen in AIDS are likely to result from a combination of immunosuppression (due to the HIV virus), deregulation of a proto-oncogene (*MYC*) and secondary viral infection (Epstein–Barr virus). Similar tumours may follow organ transplantation.

Classification

This is complex and ever-changing with a real risk of 'heart-sink' for the uninitiated. In simplest terms NHL can be divided into 'high-grade' and 'low-grade' types. High-grade tumours are composed of large poorly differentiated lymphoid cells. They have an aggressive

Table 30.1 **The WHO classification of lymphoid malignancy**[1]
With respect to NHL, approximately 90% of cases are of B-cell type and 10% of T-cell type. The commonest NHL entities are follicular (20–25% of all cases) and diffuse large B-cell (30–35%)
B-cell neoplasms
Precursor B-cell neoplasms
Precursor B-lymphoblastic lymphoma/leukaemia
Mature B-cell neoplasms
Chronic lymphocytic leukaemia/small lymphocytic lymphoma
Lymphoplasmacytic lymphoma
Hairy cell leukaemia
Plasma cell myeloma/plasmacytoma
Marginal zone lymphoma
Follicular lymphoma
Mantle cell lymphoma
Diffuse large B-cell lymphoma
Burkitt's lymphoma
B-cell proliferations of uncertain malignant potential
T-cell and putative NK-cell neoplasms
Precursor T-cell neoplasms
Precursor T-lymphoblastic lymphoma/leukaemia
Mature T-cell and NK-cell neoplasms
T-cell prolymphocytic leukaemia
T-cell large granular lymphocyte leukaemia
Adult T-cell lymphoma/leukaemia
Mycosis fungoides/Sezary's syndrome
Enteropathy-type T-cell lymphoma
Angioimmunoblastic T-cell lymphoma
Peripheral T-cell lymphoma unspecified
Anaplastic large cell lymphoma
Hodgkin's lymphoma (see p. 58)

[1]See text for discussion.

clinical course but are often curable. Low-grade tumours are composed of smaller, better differentiated cells. They are more indolent clinically but have a tendency to repeatedly relapse.

The current WHO classification avoids the overly simplistic high-grade/low-grade split and divides lymphomas into more specific subtypes based on clinical features, morphology, immunophenotype, karyotype and molecular characteristics. In addition to NHL and Hodgkin's lymphoma the WHO scheme contains a number of other lymphoid neoplasms occurring mainly at extranodal sites that are discussed elsewhere (e.g. myeloma, hairy cell leukaemia). Some of the major entities are shown in Table 30.1.

Clinical presentation

NHL is essentially a disease of lymph nodes but it has a more diverse presentation than Hodgkin's lymphoma with more irregular spread and a higher incidence of extranodal involvement. It may be an indolent disorder, perhaps

Fig 30.1 **Axillary lymphadenopathy in non-Hodgkin's lymphoma.**

requiring no immediate treatment, or an aggressive, rapidly fatal malignancy.

- *Nodal involvement.* Painless lymphadenopathy (Fig 30.1), often in the cervical region, is the most common presentation of NHL. Enlarged nodes may cause complications such as superior vena cava syndrome and hydronephrosis.
- *Extranodal involvement.* Intestinal lymphoma can present with vague abdominal pain, anaemia (caused by bleeding) or dysphagia. CNS disease frequently leads to headache and cranial nerve palsies and may cause spinal cord compression. Lymphoma may arise in the skin (e.g. mycosis fungoides). Bone marrow involvement is more common in low-grade lymphomas and can result in pancytopenia.
- *Systemic symptoms.* Sweating and significant weight loss occur in less than a quarter of patients and, where present, usually indicate advanced disease. Occasionally, patients present with metabolic complications such as hyperuricaemia, renal failure and hypercalcaemia.

Diagnosis and staging

Diagnosis depends on obtaining a tissue biopsy, usually a lymph node, for histological examination (Fig 30.2). Immunophenotyping is used to identify the degree of maturation of the malignant cell and determine whether it is of B- or T-cell origin. B-cell antigenic 'markers' include CD19, 20 and 22 and T-cell markers CD2, 3, 5 and 7. Gene rearrangement studies also aid identification. B-cell lymphomas have their immunoglobulin genes clonally rearranged while in T-cell lymphomas there is clonal rearrangement of the T-cell receptor genes. Molecular techniques (see p. 100) are being increasingly used to detect chromosome abnormalities and to derive prognostic information.

The *staging* system is similar to that used in Hodgkin's lymphoma. Patients are staged with CT scanning (Fig 30.3), MRI or PET, and a bone marrow aspirate and trephine. However, in NHL the stage plays a more modest role in management than in Hodgkin's lymphoma. The histological type of the tumour is more closely related to the likely clinical course and other factors impinge upon prognosis. An *international prognostic index* (IPI), based on age, stage, bulk of disease, performance status and serum lactate dehydrogenase (LDH) level, is commonly used (see Appendix III).

Management and prognosis

Only some of the commoner NHL subtypes will be discussed.

Follicular lymphoma

Follicular lymphoma is usually a 'low-grade' tumour. There is typically disseminated disease at presentation, an initial good response to therapy, but then recurrent relapses at decreasing intervals. Median survival is between 10 and 15 years. Patients may initially require no treatment. Local disease (unusual) may be treated with radiotherapy. For disseminated disease requiring intervention there is a wide range of possibilities. There is a move towards rituximab (anti-CD20 monoclonal antibody)-containing regimens (e.g. R-CVP: rituximab, cyclophosphamide, vincristine, prednisolone) but oral agents such as chlorambucil and fludarabine are still widely used. For relapsed disease in younger patients either autologous or allogeneic stem cell transplantation should be considered. Radioimmunotherapy (the combination of a monoclonal antibody with a radioisotope) is a promising alternative. Rituximab maintenance therapy for 2 years

Fig 30.2 **Section of a cervical lymph node showing extensive infiltration with large poorly differentiated lymphoid cells typical of diffuse large B-cell non-Hodgkin's lymphoma.**

Fig 30.3 **CT scan of the abdomen showing enlargement of lymph nodes in a patient with non-Hodgkin's lymphoma.**

after induction treatment appears to improve survival but cure remains elusive.

Diffuse large B-cell lymphoma

This is the commonest type of 'high-grade' NHL, the classic presentation being a rapidly enlarging nodal mass. A few cases will have transformed from previous follicular NHL. Localised disease is generally treated with a combination of shortened chemotherapy and local radiotherapy. Disseminated disease requires full course chemotherapy and an anthracycline-based regimen combined with rituximab (R-CHOP; cyclophosphamide, doxorubicin, vincristine, prednisolone) is the standard. Approximately 70–80% of patients will achieve remission and 60% will be cured. In patients with high-risk disease (based on IPI or genetic abnormalities) or relapse, use of more intensive chemotherapy with or without stem cell support can potentially improve the prognosis.

Selected other lymphoma subtypes

Mantle cell lymphoma is heterogeneous but is typically disseminated with marrow involvement and a poor response to treatment. Median survival is only 4 years. **Marginal zone lymphoma** is indolent and includes extranodal tumours of **mucosa-associated lymphoid type** (**MALT**). MALT lymphoma of the stomach is associated with *Helicobacter pylori* and antibiotic treatment to eliminate the bacterium may lead to lymphoma regression. **Burkitt's lymphoma** is treated with intensive combination chemotherapy with a good chance of cure in younger patients. There is a high risk of tumour lysis syndrome. **Peripheral T-cell lymphomas** have a high incidence of extranodal disease and, overall, a worse prognosis than B-cell NHL. The CHOP regimen is commonly used but in view of the disappointing results a number of experimental agents are under investigation.

Non-Hodgkin's lymphoma

- The term NHL encompasses solid tumours of lymphoid tissue which are not Hodgkin's lymphoma.

- Histological classification is complex. There is great clinical heterogeneity with indolent and aggressive types of disease.

- Indolent (e.g. follicular) NHL often initially responds well to chemotherapy but cure is elusive.

- Aggressive (e.g. diffuse large B-cell) NHL may be cured with conventional chemotherapy combined with rituximab (R-CHOP); autologous stem cell transplants are increasingly used for 'high-risk' and relapsed disease.

31 Myeloma

Introduction

Multiple myeloma is a malignant disorder in which there is an uncontrolled proliferation of clonal plasma cells in the bone marrow. Secretion of a variety of proteins by the malignant cells leads to characteristic symptoms and signs. Myeloma constitutes 10–15% of all haematological malignancies and is essentially a disease of the elderly – only 2% of cases are diagnosed in patients less than 40 years old.

Basic biology

The initial step in the development of myeloma is the appearance of a small number of clonal plasma cells (the clinical syndrome is 'monoclonal gammopathy of uncertain significance' (MGUS)). Approximately 50% of patients with MGUS have translocations involving the immunoglobulin heavy chain locus on chromosome 14q32. With progression to frank myeloma, more complex genetic events occur in the neoplastic plasma cells. Changes in the bone marrow microenvironment include the induction of angiogenesis, the suppression of cell-mediated immunity and increased secretion of interleukin-6, a powerful growth factor for myeloma cells. Bone lesions result from osteoclast activation. Myeloma cells secrete a monoclonal immunoglobulin or immunoglobulin fragments ('M-proteins' or 'paraproteins') composed of a single heavy chain class and a single light chain class, kappa or lambda. Most myelomas produce IgG or IgA but light chains alone are produced in over 10% of cases. Free light chain appearing in the urine is termed Bence Jones protein. Occasionally myeloma is non-secretory with no detectable M-protein. Localised plasma cell tumours in the absence of systemic myeloma are termed 'plasmacytomas'.

Clinical features

More than two-thirds of patients have bone pain at presentation. Pain is most common in the back and chest and may be attributed to 'arthritis'. More advanced bone disease can lead to pathological fractures or vertebral collapse with loss of height. Infiltration of the bone marrow by plasma cells may lead to symptoms of anaemia or bleeding due to thrombocytopenia. Infections are common due to immune paresis (low level of normal immunoglobulins) and other complications which may lead to symptoms include hypercalcaemia, amyloidosis and renal failure. The major cause of the nephropathy is deposition of obstructive tubular casts composed of immunoglobulin light chains – other possible factors include dehydration, infection and amyloid.

Diagnosis and staging

Myeloma is an easy malignancy to miss as the early symptoms such as malaise and backache are common in the population. The combination of backache and a high erythrocyte sedimentation rate (ESR) should be taken seriously as it may indicate myeloma or another metastatic malignancy.

In asymptomatic ('smouldering') myeloma there is generally a serum monoclonal protein >30 g/L and/or bone marrow clonal plasma cells >10% but no related organ or tissue impairment (Figs 31.1 and 31.2). A diagnosis of symptomatic

Fig 31.1 **The blood film in myeloma.** There is marked rouleaux formation and increased background staining.

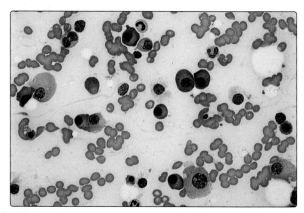

Fig 31.2 **The bone marrow in myeloma.** The malignant plasma cells show varying degrees of maturity.

Fig 31.3 **Electrophoretic strip showing serum paraprotein bands.** Patient 1 has an IgM paraprotein (Waldenström's macroglobulinaemia), patient 2 IgA myeloma and patient 3 IgG myeloma.

myeloma requires evidence of such impairment; typically increased calcium, renal insufficiency, anaemia, or bone lesions (Table 31.1 and Fig 31.3). Bony disease is increasingly assessed by MRI scanning in addition to traditional X-rays ('skeletal survey') (Fig 31.4). Patients who have a paraprotein in the serum but who do not meet the criteria for myeloma are diagnosed as having MGUS. They have a rate of progression to myeloma of 1% per year. Monoclonal gammopathy is associated with other diseases such as lymphoma, non-haematopoietic malignancies and connective tissue disorders but it is also quite common in healthy elderly people (approximately 5% over 70 years of age).

The prognosis of myeloma can be predicted from presenting clinical and laboratory features (Table 31.2). The combination of a high β_2-microglobulin level and a low albumin level

Table 31.1 **Diagnostic criteria for symptomatic myeloma**

Monoclonal protein in serum and/or urine (Fig 31.3)

Bone marrow **clonal plasma cells**[1] or plasmacytoma (Fig 31.2)

Related organ or tissue impairment (end organ damage including bone lesions)

[1]If flow cytometry is performed most plasma cells (>90%) will show a 'neoplastic' phenotype.

Table 31.2 **Myeloma: poor prognostic factors**

Low haemoglobin

High calcium

High M-protein or Bence Jones protein level

Multiple lytic lesions on X-ray

High creatinine (i.e. renal failure)

High β_2-microglobulin

Low albumin

Poor response to chemotherapy

Adverse cytogenetics (e.g. del(17p))

carries a particularly poor prognosis. Cytogenetic and molecular genetic profiles of the malignant cells also predict myeloma behaviour. Hyperdiploid and t(11;14) mutations define standard risk disease while non-hyperdiploid, t(4;14), del(17p) and del(13q) mutations indicate inferior outcome.

Management and outcome

Myeloma may be diagnosed by chance on laboratory screening in patients with limited disease and no symptoms. In this group, about 20% of all patients, the disease may remain stable for several years and there is no advantage in early intervention. Where treatment is required this generally entails drug therapy, management of specific complications, and palliation.

Drug therapy

Myeloma remains incurable with current standard treatment but there has been recent progress with the introduction of novel therapeutic agents targeting myeloma cells and their microenvironment. Treatment algorithms are evolving rapidly but the immunomodulatory agent thalidomide is frequently used in first-line regimens (often combined with dexamethasone and cyclophosphamide). In younger fitter patients (<65–70 years) induction therapy is generally followed by stem cell harvesting and intensification of treatment with high dose melphalan and autologous stem cell transplantation. This strategy gives a median survival of 5 years. Other agents increasingly used in induction and maintenance therapy include lenalidomide, pomalidomide and the proteosome inhibitor bortezomib (Velcade). All patients should

Fig 31.4 **X-rays of the skull (a) and left radius and ulna (b) in a patient with myeloma.** Numerous lytic lesions are seen.

additionally receive a bisphosphonate. In the very elderly or in patients with significant comorbidity, a gentler approach (e.g. low dose melphalan and prednisolone) may be justified. In the rare very fit young patient allogeneic stem cell transplantation is a potentially curative but very toxic option.

Management of complications

The pain of bone disease may require local radiotherapy in addition to analgesia. In spinal compression, radiotherapy and high-dose steroids usually obviate the need for laminectomy. Spinal pain may be alleviated by vertebroplasty

Fig 31.5 **The fundus in hyperviscosity syndrome complicating Waldenström's macroglobulinaemia.**

(see p. 94). Additional bisphosphonate therapy is helpful in hypercalcaemia, and anaemia can respond to erythropoietin. Renal failure often responds to rehydration and chemotherapy but haemodialysis may be required.

Palliative treatment – a team approach

Particular emphasis is placed on pain relief and the maintenance of independence (see pp. 94–95).

Waldenström's macroglobulinaemia

This disease is a form of indolent lymphoma. It is appropriately considered with myeloma as the malignant cells, which show features of lymphocytes and plasma cells, secrete an IgM paraprotein. Patients may complain only of fatigue, but high IgM levels can lead to the 'hyperviscosity syndrome', with confusion and neurological symptoms. In these cases retinal examination reveals engorged veins, haemorrhages, exudates (Fig 31.5) and rarely papilloedema. Other possible physical signs include lymphadenopathy and hepatosplenomegaly. Where treatment is required, options include chemotherapy (e.g. chlorambucil or fludarabine) and monoclonal antibodies (e.g. rituximab). Significant hyperviscosity requires plasmapheresis.

Myeloma

- Myeloma is a malignant proliferation of plasma cells.

- Diagnostic features include an 'M-protein' in the serum and/or urine, osteolytic bone lesions and infiltration of the bone marrow by malignant plasma cells.

- Bone pain is the most common presenting symptom.

- Complications include renal failure, hypercalcaemia and amyloidosis.

- Commonly used agents include thalidomide, lenalidomide and bortezomib. Autologous stem cell transplantation is performed in younger fitter patients.

- Good palliative care, especially pain relief, is crucial.

- Waldenström's macroglobulinaemia is a form of indolent lymphoma with secretion of an IgM paraprotein and possible hyperviscosity.

32 Polycythaemia

Introduction

In simple terms, polycythaemia (or erythrocytosis) means an increase in red cell count, haemoglobin and packed cell volume (PCV) above the normally accepted levels. Polycythaemia due to an absolute increase in red cell mass may occur as a myeloproliferative neoplasm (polycythaemia vera (PV)) or secondary to hypoxia or an abnormal focus of erythropoietin secretion. In 'apparent polycythaemia' the raised haemoglobin and PCV are not accompanied by a significantly raised red cell mass; usually the plasma volume is relatively reduced (Fig 32.1).

An approach to the patient with polycythaemia

The initial decision to investigate further is taken on the basis of a persisting raised PCV (haematocrit) or haemoglobin level. If true polycythaemia is confirmed by measurement of red cell mass and plasma volume then the next step is to determine whether this is primary or secondary. The full sequence of investigations is not required in all cases. For example, in a patient with known respiratory disease causing chronic hypoxia, a degree of polycythaemia is predictable and does not require investigation (Fig 32.2).

Clinical syndromes

Polycythaemia vera (PV)

PV is a myeloproliferative neoplasm; other diseases in this category are essential thrombocythaemia and myelofibrosis (see p. 66). In PV a pluripotential stem cell is mutated. Almost all patients with the disease (and some with essential thrombocythaemia and myelofibrosis) have an identical acquired point mutation in the Janus kinase 2 (*JAK2*) gene.

Clinical features. The raised red cell mass and total blood volume with associated hyperviscosity causes the symptoms and signs of the disease. Common complaints include headaches, dizziness, lethargy, sweating and pruritus (the latter particularly after a hot bath). Most importantly, there is an increased risk of arterial and venous thrombosis, particularly strokes. Paradoxically, a combination of hyperviscosity and platelet

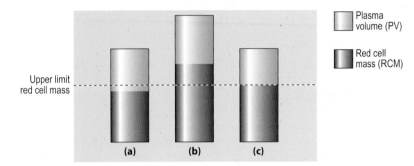

Fig 32.1 **Red cell mass and plasma volume in normality, true polycythaemia and apparent polycythaemia. (a)** Normal red cell mass (RCM) and plasma volume (PV). **(b)** True polycythaemia: there is a significant increase in RCM and total blood volume. **(c)** Apparent polycythaemia: RCM and PV are at the upper and lower limits of the normal range with a resultant increased haematocrit.

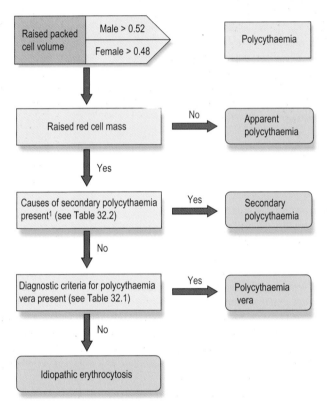

Fig 32.2 **Approach to the patient with polycythaemia.**
[1]If there is any doubt as to the secondary aetiology, investigations for polycythaemia vera (e.g. JAK2 testing) should still be performed.

dysfunction may cause a bleeding tendency. The increased cell turnover can lead to gout (Fig 32.3). Patients are characteristically plethoric and may have rosacea (Fig 32.4). Palpable splenomegaly may be present.

Diagnosis. The diagnostic challenge is to differentiate PV from a secondary polycythaemia. Splenomegaly and elevated white cell and platelet counts are suggestive of PV. Increased erythropoiesis can lead to iron deficiency. Erythropoietin estimation by radioimmunoassay is normal or low. The bone marrow aspirate and trephine in PV show

hypercellularity but there may be no pathognomonic features. Testing for the JAK2 V617F mutation is now central to the diagnosis of PV (Table 32.1). Around 95% of patients with PV are positive. In the rare negative PV cases, mutations in exon 12 of JAK2 have been found. It is likely that other genetic events (e.g. MPL, TET2 mutations) are required for disease development.

Management. The dual purpose of treatment is to relieve symptoms and to reduce the risk of complications such as thrombotic disease and bleeding. Aspirin (75 mg/day) should be given unless

Fig 32.3 **Gout complicating severe PV.**

Fig 32.4 **The face is a diagnostic clue in polycythaemia vera.** Patients are frequently plethoric and may have rosacea.

Table 32.1 **Diagnostic criteria for polycythaemia vera (PV)[1]**

The diagnosis of PV requires (1) both major criteria and one minor or (2) the first major and two minor criteria.

Major criteria

Significantly raised haematocrit[2]

Presence of *JAK2* mutation

Minor criteria

1. Bone marrow trephine biopsy showing hypercellularity for age and other features of myeloproliferation
2. Low serum erythropoietin level
3. Endogenous erythroid colony formation

[1]World Health Organization 2008.
[2]Haemoglobin level or red cell mass may also be used.

Table 32.2 **Causes of secondary polycythaemia**

Hypoxia	High altitude
	Hypoxic lung disease
	Cyanotic congenital heart disease (Fig 32.5)
	Smoking
	Abnormal Hb with increased O₂ affinity
Inappropriate secretion of erythropoietin	Renal disease (e.g. tumours, cysts, hydronephrosis)
	Hepatoma
	Cerebellar haemangioblastoma
	Phaeochromocytoma
	Uterine fibroids
Other	Androgens
	Neonatal polycythaemia
	Hypertransfusion

Note: In practice hypoxia is by far the commonest cause. Renal tumours are a rare cause but important to exclude. Neonatal polycythaemia is discussed on page 90.

Secondary polycythaemia

This is due to either a physiological response to hypoxia or an inappropriate secretion of erythropoietin. Causes are numerous and are listed in Table 32.2 (and see Fig 32.5). Treatment is essentially that of the underlying cause, although cases with very high PCVs may benefit from venesection.

Fig 32.5 **Clubbing in a patient with cyanotic congenital heart disease and secondary polycythaemia.**

Idiopathic erythrocytosis

This is a small heterogeneous group of patients who have an absolute polycythaemia without features of either PV or secondary polycythaemia. Venesection may be required.

Apparent polycythaemia

This condition has accumulated several names including spurious, stress or relative polycythaemia, pseudopolycythaemia and Gaisbock's syndrome. The usual cause is an increase in red cell mass and a decrease in plasma volume within the normally accepted limits (see Fig 32.1). Patients are most frequently male and middle-aged. Other common characteristics are excess weight, hypertension, diuretic use and significant consumption of alcohol and tobacco. The adoption of a healthier lifestyle often leads to resolution of polycythaemia. Venesection is not routine but is considered where there are thrombotic risk factors.

contraindicated. The PCV is reduced below 0.45 by venesections (up to 450 mL of blood removed) which may initially be required twice weekly. In more severe disease the need for venesection can become intolerable and cytotoxic drugs are used to suppress erythropoiesis. Hydroxycarbamide is the usual choice. Interferon alfa can be useful in younger patients and in pregnancy. Busulfan is effective given intermittently but is best limited to older patients as there is a significant risk of secondary malignancy. Drug treatment is particularly important when there is a need to control coexistent thrombocytosis or progressive splenomegaly. JAK2 inhibitors are under investigation.

PV is a relatively benign disorder and if well controlled is compatible with a median survival of greater than 10 years. However, it is a clonal disease and a few patients eventually transform to myelofibrosis (10%) or even acute leukaemia (5%). The risk of the latter is increased by treatment with alkylating agents.

> ### Polycythaemia
>
> - Polycythaemia means an increase in haemoglobin and PCV above normally accepted limits.
> - Polycythaemia can be absolute (with an increased red cell mass) or apparent (with a normal red cell mass). The absolute form can be primary or secondary.
> - Polycythaemia vera is a myeloproliferative neoplasm associated with mutations in the JAK2 gene. Secondary polycythaemia arises from a physiological response to hypoxia or inappropriate secretion of erythropoietin.
> - Management of PV is by venesection alone or with cytotoxic drugs.
> - Treatment of secondary polycythaemia is essentially that of the underlying cause.
> - Apparent polycythaemia may respond to adoption of a healthier lifestyle.

33 Essential thrombocythaemia and myelofibrosis

Essential thrombocythaemia

Essential thrombocythaemia (ET) is a chronic myeloproliferative neoplasm characterised by a persistent increase in platelet count. It is thought to be a clonal stem cell disorder although recent studies suggest that it is heterogeneous. Almost half of ET patients are positive for the *JAK2 V617F* mutation (see p. 64). They appear to have distinct clinical features including a closer link to polycythaemia vera and a higher incidence of thrombosis. ET may be associated with either thrombotic or haemorrhagic complications, the latter caused by abnormal platelet function. The average age of presentation is around 60 years. The prognosis is generally good although there is a risk of transformation to myelofibrosis, polycythaemia and acute myeloid leukaemia.

Clinical features

ET may be asymptomatic and discovered accidentally on routine blood testing. Symptoms commonly arise from disturbances of the microcirculation. Patients may complain of burning sensations in the soles and palms, cold peripheries and varied neurological symptoms including headache and dizziness. Arteriolar occlusion can cause ischaemia, gangrene or acrocyanosis. Thrombosis of large arteries is of even greater concern. Haemorrhagic problems are less common but include ecchymoses, epistaxis, menorrhagia and bleeding into the mouth and gut. Splenomegaly is unusual at least in part because of splenic infarction, which can be painful.

Diagnosis

Platelet counts can be as high as 2000×10^9/L and usually exceed 450×10^9/L (the normal range is $150–400 \times 10^9$/L) (Fig 33.1). In practice, there is no single test to specifically identify ET – diagnosis is often a process of exclusion. As thrombocytosis may accompany a wide range of disorders including infections, inflammatory conditions, malignancy and iron deficiency, a thorough history and examination is mandatory. The lack of a measurable 'acute phase response' (i.e. normal erythrocyte sedimentation rate, plasma viscosity and fibrinogen) increases the likelihood of

ET as opposed to a 'reactive' thrombocytosis. Even where there is an acquired *JAK2* gene mutation, other myeloproliferative disorders must be excluded. Bone marrow examination is worthwhile to exclude chronic myeloid leukaemia (absence of Philadelphia chromosome), myelofibrosis or myelodysplasia, and to check iron stores. Patients with polycythaemia vera may have thrombocytosis, while patients with ET can have an increased red cell mass. In practice such patients are better diagnosed as having myeloproliferative neoplasms rather than forced into either category. Only about 5% of all raised platelet counts are due to ET, but persistence of the count above 1000, particularly with coexistence of thrombosis or haemorrhage, makes it the likely diagnosis. Abnormal platelet function tests suggest ET rather than a reactive thrombocytosis.

Management

Management is not straightforward. The decision whether to treat at all must follow consideration of the patient's age, the degree of thrombocytosis and the presence or perceived risk of significant thrombotic or haemorrhagic events. Any clinical benefit must be weighed against potential toxicity of cytotoxic drugs. In a patient of more advanced age (>60 years) or with a very high platelet count (>1500) or a history of thromboembolic disease, the treatment of choice is hydroxycarbamide and low-dose aspirin. Anagrelide or interferon alfa may be preferred where hydroxycarbamide is not tolerated. The objective of treatment is to maintain the platelet count in the normal range and prevent thrombosis and haemorrhage. Low-dose aspirin alone is a reasonable option in patients at lower risk of these complications. Interferon is the usual drug of choice in pregnancy.

Myelofibrosis

Primary myelofibrosis is a myeloproliferative neoplasm characterised by bone marrow fibrosis and splenomegaly. It may develop de novo or in the setting of polycythaemia vera or essential thrombocythaemia. Most patients are over 50 years.

Myelofibrosis is a neoplastic clonal disorder originating in a single

pluripotential stem cell. Abnormal megakaryocytes are produced in increased numbers and it is these cells which release cytokines such as platelet-derived growth factor (PDGF) and transforming growth factor-β, which stimulate fibroblast proliferation and build-up of collagen in the bone marrow. The scarred marrow is unable to function normally and haematopoietic stem cells move to the spleen and liver (extramedullary haematopoiesis).

Fig 33.1 **Blood film in essential thrombocythaemia showing increased numbers of platelets of varying size.**

Fig 33.2 **Blood film in myelofibrosis showing a myelocyte and nucleated red cell (i.e. leucoerythroblastic film) and tear-drop poikilocytes.**

Fig 33.3 **Bone marrow trephine biopsy in myelofibrosis. (a)** Marked fibrosis and osteosclerosis. **(b)** Increased reticulin fibres (stained by silver impregnation).

Fig 33.4 **Massive splenomegaly in myelofibrosis.**

Leukaemic transformation occurs in about 15% of patients. Asymptomatic patients may require no treatment. For anaemia a trial of a corticosteroid, androgen or erythropoietin is worthwhile but regular transfusion is usually needed. Oral chemotherapeutic agents such as hydroxycarbamide may improve quality of life by reducing systemic upset and shrinking the spleen. There is abnormal bone marrow angiogenesis in myelofibrosis and the anti-angiogenic agents thalidomide and lenalidomide can improve blood counts and reduce splenomegaly with some durable responses. The JAK2 inhibitor ruxolitinib is a promising new agent. Its major benefits are reduced splenomegaly and constitutional symptoms. Other JAK2 inhibitors are under investigation.

Splenic irradiation can alleviate splenic pain. Splenectomy must not be undertaken lightly as it is associated with considerable mortality (around 5–10%). However, it is considered for painful splenomegaly, unacceptable transfusion requirements, life-threatening thrombocytopenia, profound cachexia or complications of portal hypertension.

Allogeneic stem cell transplantation is the only potentially curative procedure. Use of reduced intensity conditioning regimens (see p. 57) may allow its wider application.

Clinical features

The disease is often insidious in onset with fatigue and weight loss. Splenomegaly is present in all cases and massive in 10% (Fig 33.4). Splenic pain is common and a bulky spleen may lead to portal hypertension, bleeding varices and ascites. Hepatomegaly is seen in two-thirds of cases.

Diagnosis

Anaemia is almost universal and the blood film shows teardrop poikilocytes and a 'leucoerythroblastic' picture (Fig 33.2). In the early stages, thrombocytosis and neutrophilia may occur but in more advanced disease low counts are the rule. Bone marrow aspiration characteristically results in a 'dry tap' (i.e. only peripheral blood aspirated), and a marrow trephine showing dense reticulin fibres on silver staining, fibrosis and osteosclerosis is needed for diagnosis (Fig 33.3). There is usually megakaryocytic hyperplasia. The *JAK2* gene mutation is present in approximately 50% of cases. X-rays often show bone sclerosis. The major differential diagnosis is from other myeloproliferative disorders and myelodysplastic syndromes which may be associated with a degree of marrow fibrosis. Systemic causes of marrow fibrosis such as marrow infiltration by carcinoma or lymphoma and disseminated tuberculosis should also be considered.

Prognosis and management

Average survival is 4–7 years but this is very variable. Management is increasingly guided by prognostic scoring systems.

> ### Essential thrombocythaemia and myelofibrosis
>
> - ET is a chronic myeloproliferative neoplasm characterised by a persistent increase in platelet count.
> - Patients with ET may be asymptomatic or have either thrombotic or haemorrhagic complications.
> - Patients with ET at high risk of complications are usually treated with hydroxycarbamide and low-dose aspirin.
> - Myelofibrosis is a myeloproliferative neoplasm characterised by bone marrow fibrosis and splenomegaly.
> - Common symptoms in myelofibrosis are fatigue, weight loss and splenic pain.
> - Treatment of myelofibrosis is problematic. Regular transfusion is often needed for anaemia. Cautious chemotherapy, splenic irradiation and splenectomy can relieve symptoms in some patients. JAK2 inhibitors show promise.

34 Thrombocytopenia

Thrombocytopenia can be simply defined as a blood platelet count of below $150 \times 10^9/L$. With the routine measurement of platelet number by automated cell counters it is a relatively common laboratory finding. Before initiating further investigations it is important to confirm that a low platelet count is genuine by careful inspection of the blood sample and film. Either a small clot in the sample or platelet clumping (Fig 34.1) can cause artefactual thrombocytopenia.

Causes

Major causes of thrombocytopenia are listed in Table 34.1. Many of the diseases and syndromes are discussed elsewhere.

In general terms there are four possible processes leading to thrombocytopenia:

- *Failure of marrow production.* The bone marrow failure of haematological disease (e.g. aplastic anaemia, leukaemia) usually causes pancytopenia. However, thrombocytopenia may be the only sign of intrinsic marrow disease or marrow suppression associated with infection or chemotherapy.
- *Shortened lifespan.* Platelets can be destroyed in the circulation. The most common mechanism is an immunological reaction in clinical syndromes such as immune thrombocytopenia.
- *Sequestration.* Splenomegaly can cause low platelet counts because of pooling in the enlarged organ. The spleen is not necessarily massively enlarged.
- *Dilution.* Normal platelets are diluted by massive blood transfusion.

Clinical presentation

Patients with thrombocytopenia are particularly prone to bleeding from mucous membranes. It should be emphasised that spontaneous bleeding is usually only seen with platelet counts of less than $10-20 \times 10^9/L$, although patients with associated platelet dysfunction may bleed at higher counts. Conjunctival haemorrhage, nose and gum bleeding and menorrhagia are all relatively common, with haematuria and melaena less frequent. Intracranial bleeding is of serious import but, thankfully, is rare. Possible examination findings include purpura and more extensive petechial haemorrhages involving the skin and mucous membranes (Fig 34.2). The retina should be routinely inspected for haemorrhages.

Clinical syndromes

Immune thrombocytopenia (ITP)

ITP is a disease characterised by immune thrombocytopenia mediated by platelet antibodies that accelerate platelet destruction and inhibit their production. It is a heterogeneous disorder but it is conventional to divide it into two discrete entities: acute ITP and chronic ITP (Table 34.2). This division is convenient for discussion of pathogenesis and apt for most patients, but in 'real life' there is overlap between the two syndromes.

Acute ITP

The acute form of the disease is usually seen in childhood. It typically has an abrupt onset a week or so following a trivial viral illness. It is likely that in post-viral cases IgG antibody attaches to viral antigen absorbed onto the platelet surface. The resultant sudden fall in platelet count (often to below $20 \times 10^9/L$) can lead to all the symptoms and signs quoted above. Despite this, serious complications such as intracranial bleeding are very rare and the disease is self-limiting in around 90% of cases. Often only observation is required, but where the bleeding tendency is unusually severe, oral corticosteroids or intravenous immunoglobulin can be given as in chronic ITP (see below). A few children go on to develop chronic thrombocytopenia, but even here the disease is relatively benign and may eventually spontaneously remit.

Table 34.1 **Causes of thrombocytopenia**	
Pathogenesis	**Disease examples**
Failure of production	Leukaemia, myelodysplasia, aplastic anaemia, megaloblastic anaemia, myelofibrosis, malignant infiltration, infection, drugs[1]
Shortened lifespan	
Immune	ITP, drugs[1], connective tissue disorders, antiphospholipid antibody syndrome, infection, post-transfusion purpura, neonatal alloimmune thrombocytopenia
Non-immune	DIC, thrombotic thrombocytopenic purpura
Sequestration	Hypersplenism, cardiopulmonary bypass surgery
Dilution	Massive blood transfusion

[1]See Table 34.3.
ITP, immune thrombocytopenia; DIC, disseminated intravascular coagulation.

Table 34.2 **Comparison of classic acute and chronic ITP**		
Characteristic	**Acute ITP**	**Chronic ITP**
Age	Childhood	Adult life
Previous viral infection	Frequent	Unusual
Platelet count (μ $10^9/L$)	Often <20	Variable
Onset	Sudden	Insidious
Duration	Few weeks	Years/lifelong
Spontaneous remission	Around 90%	Rare

ITP, immune thrombocytopenia.

Fig 34.1 **Blood film showing clumping of platelets.** This phenomenon causes an artefactual thrombocytopenia in the automated blood count.

Fig 34.2 **Purpuric rash in a patient with acute ITP.**

Fig 34.3 **Blood film in ITP.** The platelets are reduced in number and increased in size.

Table 34.3 **Some drugs associated with thrombocytopenia**	
Heparin	Penicillin
Quinine/quinidine	Diazepam
Gold salts	Tolbutamide
Sulphonamides	Aspirin
Thiazides	Cephalosporins
Rifampicin	Ranitidine

Chronic ITP

There has been recent change in our understanding of the pathophysiology of chronic ITP. Antibodies that mediate platelet destruction also impact platelet production by damaging megakaryocytes and/or blocking the release of proplatelets. A few cases may not be antibody-mediated and will not respond to standard immunosuppressive therapies.

Chronic ITP is most common in adult life. Patients may be asymptomatic or have insidious onset of bleeding problems. Serious spontaneous bleeding is generally limited to platelet counts below $10 \times 10^9/L$ and even then it is unusual. Fatigue is common. Paradoxically, it appears that the disorder may have a pro-thrombotic element where platelet counts are restored to normal. A palpable spleen suggests a diagnosis other than ITP.

The blood film confirms thrombocytopenia; often the platelets are increased in size (Fig 34.3). There is no single specific test for ITP. A bone marrow aspirate and trephine biopsy will show increased megakaryocytes but it is often not necessary if other features are typical. Further investigations are designed to exclude other causes of isolated thrombocytopenia such as connective tissue disorders and antiphospholipid antibody syndrome. Apparent 'primary' ITP may be secondary to subclinical viral infections such as hepatitis C, cytomegalovirus, HIV and *Helicobacter pylori*. In younger patients congenital thrombocytopenias may be confused with ITP. A thorough drug history is essential.

Patients with asymptomatic mild thrombocytopenia can be merely observed. It is difficult to state a platelet count below which treatment is mandatory. In practice, serious bleeding is rare even at lower platelet counts and drug side-effects are common so treatment should generally be reserved for patients who have symptoms or signs. The normal first-line treatment is prednisolone (1 mg/kg body weight). About two-thirds of patients have a significant increase in platelet count within weeks but subsequent dose reduction often leads to relapse. Where there is no response to steroids, immunoglobulin (IVIg) can be efficacious. Platelet transfusions are seldom indicated as the platelets are rapidly destroyed but they may be considered in severe haemorrhage.

If the platelet count cannot be adequately maintained on non-toxic doses of corticosteroid then splenectomy is considered. About two-thirds of patients have a good response. The management of severe/symptomatic thrombocytopenia post-splenectomy is improving as new agents are introduced. The monoclonal antibody rituximab may give durable responses. Second-generation thrombopoietin receptor (TPO-R) agonists stimulate platelet production via megakaryocyte proliferation and maturation. Two TPO-R agonists in current use are romiplostim and eltrombopag. There remains a need for other approaches including relatively non-toxic doses of corticosteroids (e.g. prednisolone 10 mg), pulsed high dose corticosteroids, intermittent IVIg, danazol, vinca alkaloids, ciclosporin, azathioprine and mycophenolate. All give some responses reflecting the heterogeneity of the disease.

Drug-induced thrombocytopenia

Many drugs have been linked with isolated thrombocytopenia (Table 34.3). The mechanism is usually the formation of antiplatelet antibodies. General management is withdrawal of the offending drug and platelet transfusion for significant bleeding.

Heparin-induced thrombocytopenia (HIT) is an immune-mediated disorder caused by the development of antibodies to platelet factor 4 and heparin. The thrombocytopenia is typically non-severe and occurs 5–10 days after starting heparin. Unlike other drug-induced thrombocytopenias, HIT leads to increased risk of thromboembolism. Heparin should be stopped and an alternative anticoagulant substituted.

Post-transfusion purpura

In this very rare syndrome severe thrombocytopenia develops approximately 1 week after a blood transfusion. In most cases the patient's platelets are negative for the platelet antigen HPA-1a and the transfused platelets are HPA-1a positive. In a way incompletely understood an anti-HPA-1a isoantibody destroys the patient's own platelets. Bleeding may be severe. IVIg is an effective treatment.

Thrombocytopenia

- Thrombocytopenia (a low platelet count) is a relatively common laboratory finding. It is important that it is confirmed by inspection of a blood film.

- In general thrombocytopenia can be caused by failure of marrow production, shortened platelet lifespan, sequestration in the spleen and dilution by massive blood transfusion.

- Immune thrombocytopenia (ITP) is a heterogeneous disease characterised by platelet antibodies which accelerate platelet destruction and inhibit their production.

- Acute ITP is usually seen in childhood and is typically self-limiting. Chronic ITP classically occurs in adult life. There is often an initial response to steroid treatment but splenectomy may ultimately be required. Newer agents include rituximab and thrombopoietin receptor agonists.

35 Disorders of platelet function and vascular purpuras

Platelet dysfunction should be considered wherever there are the clinical symptoms and signs of thrombocytopenia (p. 14) in the presence of a normal or only moderately reduced platelet count. Disorders of platelet function can be divided into inherited disorders which are rare but well characterised in the laboratory, and acquired disorders which are much more common but often of obscure aetiology. Bleeding problems may also arise in a number of inherited and acquired disorders of the vasculature and its supporting connective tissue – the vascular purpuras.

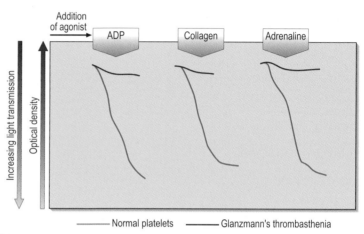

Fig 35.1 **Platelet aggregation studies.** When compared with the normal control it can be seen that in Glanzmann's thrombasthenia there is loss of aggregation with all the agonists used.

Laboratory testing of platelet function

Ideally, blood samples for testing of platelet function should be taken from fasting and resting subjects who have not smoked, ingested caffeine or drugs known to affect platelet function. A blood count and blood film are routinely performed. The *bleeding time*, where a small incision is made in the forearm skin and the time to cessation of bleeding recorded, is now less used as it is subjective and has poor reproducibility. A number of dedicated platelet function instruments (e.g. PFA-100) allow screening tests but the results must be interpreted with caution as they are not diagnostic or sensitive for mild platelet disorders.

Platelet aggregation studies assess the ability of platelets to aggregate in response to the addition of a variety of agonists (e.g. ADP, adrenaline (epinephrine), collagen, arachidonic acid, ristocetin). The tracings produced (Fig 35.1) require expert interpretation. The methodology remains the gold standard with the response to agonists giving characteristic patterns in inherited disorders. Other tests of platelet function include flow cytometry for the quantitation of glycoprotein receptor density, and the measurement of total and/or released adenine nucleotides. The latter tests may confirm the findings from platelet aggregation studies (e.g. in Bernard–Soulier syndrome) or reveal abnormalities where aggregation studies are normal or equivocal (e.g. in a storage pool disease or release defect).

Inherited disorders of platelet function

The commonest inherited platelet function and coagulation disorder, von Willebrand disease, is described on page 74.

Bernard–Soulier syndrome

This is a rare autosomal recessive bleeding disorder. There is a combination of platelet dysfunction, thrombocytopenia and abnormal platelet morphology. The mild thrombocytopenia is probably caused by reduced platelet survival. The functional platelet defect arises from mutation in the polypeptides of the glycoprotein (GP) Ib/IX/V complex. This complex is crucial for the initial adhesion of platelets to exposed subendothelium at high shear flow and for binding of platelets to von Willebrand factor. In platelet aggregation studies there is failure to aggregate with ristocetin. Bleeding can be severe and particularly complicates other predisposing events such as peptic ulcers and pregnancy. Patients require platelet transfusion for severe bleeding and prior to surgery. Antifibrinolytic agents and DDAVP (see p. 73) are useful in some cases.

Glanzmann's thrombasthenia

This rare autosomal recessive disease is also caused by loss or dysfunction of a platelet glycoprotein complex – GP IIb/IIIa. This normally acts as a receptor for adhesive proteins such as fibrinogen and von Willebrand factor. Platelet numbers and morphology are normal but the platelets fail to aggregate with all agonists except ristocetin (see Fig 35.1). Clinical manifestations are variable but there is typically onset in the neonatal period and subsequent cutaneous and gastrointestinal bleeding, and menorrhagia. Platelet transfusions are indicated where local haemostatic measures fail. If there is platelet refractoriness, recombinant factor VIIa can be used.

Other disorders

Hereditary diseases of platelet function may also result from deficiency of platelet storage organelles (storage pool disorders) or release defects where there is failure to successfully release granule contents upon platelet activation. These disorders usually cause only mild bleeding problems.

Acquired disorders of platelet function

These disorders are common. Causes include foods, drugs, systemic disorders and diseases of the blood (Table 35.1).

Aspirin

Many drugs can affect platelet function but aspirin is the best documented and the most frequently prescribed. At lower doses aspirin selectively acetylates and irreversibly inactivates the enzyme cyclooxygenase-1 (COX-1), preventing the production of thromboxane A_2 from arachidonic acid and inhibiting aggregation for the remainder of the platelet's lifespan. Responses are variable but aspirin can dramatically prolong the bleeding time and cause haemorrhage in patients with thrombocytopenia or other coexistent bleeding problems.

Chronic renal failure

Uraemia can lead to multiple platelet defects. Elevated levels of nitric oxide may inhibit platelet adhesion, activation and aggregation. Anaemia contributes to uraemic bleeding as fewer red cells mean that fewer platelets are displaced towards an injured vessel wall. Dialysis reduces haemorrhagic symptoms. This can be supplemented by correction of severe anaemia, DDAVP and platelet transfusions.

Cardiopulmonary bypass

Platelets are activated and degranulated in the extracorporeal circuit, impairing their effectiveness in vivo. This may be exacerbated by hypothermia and large doses of heparin. Excessive bleeding is uncommon but where this happens platelet transfusion is efficacious.

Haematological diseases

Platelet function is impaired in a number of blood diseases, including acute myeloid leukaemia, myelodysplastic syndromes, myeloproliferative disorders and myeloma.

Vascular purpuras

A bleeding tendency caused by a local or general vascular abnormality is referred to as a vascular purpura (Table 35.2). Diagnosis of these diseases is made mainly on clinical grounds with laboratory exclusion of other haemostatic defects.

Inherited disorders

Hereditary haemorrhagic telangiectasia (HHT)

The hallmark of this rare autosomal dominant disease is the development of multiple ateriovenous malformations (AVMs). Small AVMs are referred to as telangiectasia. Close to the surface of the skin and mucous membranes, they often rupture and bleed. Two mutated genes, endoglin and *ALK1*, have been implicated. Clinical problems include recurrent epistaxes (90% of cases), gastrointestinal haemorrhage, haematuria and larger pulmonary arteriovenous malformations (PAVMs). Chronic bleeding from the gut causes iron deficiency anaemia. On examination there are the characteristic telangiectasia (Fig 35.2). Management includes local control of bleeding (e.g. laser treatment of telangiectasia), iron supplements and embolisation of PAVMs.

Table 35.1 **Causes of abnormal platelet function**	
Inherited	Bernard–Soulier syndrome
	Glanzmann's thrombasthenia
	Storage pool disorders
	Release defects
	Other (e.g. von Willebrand disease)
Acquired	Drugs (e.g. aspirin)
	Foods (e.g. garlic)
	Chronic renal failure
	Cirrhosis
	Cardiopulmonary bypass surgery
	Blood diseases: acute myeloid leukaemia, myelodysplastic syndromes, myeloproliferative disorders, myeloma
	Various systemic disorders[1]

[1]These include disseminated intravascular coagulation (DIC) and thrombotic thrombocytopenic purpura (TTP).

Table 35.2 **The vascular purpuras**	
Inherited	Hereditary haemorrhagic telangiectasia[1]
	Connective tissue diseases
	Ehlers–Danlos syndrome
	Pseudoxanthoma elasticum
	Marfan syndrome
Acquired	Henoch–Schönlein purpura
	Various infections
	Drug reactions (allergic purpuras)
	Senility
	Prolonged corticosteroid treatment
	Scurvy
	Mechanical

[1]Sometimes known as Rendu–Osler–Weber disease.

Inherited diseases of connective tissue

Several rare inherited disorders of connective tissue predispose to bleeding. The mechanism is either a general failure of support of blood vessels or defective interaction between platelets and abnormal collagen. Specific diseases include Ehlers–Danlos syndrome, pseudoxanthoma elasticum and Marfan syndrome.

Acquired disorders

This is a very heterogeneous group. Henoch–Schönlein purpura is a syndrome usually seen in childhood where an itchy purpuric rash typically follows an infection. Spontaneous remission is

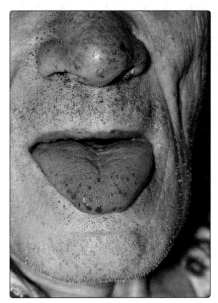

Fig 35.2 **Telangiectasia in hereditary haemorrhagic telangiectasia.**

Fig 35.3 **Senile purpura.**

the rule but renal failure may result. Other causes of acquired purpuric rashes include infections, drug reactions, scurvy, trauma, prolonged steroid therapy and simple old age (senile purpura, Fig 35.3).

> ### Disorders of platelet function and vascular purpuras
>
> - Platelet dysfunction should be considered where there are the clinical features of thrombocytopenia in the presence of a normal or only moderately reduced platelet count.
> - Laboratory testing of platelet function normally includes a blood count, a blood film and platelet aggregation studies. Careful collection of the sample is crucial.
> - Inherited disorders of platelet function are generally well characterised but rare (e.g. Bernard–Soulier syndrome), whereas acquired disorders are more frequent but often of obscure aetiology.
> - Aspirin is a common cause of acquired platelet dysfunction.
> - A 'vascular purpura' is a disorder with a bleeding tendency caused by a local or general vascular abnormality. Diseases may be inherited (e.g. hereditary haemorrhagic telangiectasia) or acquired (e.g. Henoch–Schönlein purpura).

36 Haemophilia

Haemophilia is an inherited disorder of coagulation. The general term haemophilia is usually taken to mean haemophilia A, a deficiency of factor VIII, but a smaller number of cases are caused by a deficiency of factor IX (haemophilia B).

Haemophilia A

Haemophilia A is transmitted as an X-linked recessive disorder. Thus, all males with the defective gene have haemophilia, all sons of haemophiliac men are normal, all daughters are obligatory carriers and daughters of carriers have a 50% chance of also being carriers. The disease prevalence is 1 in 10 000 people. The gene for factor VIII is situated at the tip of the long arm of the X chromosome. A wide variety of mutations of the gene can lead to underproduction of factor VIII and the clinical syndrome of haemophilia. In about half of haemophilia families an unusual molecular genetic abnormality involving inversion of the factor VIII gene at intron 22 has been found. A family history is not inevitably present, as up to 30% of all new cases of haemophilia are due to recent sporadic mutations.

Clinical features

As factor VIII is a critical component of the blood coagulation pathway (see p. 12), low levels predispose to recurrent bleeding. The likelihood of bleeding can be roughly predicted from the factor VIII level, which may be expressed as units/dL or as percentage activity (Table 36.1).

Bleeding in haemophilia

The disease usually becomes apparent when the child begins to crawl. Severely affected patients not receiving prophylactic treatment experience 30–50 bleeding episodes each year. The most common problems are spontaneous bleeds into joints, often elbows or knees, although any joint can be involved. Patients may develop particular *target joints* which bleed frequently. They often have an innate feeling that a bleed has started prior to any objective signs. Recurrent or inadequately managed joint bleeds lead to chronic deformity of the joint with swelling and pain (Fig 36.1).

Bleeding may also afflict deep-seated muscles, often the flexor muscle groups. If ignored, the enlarging haematoma

Table 36.1 **Factor VIII level and clinical severity of haemophilia**	
Factor VIII level	**Clinical severity**
Less than 2 units/dL	**Severe:** frequent spontaneous bleeds into joints and muscles
2–5 units/dL	**Moderate:** some spontaneous bleeds, bleeding after minor trauma
5–45 units/dL	**Mild:** bleeding only after significant trauma or surgery

can compress adjacent nerves and vessels with serious consequences (Fig 36.2). Haematuria is not unusual and, until recently, intracranial bleeding was the most common cause of death in haemophilia.

Complications of treatment

In affluent countries, factor VIII replacement treatment as described below has been enormously beneficial in allowing early control of bleeding and the avoidance of chronic joint damage. Unfortunately, most haemophiliac patients treated before 1985 became infected with pathogenic viruses contaminating factor VIII concentrate, notably HIV and hepatitis C. There are now improving therapies for both HIV and hepatitis C infection and younger patients receiving only virus-free factor products have avoided these complications. Approximately 25% of patients with severe haemophilia will develop antibodies to factor VIII ('inhibitors'). They tend to appear in childhood but may occur after years of treatment.

Diagnosis

Haemophilia is associated with a prolonged activated partial thromboplastin time (APTT) in the routine clotting screen. The diagnosis is confirmed by a factor VIII assay. In the presence of a family history there are usually few problems in diagnosis. Tests can be

Fig 36.2 **Psoas muscle bleed in haemophilia A.** There was sensory loss in the outlined area caused by pressure on the femoral nerve.

performed on umbilical cord blood. In the absence of a family history the disease may present in a young child with bruising and a swollen joint and be mistakenly regarded as non-accidental injury. Mild haemophilia may only cause problems after trauma or surgery. All patients with bleeding or bruising of a severity disproportionate to the trauma sustained should be investigated to exclude a bleeding disorder.

Management

Treatment of haemophilia is complex, and severe disease is best managed in haemophilia centres where an experienced team of doctors, nurses, physiotherapists and social workers can help patients and their families to lead a relatively normal life.

Treatment of bleeding

Most haemophiliac patients require replacement therapy with factor VIII concentrate and this is often self-administered at home when a bleed occurs ('on demand' treatment). The

Fig 36.1 **Chronic knee damage in severe haemophilia A. (b)** Shows bilateral osteoporosis, narrowing of the joint space and joint deformity.

Fig 36.3 **Typical response to factor VIII infusion in a patient with severe haemophilia.** An infusion of 3500 units will increase the level to around 100% in a 70 kg man. As factor VIII has a half-life of 12 hours, the level falls to 50% at this time – an infusion of 1750 units increases the level from 50 to 100%.

Fig 36.4 **Southern blotting illustrating the factor VIII gene inversion.** Lane 1, normal male; Lane 2, female heterozygous for proximal inversion; Lane 3, male with distal inversion; Lane 4, female heterozygous for distal inversion; Lane 5, normal female.

dose and duration of treatment depends on the patient's size and the locality and magnitude of the bleed. One unit of factor VIII is the amount contained in 1 mL of normal plasma. For spontaneous haemarthroses it is sufficient to raise the factor VIII level to 30% of normal; in a 70 kg man this entails a dose of around 1000 units. More serious bleeding or surgery requires levels of 70–100% maintained until the risk subsides (Fig 36.3). Factor VIII products undergo processing to maximise quality, purity and viral safety. Plasma-derived factor VIII is being increasingly replaced by recombinant factor VIII. Third-generation recombinant factor VIII is free of any animal or human protein. Prophylactic (alternate day) recombinant factor VIII treatment in children eradicates bleeding and improves quality of life. Periods of 'secondary prophylaxis' may be considered in older patients with problematic joint bleeds.

Treatment of inhibitors is highly specialised. Acute bleeds can be treated with recombinant factor VII$_a$ or a concentrate of activated vitamin K derived clotting factors (FEIBA). Eradication of the inhibitor may be achieved by immune tolerance regimens where factor VIII is given regularly in high doses with or without immunomodulatory agents.

In patients with mild disease, 1-amino-8-D-arginine vasopressin (DDAVP), given intravenously or by nasal spray, mobilises factor VIII from stores and may avoid the need for concentrate. The antifibrinolytic agent tranexamic acid can also be used to reduce bleeding – it should, however, be avoided in haematuria where it can induce clot colic.

Likely advances in haemophilia drug therapy are pegylated recombinant factor VIII allowing less frequent administration and novel approaches including non-peptide haemostatic agents which reduce reliance on replacement coagulation factor.

Treatment of viral infection
Haemophiliac patients with HIV infection require state-of-the-art management of the physical and social problems which can arise. Hepatitis C infection carries a long-term risk of cirrhosis (20–30%) and hepatocellular cancer. The combination of pegylated interferon and ribavirin eradicates the virus in 50–80% of cases dependent on the viral genotype.

Gene therapy
Gene therapy is a potentially curative treatment for haemophilia and is discussed on page 103.

The carrier state and genetic counselling
Female carriers are generally asymptomatic but some will have low enough

levels of factor VIII (10–30%) to cause excessive bleeding after trauma. In families with inversion of the factor VIII gene (see above), first-generation molecular biology methods have been used in carrier and prenatal diagnosis (Fig 36.4). The more recent development of polymerase chain reaction (PCR)-based screening and sequencing technology has allowed identification of the mutation in nearly all patients with haemophilia A. Large databases of the known mutations are freely available.

Haemophilia B

Haemophilia B is an X-linked recessive bleeding disorder in which there is a deficiency of factor IX. There are many clinical similarities to haemophilia A – severely affected patients suffer recurrent spontaneous joint bleeds. However, inhibitors (antibodies to factor IX) are less common than in haemophilia A. Earlier factor IX concentrates were associated with thromboembolic complications but safer high purity preparations and recombinant products are now available for treatment. The half-life of infused factor IX is around 18 hours and thus it can often be given just once daily to maintain levels after spontaneous bleeding or surgery. Prophylactic treatment can be given once or twice weekly.

Haemophilia

- Haemophilia A is an X-linked recessive disorder characterised by deficiency of factor VIII.
- Severely affected patients suffer recurrent spontaneous bleeds, most often into joints.
- Replacement therapy with factor VIII concentrate is needed in all but mild cases; previous contamination of plasma-derived concentrates has led to HIV and hepatitis C infection.
- DDAVP and tranexamic acid can help control bleeding in mild disease.
- The management of choice in severely affected children is prophylactic treatment with genetically engineered recombinant factor VIII.
- Haemophilia B is characterised by deficiency of factor IX; inheritance and clinical features are similar to haemophilia A.

37 Von Willebrand disease and other inherited coagulation disorders

Von Willebrand disease

Von Willebrand disease (vWD) is the most common inherited bleeding disorder. The prevalence of symptomatic vWD is approximately 0.01%. Identification of milder forms is complicated by the broad range of von Willebrand factor (vWF) levels in the normal population; it is important to recognize that the diagnosis of vWD requires the presence of bleeding symptoms (see Fig 37.1).

All vWD is caused by mutations in the gene for vWF. vWF is an adhesive glycoprotein secreted by endothelium and megakaryocytes (see also p. 12). It is a multimeric protein with a characteristic normal distribution of multimer sizes in plasma. vWF has two key functions: promotion of platelet adhesion to damaged endothelium and other platelets (Fig 37.2) and the transport and stabilisation of factor VIII. Thus, the clinical disorder of vWD is associated with excessive bleeding due to abnormal platelet function and low factor VIII activity. The relationship between the risk of bleeding and vWF level is not strong until the level is very low. The clinical and laboratory heterogeneity of vWD necessitates the definition of several subtypes.

Classification (Table 37.1 and Fig 37.3)

The current classification of vWD depends on electrophoretic analysis of vWF multimers. In type 1 vWD, the multimers appear to be normal in structure and function but decreased in concentration. In type 2 vWD there is a qualitative deficiency of vWF divisible into four subtypes. In type 2A there is an absence of high molecular weight vWF multimers and markedly reduced vWF binding to platelets. 2B refers to a variant where defective platelet adhesion results, paradoxically, from increased binding of vWF to platelets. In 2M there is decreased platelet-dependent vWF function despite a relatively normal multimer pattern while 2N is characterised by failure of vWF to bind factor VIII. In the rare type 3 form, there is an almost complete deficiency of vWF and the factor VIII level is markedly decreased.

There is correlation between the subtype and the mode of inheritance. Type 1 vWD is the most common form of the disease (80% of cases) and inheritance is often autosomal dominant. Type 2 vWD (15% of cases) may be dominant or recessive and the type 3 variant is recessive. Because inherited deficiencies of vWF function are common the accidental co-inheritance of otherwise recessive vWD alleles may occur ('compound heterozygosity'). There is currently no genotypic classification of vWD. More than 250 mutations of all types have been identified. These include large and small deletions, nonsense and missense mutations and splicing abnormalities.

Clinical features

Severe vWD is characterised by spontaneous bleeding, particularly epistaxes, gum bleeding and menorrhagia. Easy bruising is also common but (with the exception of type 3) haemarthroses and muscle haematomas are rare. Milder disease often presents with excessive bleeding following trauma or surgical procedures and the diagnosis can easily be

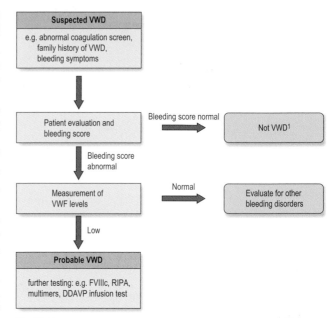

Fig 37.1 **One approach to vWD diagnosis.** In practice, this has to be individualised (see text). vWD, von Willebrand disease; vWF, von Willebrand factor; FVIIIc, factor VIII; RIPA, ristocetin-induced platelet aggregation.
[1]In children should have lower threshold for measuring vWF levels.

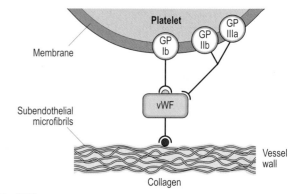

Fig 37.2 **The role of von Willebrand factor in platelet adhesion.** Following vessel wall injury, large multimers of vWF bind to subendothelial microfibrils and also to glycoprotein (Gp) Ib on the platelet membrane thus mediating platelet adhesion. A secondary binding site with platelet Gp IIb/IIIa promotes further adhesion.

Fig 37.3 **SDS–PAGE multimer analysis of von Willebrand factor.** Typical multimer patterns in normal plasma and types 1, 2A, 2B and 3 vWD are shown diagrammatically.

missed. A thorough history is crucial and must include assessment of the severity of recent bleeding, the existence of previous bleeding problems (particularly after surgery, dental extractions and childbirth) and the presence of a family

Table 37.1 **Summary of classification of vWD**

- Type 1 vWD is a partial quantitative deficiency of vWF
- Type 2 vWD is a qualitative deficiency of vWF
- Type 3 vWD is a virtually complete deficiency of vWF
- Type 2A vWD is a qualitative variant with an absence of high molecular weight vWF multimers
- Type 2B vWD is a qualitative variant with *increased* affinity of vWF for platelet glycoprotein Ib (reduced in other types)
- Type 2M vWD is a qualitative variant *not* caused by absence of high molecular weight multimers
- Type 2N vWD is a qualitative variant with reduced affinity of vWF for factor VIII

Note: Mixed phenotypes may be caused by compound heterozygosity.

history of easy bleeding. A standard questionnaire can be used to generate a quantitative 'bleeding score'. Death from bleeding is rare but it may follow massive gastrointestinal haemorrhage.

Laboratory diagnosis

Diagnosis can be complicated and tests often have to be repeated. It is not clear which laboratory measurement best correlates with the severity of bleeding.

1. **Blood count.** The platelet count is normal except for a moderate reduction in some cases of type 2B disease.
2. **Activated partial thromboplastin time (APTT).** Usually prolonged due to low factor VIII:C levels. The prothrombin time (PT) is normal.
3. **Quantitative immunoassay for vWF antigen.**
4. **Functional assay of vWF.** The commonest methodology is the 'ristocetin cofactor assay'. Collagen binding assays are also used.
5. **Factor VIII:C assay.** Often low. May be borderline or normal in mild type 1 disease.
6. **Multimer analysis.** The multimer composition of circulating VWF is assessed by either crossed immunoelectrophoresis or sodium dodecyl sulphate electrophoresis (see Fig 37.3).
7. **Platelet aggregation studies.** Ristocetin (an obsolete antibiotic) induces platelet aggregation in normal plasma but not in severe vWD. An exception is the type 2B variant where platelets aggregate at unusually low concentrations of ristocetin.
8. **Blood group.** Normal plasma vWF levels tend to be lower in group O individuals.
9. **General tests of primary haemostasis.** The bleeding time is

now little used. The PFA-100 (see p. 70) is a useful screening test but is also abnormal in other platelet disorders.

Management

Very mild bleeding problems may require little intervention, perhaps just local measures and the prescription of an antifibrinolytic drug such as tranexamic acid. More significant bleeding generally responds to an infusion or intranasal spray of DDAVP (desmopressin) which stimulates release of vWF from stores. DDAVP is predictably most effective in patients with a partial quantitative impairment of vWF (type 1). It is less effective in most type 2 variants and is generally contraindicated in type 2B. Patients with type 3 disease do not respond to DDAVP as they lack any capacity to secrete vWF. Where DDAVP is ineffective or contraindicated, then selected plasma-derived factor VIII concentrates containing sufficient vWF are used. An unusually sustained rise in factor VIII levels can be obtained as the vWF in the concentrate prolongs survival of the patient's own factor VIII. Recombinant vWF is under development. Patients with vWD normally require treatment with either DDAVP or factor VIII concentrate prior to surgery.

Effective genetic counselling in vWD demands a full understanding of the disease subtype and mode of inheritance.

Other inherited coagulation disorders

Factor deficiencies

Factor VIII and factor IX deficiencies

See section on haemophilia (pp. 72–73).

Factor XI deficiency

This bleeding disorder occurs most commonly in Ashkenazi Jews. There is a variable relationship between the factor XI level and the bleeding tendency. Treatment options for significant

bleeding include factor XI concentrate and recombinant factor VIIa.

Factor VII deficiency

This is inherited as an autosomal recessive disorder. The bleeding tendency is very variable with central nervous system haematoma a real risk in severe cases. The diagnosis is confirmed by factor VII assay and recombinant factor VII concentrate is available for treatment.

Factor V deficiency

This is a very rare autosomal recessive condition. Bleeding episodes are treated with virally inactivated fresh frozen plasma.

Factor XIII deficiency

Another rare autosomal recessive disorder, factor XIII deficiency causes a severe haemorrhagic tendency and poor wound healing. Most sufferers present early in life, often with profuse bleeding from the umbilical cord, and death may result from intracranial haemorrhage. Screening coagulation tests are normal. Diagnosis requires the laboratory demonstration of solubility of patient plasma clots in urea (there is defective crosslinking of fibrin). Factor XIII concentrate is available for treatment.

Abnormalities of fibrinogen

Inherited disorders of fibrinogen are broadly divisible into quantitative deficiencies (afibrinogenaemia and hypofibrinogenaemia) and qualitative abnormalities (dysfibrinogenaemia). Afibrinogenaemia is an autosomal recessive disease in which blood fails to clot in all coagulation screening tests and plasma fibrinogen is barely detectable by radioimmunoassay. The bleeding tendency can be severe with spontaneous haemorrhage and excessive blood loss after surgery. Fibrinogen concentrate is the treatment of choice. Many patients with hypofibrinogenaemia and dysfibrinogenaemia are asymptomatic.

Von Willebrand disease and other inherited coagulation disorders

- vWD is a relatively common and very heterogeneous inherited bleeding disorder. Deficiency of von Willebrand factor (vWF) causes abnormal platelet function and low factor VIII activity.
- Classification of vWD relies on electrophoretic analysis of vWF multimers.
- Mild bleeding problems in vWD require little intervention. More significant bleeding is treated with either DDAVP or factor VIII concentrates containing vWF.
- There are various other inherited coagulation factor deficiencies. In most there are specific concentrates available for treatment.
- Inherited disorders of fibrinogen include quantitative deficiencies (afibrinogenaemia and hypofibrinogenaemia) and qualitative abnormalities (dysfibrinogenaemia).

38 Acquired disorders of coagulation

Disseminated intravascular coagulation (DIC)

DIC is a complex clinical syndrome which complicates many serious illnesses (Table 38.1). It is characterised by intravascular deposition of fibrin and accelerated degradation of fibrin and fibrinogen caused by excess activity of proteases, notably thrombin and plasmin, in the blood (Fig 38.1). DIC is heterogeneous both in its pathophysiology and clinical manifestations. In most cases it probably begins when circulating blood is exposed to tissue factor released from damaged tissues, malignant cells or injured endothelium. This in turn leads to generation of thrombin which causes formation of soluble fibrin, activation of circulating platelets, and secondary fibrinolysis.

DIC can cause bleeding, large vessel thrombosis and haemorrhagic tissue necrosis (Fig 38.2). The coagulation defect arises from consumption of coagulation factors and platelets and increased fibrinolytic activity. In clinical practice acute DIC usually presents as widespread bleeding in an ill patient. Oozing of blood from cannulation sites is characteristic. Microthrombus formation can lead to irreversible organ damage; the kidney, lungs and brain are frequent targets. DIC is not necessarily a fulminant syndrome; more chronic forms may be seen particularly in association with malignancy (e.g. prostatic carcinoma).

Diagnosis depends on the laboratory demonstration of accelerated fibrinolysis accompanied by falling levels of coagulation factors in an ill patient. The following combination of laboratory test abnormalities is typical:

- reduced platelet count
- prothrombin time (PT) prolonged and activated partial thromboplastin time (APTT) usually prolonged
- thrombin time prolonged
- fibrinogen level reduced
- high levels of fibrin(ogen) degradation products (FDPs) and cross-linked fibrin degradation products ('D-dimers').

The cornerstone of management of DIC is the treatment of the underlying disease. Patients are more likely to die from this than from thrombosis or bleeding. However, specific treatment of DIC may be life-saving and if bleeding occurs support with blood products is indicated. Platelets, fresh frozen plasma (FFP – a source of coagulation factors) and cryoprecipitate (a source of fibrinogen) may all be used. Wherever possible the choice of blood products should be guided by the platelet count and coagulation tests. More controversial is the use of pharmacological inhibitors of coagulation and fibrinolysis. Although heparin can reduce clotting factor consumption and secondary fibrinolysis, it

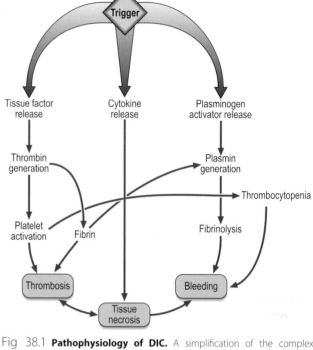

Fig 38.1 **Pathophysiology of DIC.** A simplification of the complex interactions.

Fig 38.2 **Haemorrhagic bullae and gangrene in severe DIC.**

Fig 38.3 **Spontaneous bruising in acquired haemophilia.**

Table 38.1 **Common causes of DIC**
■ Infections – particularly septicaemia
■ Malignancy – disseminated carcinoma or acute leukaemia
■ Obstetric emergencies – septic abortion, abruptio placentae, etc. (see p. 89)
■ Shock – surgical trauma, burns
■ Severe haemolytic transfusion reaction
■ Liver disease

can also increase the haemorrhagic risk by its anticoagulant action. Its use should be considered where thrombosis predominates. Recombinant activated protein C may be beneficial in patients with severe sepsis and DIC.

Vitamin K deficiency

Vitamin K in the body is derived from dietary vegetables and intestinal flora.

Once absorbed it is stored in the liver and following further metabolism it acts as a cofactor for γ-glutamyl carboxylation of coagulation factors II, VII, IX and X and proteins C and S. Vitamin K deficiency is probably the most common acquired coagulation disorder encountered in hospital patients. The vitamin K antagonist effect of warfarin is discussed on page 80 and the vitamin K deficiency of liver disease later in this section.

Dietary deficiency

Normal dietary requirements for vitamin K are low (0.1–0.5 g/kg) and thus patients must be considerably malnourished before overt deficiency occurs. This most commonly occurs in patients receiving intensive medical care, particularly where broad-spectrum antibiotics are used. Deficiency is suggested clinically by excessive bleeding and in the laboratory by a prolonged prothrombin time. Supplemental vitamin K should ideally be given before bleeding problems occur.

Malabsorption

Malabsorptive conditions such as coeliac disease and tropical sprue may lead to vitamin K deficiency. Vitamin K can also be lost in chronic biliary obstruction due to failure of bile salts necessary for fat absorption to reach the bowel.

In the newborn

Vitamin K deficiency may arise in the first weeks or months of life, most commonly in breast-fed, full-term and otherwise healthy babies. Contributory factors include low placental transfer of vitamin K, low concentrations of vitamin K in breast milk, low intake of milk and a sterile gut. The time of onset is variable but haemorrhage most commonly occurs on the 2nd to 4th day. A coagulation screen is abnormal with the prothrombin time and APTT both prolonged. In most countries prophylactic vitamin K (1 mg intramuscular injection) is given to newborn babies. Affected babies respond to parenteral vitamin K but fresh frozen plasma or prothrombin complex concentrate may be needed for severe haemorrhage.

Liver disease

The liver is vital to normal haemostasis. It produces all the factors of the intrinsic and extrinsic coagulation pathway and clears potentially damaging products of coagulation such as fibrin degradation products and activated clotting factors. In advanced liver disease there are often multiple haemostatic abnormalities including reduced synthesis of clotting factors, increased consumption of clotting factors (DIC), qualitative and quantitative platelet abnormalities, qualitative fibrinogen abnormalities and accelerated clot lysis. Where bleeding occurs, therapy is guided by the dominant haemostatic problems. Possible interventions include parenteral vitamin K, fresh frozen plasma, cryoprecipitate and platelet infusions.

Acquired haemophilia

Antibodies ('inhibitors') that block the action of coagulation factors may appear in patients who have no hereditary disorder of coagulation. Such autoantibodies most commonly target factor VIII and the clinical syndrome is termed 'acquired haemophilia'. Acquired haemophilia may be associated with a number of conditions including rheumatoid arthritis and other autoimmune disorders, skin disorders, malignancy, drug therapy (particularly penicillin) and pregnancy. However, the most common presentation is in an elderly patient with no associated condition. Possible clinical problems include haemorrhage into soft tissues and muscles (Fig 38.3), haematuria, haematemesis and prolonged bleeding postpartum or postoperatively. Bleeding can be difficult to control and death occurs in approximately 10% of cases.

In the laboratory, the diagnosis of acquired haemophilia is suggested by a prolonged APTT worsening with incubation and not corrected by the addition of normal plasma, and a low factor VIII level. Laboratory assay of the inhibitor is based on the ability of the patient's plasma to neutralise the activity of a known amount of factor VIII.

Management is complex and controversial but can be divided into the treatment of the acute bleeding episode and subsequent attempts to eliminate the autoantibody by immunosuppressive treatment. Possible approaches to the acute episode include activated prothrombin complex concentrate (such as FEIBA, which contains activated factors VII, IX, and X) and recombinant factor VIIa. Immunosuppressive strategies include intravenous immunoglobulin and plasmapheresis in the acute episode and longer-term steroids or cyclophosphamide. The usual approach is summarised in Figure 38.4.

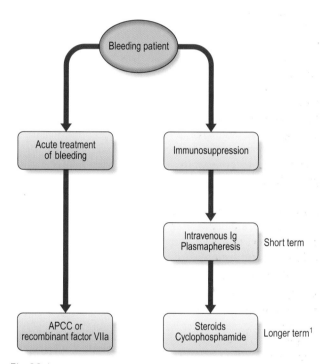

Fig 38.4 **The management of acquired haemophilia.** APCC, activated prothrombin complex concentrate; Ig, immunoglobulin; a, activated.
[1]In refractory cases other immunosuppressive agents such as ciclosporin or rituximab (anti-CD20) may be considered.

Acquired disorders of coagulation

- Disseminated intravascular coagulation (DIC) is a complex clinical syndrome which complicates serious illness. It causes both haemorrhage and thrombosis. Laboratory tests are needed to confirm the diagnosis.

- Treatment of DIC is essentially that of the underlying cause. Blood products are often indicated where bleeding occurs.

- Vitamin K deficiency is a common acquired coagulation disorder.

- Advanced liver disease can cause multiple haemostatic abnormalities.

- Acquired haemophilia is generally caused by an autoantibody targeted against factor VIII. It may be idiopathic or associated with other autoimmune diseases, malignancy, pregnancy or drug treatment.

39 Thrombophilia

Patients who are predisposed to thrombosis generally either have a disorder of the blood or an abnormality of the vessel wall. Where enhanced coagulation is the major mechanism, the disorder is referred to as 'thrombophilia'. Patients with thrombophilia either tend to have thrombosis at an unusually early age or to develop recurrent thrombotic problems. Venous thrombosis predominates with the chance of thrombosis increased by the coexistence of other risk factors. Thrombophilia can be inherited or acquired.

Which patients should be investigated for thrombophilia?

Testing for heritable thrombophilia is not indicted in unselected patients presenting with venous thrombosis. Table 39.1 summarises factors which should prompt consideration of thrombophilia. Accurate history taking is essential; particular attention should be given to the nature of the recent thrombotic event, the presence of known risk factors (Table 39.2), a previous history of thrombosis and the family history. Definition of a 'positive' family history of thrombosis is problematic. If we use the simple definition of a history of deep vein thrombosis (DVT) or pulmonary embolus (PE) in a first or second degree relative, then approximately 25% of all patients will have a positive family history. Even among those with a strong family history only a small minority will have a cause of inherited thrombophilia identified.

Basic investigations of thrombophilia should include a blood count (to exclude polycythaemia and other myeloproliferative disorders) and a coagulation screen. Further laboratory testing is dictated by the possible causes of familial and acquired thrombophilia detailed below. Testing for thrombophilia should not be undertaken during an acute episode of venous thromboembolism when low levels of coagulation inhibitors are routinely found. Systemic disorders such as liver disease or disseminated intravascular coagulation (DIC) can depress the levels of coagulation inhibitors and thus simulate the laboratory abnormalities found in familial thrombophilia.

Table 39.1 **Characteristics suggesting possibility of thrombophilia**
■ Venous thrombosis in patient less than 40 years old
■ Recurrent venous thrombosis or thrombophlebitis
■ Venous thrombosis in unusual site
■ Arterial thrombosis in patient less than 30 years old
■ Strong family history of venous thrombosis
■ Recurrent fetal loss
■ Skin necrosis in patient receiving warfarin
■ Purpura fulminans

Table 39.2 **Major risk factors for thrombosis**

Venous	Arterial
Increasing age	Increasing age
Immobility	Smoking
Obesity	Male sex
Oral contraceptive pill	Hypertension
Trauma/surgery	Strong family history
Thrombophilia (see text)	Hyperlipidaemia
Pregnancy	Diabetes mellitus
Malignancy	Raised fibrinogen

Familial thrombophilia

In theory, familial thrombophilia could be caused by any genetically determined defect of the coagulation or fibrinolytic systems that causes accelerated thrombin formation or impaired fibrin dissolution. In practice, the well-defined causes are associated with accelerated thrombin formation either due to a shortage or failure of activation of one of a number of circulating inhibitors of coagulation (Fig 39.1). Inherited thrombophilia defects are only important in venous thrombosis.

Fig 39.1 **Actions of proteins C and S.** Thrombin and protein C bind to thrombomodulin (TM), an endothelial membrane protein (steps 1 and 2). Protein S then binds to this complex and also endothelial phospholipid (PL) (step 3). The resulting complex proteolytically degrades activated factors V and VIII (step 4). Protein C is activated by proteolytic cleavage by thrombin. In APCR, factor V is relatively resistant to inactivation by the protein C complex.

Factor V Leiden (FVR506Q)

The anticoagulant property of activated protein C (APC) lies in its capacity to inactivate the activated cofactors Va and VIIIa by limited proteolysis. Inherited resistance to the anticoagulant action of APC (APCR) is an important cause of thrombophilia. In most cases resistance is caused by a single point mutation in the factor V gene (factor V Leiden) with replacement of Arg_{506} with Gln. Arg_{506} is located at one of the APC cleavage sites in factor Va and the mutated Va is less sensitive than normal Va to APC-mediated inactivation.

APCR has an autosomal dominant mode of inheritance and is the most common known cause of familial thrombophilia. The increased risk of venous thrombosis in APCR has been estimated as 4–8-fold in heterozygotes and 50–100-fold in homozygotes. The prevalence of the disorder in Western Europe is 3–7% with an incidence of around 15% in unselected cases of venous thrombosis. The risk of venous thrombosis is highest in patients homozygous for the mutation or in heterozygotes with other risk factors.

Prothrombin G20210A

This prothrombin gene polymorphism is the second most common known cause of familial thrombophilia. It is found in approximately 4% of unselected patients with DVT. Both APCR and the prothrombin gene polymorphism are associated with a small increased risk of recurrent fetal loss.

Protein C and S deficiencies

Hereditary deficiency of protein C is an autosomal dominant disorder found in 2–5% of patients with thromboembolic disease. An acquired deficiency of protein C can occur in liver disease, DIC and warfarin treatment. Familial protein C deficiency manifests as an increased incidence of venous thromboembolism. Thrombotic events vary from a superficial thrombophlebitis to DVT and PE. They may be spontaneous or triggered by other factors such as surgery or pregnancy. In the rare homozygous form, the infant can be born with undetectable levels of protein C and quickly develop DIC and skin necrosis due to microvascular thrombosis of subcutaneous vessels (*purpura fulminans*). Protein S is the non-enzymatic cofactor of protein C. Hereditary deficiency has similar clinical features to protein C deficiency.

Antithrombin deficiency

Antithrombin (AT) is the major physiological inhibitor of thrombin and clotting factors IXa, Xa, XIa and XIIa. Deficiency can be inherited in an autosomal dominant manner. Its prevalence is unclear but AT deficiency probably contributes to venous thrombosis in around 2–5% of younger patients. The risk of thrombosis varies between disease subtypes, being greater for an abnormality affecting the reactive (thrombin binding) site than for an abnormality affecting the heparin binding site. Overall, it seems that the risk of venous thrombosis is larger in heterozygotes for AT deficiency than for those with APCR, protein C or protein S deficiency. The risk increases with age, with up to 80% developing venous thrombosis by 55 years.

Other forms of familial thrombophilia

High levels of the amino acid homocysteine are associated with atherosclerosis and venous thrombosis and high factor VIII concentrations have been linked with an increased risk of venous thrombosis. The mechanisms involved and the degree to which they are genetically determined is unclear. Other candidates for familial thrombophilia status include the dysfibrinogenaemias (p. 75) and factor XII deficiency.

Management of familial thrombophilia

The precise role of laboratory thrombophilia testing in clinical decision making remains unclear.

Acute venous thrombosis

This should be treated with heparin and warfarin as in patients without heritable thrombophilia (p. 80). Patients with protein C (and occasionally protein S) deficiency can rarely develop warfarin-associated skin necrosis; this may be caused by an initial rapid fall in protein C levels after warfarin commencement leading to a hypercoagulable state and thrombosis in the subcutaneous circulation. The risk can be minimised by ensuring full heparinisation before introducing warfarin. Protein C concentrates have been given to treat purpura fulminans in homozygous disease.

Other situations

Case finding of asymptomatic relatives with low risk thrombophilia (e.g. factor V Leiden) is not indicated. Asymptomatic patients with familial thrombophilia detected on laboratory tests do not usually need anticoagulation. Patients with recurrent thrombosis or a single thrombosis with a high risk of recurrence (e.g. multiple thrombophilic defects) should be considered for long-term anticoagulation. Management of thrombophilia in pregnancy is complex. Warfarin is potentially teratogenic and subcutaneous low molecular weight heparin is given where anticoagulation is necessary.

Counselling

Counselling is frequently not straightforward. Any doubts relating to diagnosis and the probability of thrombosis in asymptomatic family members must be acknowledged. Known acquired risk factors such as immobility, obesity and the oestrogen-containing oral contraceptive should be avoided wherever possible. There is a two to four times increased risk of venous thromboembolism in women receiving hormone replacement therapy (HRT).

Acquired forms of thrombophilia

Antiphospholipid antibody syndrome

Diagnosis of this syndrome requires either venous and/or arterial thromboembolism or adverse outcomes in pregnancy in the presence of a persisting antiphospholipid antibody (Table 39.3). The syndrome can be 'primary', where the patient has no obvious autoimmune disease, or 'secondary' if the patient also has systemic lupus erythematosus (SLE) or a lupus-like disease. About half of all patients have the primary form of the disorder. Up to 2% of the general population have detectable antiphospholipid antibodies – the probability of clinical problems is greatest where the antibody titre is high.

The cause of thrombophilia in antiphospholipid antibody syndrome is not entirely understood. Antiphospholipid antibodies have been shown to play a direct role in the development of thrombosis in experimental animal models. Management must be individualised. Where there has been an episode of major thrombosis, warfarin appears to offer the best protection against recurrent thrombosis. Aspirin may give additional benefit in arterial thrombosis. Women with a history of morbidity in pregnancy are best treated in future pregnancies with a combination of aspirin and heparin.

Other acquired forms of thrombophilia

Myeloproliferative disorders are discussed elsewhere (pp. 64–67). Increased levels of plasma fibrinogen, and D-dimers may be predictors for coronary artery disease. Whether these and other haemostatic abnormalities are constitutional changes predisposing to coronary atherosclerosis and thrombosis or whether they are markers of pre-existing inflammation and endothelial dysfunction is unclear.

Table 39.3 **Clinical and laboratory criteria for a diagnosis of antiphospholipid antibody syndrome (at least one clinical and one laboratory feature must be present)**
Clinical features
Vascular thrombosis
Pregnancy morbidity (e.g. unexplained late fetal death, prematurity due to placental insufficiency/eclampsia, recurrent first trimester spontaneous abortion)

Laboratory tests	
Antiphospholipid antibodies:	lupus anticoagulant and/or anticardiolipin/β2-glycoprotein 1 antibodies

---

Thrombophilia

- The term 'thrombophilia' describes a predisposition to thrombosis caused by abnormally enhanced coagulation. Patients often have venous thrombosis at an early age or develop recurrent thrombotic problems.

- Classic familial thrombophilia disorders are deficiencies of the naturally occurring inhibitors of coagulation, protein C, protein S and antithrombin.

- Factor V Leiden is a thrombophilia disorder caused by an inherited mutation in the factor V gene. Heterozygosity is common (3–7% in Western European population).

- The clinical role of laboratory thrombophilia testing is not well defined.

- Antiphospholipid antibody syndrome is an acquired disorder characterised by laboratory identification of antiphospholipid antibodies and clinical features including thrombophilia and morbidity in pregnancy.

40 Anticoagulation and thrombolytic therapy

Two major classes of drugs are commonly used in the management of thromboembolic disease. The anticoagulants heparin and warfarin are used to prevent thrombosis and limit the extension of an established clot, while thrombolytic agents such as streptokinase are used to dissolve thrombus.

Anticoagulation

Heparin
Unfractionated heparin is a naturally occurring glycosaminoglycan produced by mast cells. Low molecular weight (LMW) heparin is prepared by controlled depolymerisation of the unfractionated form. Both unfractionated and LMW heparin exert their anticoagulant properties by binding to antithrombin (AT) and potentiating its activity. AT is a normal circulating anticoagulant which inhibits the actions of factor Xa and thrombin. LMW heparin differs from unfractionated heparin in having a relatively greater anti-Xa than antithrombin activity.

Unfractionated heparin
Standard unfractionated heparin may be used therapeutically to treat established thrombosis (usually intravenously at higher dosage) or prophylactically to prevent thrombosis (usually subcutaneously at lower dosage). Most common indications for therapeutic use are deep vein thrombosis (DVT) and pulmonary embolism (PE) (Fig 40.1). A typical regimen is an intravenous loading dose of 5000 units followed by an infusion of 1000–2000 units/hour. The anticoagulant response varies as the drug binds non-specifically to plasma and cellular proteins. Laboratory monitoring using the APTT (see p. 20) is required; the therapeutic range is usually 1.5–2.5, these values being the ratio of the patient's APTT to a control sample. As the half-life is short, high APTTs are managed by stopping the heparin but in the event of bleeding (in up to 7% of cases) the antidote protamine can be given. When the APTT is too low the heparin dose should be promptly increased. Heparin is normally continued until oral anticoagulation is therapeutic.

Prophylactic heparin is most commonly given to prevent DVT and PE in patients undergoing surgery. It is particularly indicated in patients with known risk factors for venous thrombosis (see p. 78) and in major procedures. A typical prophylactic regimen is 5000 units subcutaneously preoperatively and 5000 units 8- to 12-hourly after surgery, for 7 days or until the patient is mobile. No laboratory monitoring is necessary in routine cases – where required anti-X_a assays are used.

Apart from haemorrhage, patients on heparin may develop thrombocytopenia (see p. 69) and prolonged use can cause osteoporosis. It should be prescribed cautiously where there is any bleeding tendency.

LMW heparin
LMW heparins are now preferred for treatment of DVT and PE and prophylaxis. They appear to have superior efficacy, a better safety profile and to be more cost-effective than unfractionated heparin. LMW heparins cause less bleeding and a lower incidence of thrombocytopenia and osteoporosis. The more predictable dose response precludes the need for routine monitoring and the long half-life allows once or twice daily subcutaneous administration. Where monitoring is indicated (e.g. in renal failure), the anti-Xa effect is measured. LMW heparin treatment allows outpatient management of uncomplicated DVT.

Fondaparinux is a synthetic form of the heparin pentasaccharide molecule with a specific anti-Xa effect. It has similar indications to LMW heparin.

Warfarin
Oral anticoagulant drugs are derived from 4-hydroxycoumarin and the standard agent is warfarin. Warfarin works by antagonising vitamin K, which is needed for the gamma carboxylation of certain glutamic acid residues that facilitate calcium binding of coagulation factors II, VII, IX and X (Fig 40.2).

Some indications for warfarin are shown in Table 40.1. Where rapid anticoagulation is required a reasonable starting regimen is a single 10 mg dose and then protocol-guided adjustment according to the international normalised ratio (INR). A coagulation screen should always be checked before

Fig 40.1 **Large pulmonary embolus at the bifurcation of the main pulmonary trunk.**

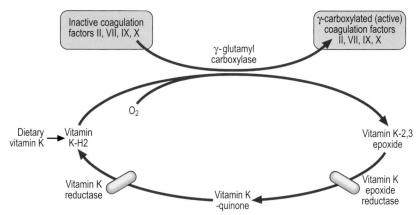

Fig 40.2 **The vitamin K cycle and the action of warfarin.** The major site of warfarin action is not a direct effect on the carboxylation step needed for coagulation factor activation but on steps needed for resynthesis of active vitamin K from its epoxide form.

Table 40.1 Warfarin: common indications and recommended INRs

Indication	Target INR[1]
Deep vein thrombosis	2.5
Pulmonary embolus	2.5
Atrial fibrillation	2.5
Mural thrombosis	2.5
Cardioversion	2.5
Mechanical prosthetic heart valves	2.5–3.5[2]
Recurrent venous thromboembolism on warfarin therapy	3.5
Thrombosis in antiphospholipid antibody syndrome	2.5

[1]An INR within 0.5 units of the target is usually satisfactory.
[2]Depending on valve.

Table 40.2 Drugs interacting with warfarin[1]

Potentiating	Antagonising
Alcohol	Oral contraceptives
Cimetidine	Spironolactone
Allopurinol	Antihistamines
Quinine	Barbiturates
Amiodarone	Rifampicin
Co-trimoxazole	Sucralfate
Metronidazole	Anti-epileptics
Tricyclics	
Aspirin and salicylates	
Anabolic steroids	
Thyroxine	
Sulfinpyrazone	

[1]These are some commonly implicated agents – this is not a comprehensive list.

warfarin is prescribed. The maintenance dose is usually between 3 and 9 mg. Laboratory monitoring depends on the prothrombin time (see p. 20). As thromboplastin reagents used in this test vary, their sensitivity is labelled with an international sensitivity index (ISI) which permits reporting as an INR such that INR=(prothrombin time)^{ISI}.

As it takes several days for warfarin to become therapeutic, the conventional treatment of established thrombosis is to start heparin and warfarin simultaneously and only to stop heparin when the desired INR has been achieved. Warfarin should be used with caution in patients with a bleeding tendency. The most common side-effect is haemorrhage, the risk of serious bleeding correlating with the height of the INR. Poor control of anticoagulation and bleeding may arise from poor prescribing or compliance, intercurrent illness and interaction with a potentiating drug (Table 40.2). A prolonged INR in a non-haemorrhagic patient may only require withdrawal of the drug for a few days. Where there is haemorrhage, warfarin can be reversed within hours by oral/intravenous vitamin K (0.5–5 mg) and instantly by infusion of a concentrate of prothrombin complex. Guidelines are complex and significant warfarin overdosage should be discussed with a haematologist. The duration of warfarin treatment depends on the indication. Anticoagulation may be needed for only 3 months in a patient with a limited DVT and reversible risk factors (e.g. post-surgery). Longer periods are indicated in idiopathic venous thrombosis, and lifelong warfarin treatment may be justified following recurrent episodes of venous thrombosis or where there is a known ongoing thrombotic risk such as a prosthetic heart valve, atrial fibrillation or a thrombophilic state.

Community and outpatient warfarin treatment is best monitored in specialist clinics where control is audited and technologies such as computerisation exploited.

New oral anticoagulant agents
There is a need for oral anticoagulant agents with more predictable pharmacokinetics than warfarin. A number of new drugs have been tested in clinical trials and are now entering clinical practice for both prophylaxis and treatment of thromboembolic disease. Examples include the direct thrombin inhibitor dabigatran exilate and the factor X inhibitor rivaroxaban. This is a fast moving area of medicine and new anticoagulants are further discussed on page 102.

Thrombolytic therapy
Thrombolytic agents dissolve fresh clots and therefore restore vascular patency more quickly than anticoagulants. The commonly used agents – streptokinase, urokinase and tissue plasminogen activator (alteplase) – work by activating the fibrinolytic system (see p. 13 and Fig 40.3). They convert plasminogen, the inactive proenzyme of the system, to the proteolytic enzyme plasmin. Thrombolytic drugs are indicated in any patient with acute myocardial infarction in which the benefit is likely to outweigh the risk of treatment. Early administration gives the best results. Other possible uses for this class of drugs include treatment of complicated venous thrombosis, acute ischaemic stroke and the unblocking of occluded venous catheters. The major side-effect is excessive bleeding.

Fig 40.3 **Action of thrombolytic agents.**

> ### Anticoagulation and thrombolytic therapy
>
> - The anticoagulant drugs heparin and warfarin are used to prevent thrombosis and limit the extension of an established clot.
> - Unfractionated heparin is given intravenously and low molecular weight heparin, now generally preferred, is given subcutaneously.
> - Warfarin is given orally and acts by inhibiting vitamin K.
> - Therapeutic treatment with both unfractionated heparin and warfarin requires careful laboratory monitoring.
> - New oral anticoagulant drugs (e.g. dabigatran, rivaroxaban) are entering clinical practice.
> - Thrombolytic agents are used to dissolve thrombus. They act by converting plasminogen to the proteolytic enzyme plasmin.

41 Blood groups and blood testing

The blood groups

Blood group antigens exist on the surface of the red cell membrane (see also p. 4). There are numerous blood group systems encoded by genes on different chromosomes. They are highly variable in their polymorphism and clinical significance.

The most important blood group is the ABO system. The genes encoding the ABO antigens are located on chromosome 9 and are inherited in an autosomal dominant fashion. Each antigen is a sugar residue made by a specific glycosyl transferase. The ABO system is crucial in clinical blood transfusion as there are naturally occurring IgM antibodies in the serum targeted against the non-present ABO antigens (Table 41.1). These antibodies necessitate the use of ABO 'compatible' blood for transfusion. For example, the administration of incompatible group A blood to a group B patient would engender a potentially fatal haemolytic transfusion reaction due to the destruction of the donor's group A red cells by the recipient's anti-A antibody.

In other blood group systems 'naturally occurring' antibodies are rare. However, 'immune antibodies', usually of IgG type, may be induced by transfusion of blood expressing different blood group antigens or maternal exposure to fetal red cell antigens. Where such immune antibodies are present, transfused blood must be matched for the relevant blood group system in addition to ABO. Maternal formation of immune antibodies against antigens of the Rhesus (Rh) blood group system, particularly the strongest antigen D, accounts for most cases of haemolytic disease of the newborn (p. 90).

The testing of blood

Donor blood

The safety of blood transfusion is maximised by careful selection of donors. All donors should be in good health and, wherever possible, unpaid volunteers. Particular care is taken to exclude potential donors who may harbour infective diseases which are transmissible by blood transfusion – thus people with recent jaundice (? hepatitis), a history of recent travel to malarial areas or risk factors for HIV or Creutzfeldt–Jakob

Table 41.1 The occurrence of ABO antigens and antibodies

	ABO blood group			
	O	A	B	AB
Antigens on red cells	None	A	B	A+B
Antibody in serum	Anti-A+B	Anti-B	Anti-A	None
Frequency (%)[1]	47	42	8	3

[1]In the United Kingdom.
Incidences vary greatly in different populations.

Table 41. 2 Routine testing of donated blood

ABO group
Rhesus group
Red cell antibody screen
Hepatitis B surface antigen, HBV DNA
Antibody to syphilis
Anti-HIV-1 and anti-HIV-2, HIV-1 antigen, HIV RNA
Anti-Hepatitis C, HCV RNA
Anti-HTLV

disease (CJD) infection are not suitable donors.

The objective of routine testing of donated blood is to provide blood which can be selected for likely compatibility with a patient and which contains no identifiable infectious agent (Table 41.2). Antibody testing (e.g. for HIV and hepatitis C) is now supplemented by molecular techniques sensitive enough to trace the virus in the blood before the development of antibodies (i.e. during the 'window period').

Testing before transfusion

Most incompatible transfusions are caused not by errors in the transfusion laboratory but by giving blood to the 'wrong' patient (i.e. not the patient whose serum was tested prior to the transfusion). The source of such mistakes is usually inaccurate documentation on forms and specimens or inadequate procedures for identifying patients prior to transfusion (see also p. 84).

If tests on donor and recipient blood confirm matching for ABO and Rhesus groups, the transfusion will be compatible in around 98% of cases. The sequence of tests prior to transfusion

> **Most incompatible blood transfusions arise from clerical errors and mistaken patient identity.**

includes antibody screening of the patient's serum and crossmatching to ensure compatibility in the remaining 2%.

Blood grouping

The recipient's red cells are tested for ABO and Rhesus antigens and the

Fig 41.1 **ABO blood grouping on a microplate.**

Fig 41.2 **Blood grouping using a gel system. (a)** ABO and RhD grouping. **(b)** Rh and Kell grouping. Unagglutinated red cells pass through the gel (after centrifugation) whereas agglutinated cells do not.

Fig 41.3 **The antiglobulin test.** In the *direct* test red cells are sensitised in vivo, in the *indirect* test they are sensitised in vitro.

serum tested for naturally occurring antibodies to confirm the ABO group. Blood grouping tests traditionally rely on the visual identification of agglutination of red cells induced by the presence of antibodies against antigens present on the cell surface (Fig 41.1). Gel technology (see Fig 41.2) is widely used and increasingly automated. DNA-based tests may be employed as an adjunct to haemagglutination but they are not currently indicated for routine ABO and Rh group testing.

Antibody screening
The patient's serum is tested against three standard sets of screening red cells of known antigenic type. This is to detect immune or 'atypical' antibodies (i.e. non-ABO) which might destroy donor red cells. Clinically relevant antibodies are generally reactive at 37°C. A sensitive indirect antiglobulin test technique is used (see Fig 41.3). If an antibody is detected by this screen then a larger panel of red cells is tested to indentify it. The blood selected for the patient must be negative for the relevant antigen.

Crossmatching
The final compatibility check is to mix the patient's serum with red cells from each donor unit. The aim is to highlight any earlier errors in grouping or antibody screening and to identify the presence of antibodies against rare antigens not present on the screening cells. The minor crossmatch – mixing of donor serum with patient red cells – is not routinely performed. With the integration of sophisticated computer systems into laboratories, the serological crossmatch is being selectively replaced by 'electronic crossmatching'. This relies on

a combination of repeat group and antibody testing, specialised software and stringent standard operating procedures to detect any incompatibility.

Practicalities of blood ordering

Where blood transfusion is required and adequate time is available, tests proceed as above and compatible units are issued. In emergencies, blood is sometimes needed more quickly than this routine testing allows. Normal procedures may be adapted to speed up issue of group specific blood. If there is insufficient time to determine the patient's ABO group, then group O Rhesus-negative blood may be used.

The bulk of blood is crossmatched for use in elective surgical procedures. Where there is only a small chance (less than 10%) that transfusion will be required it is reasonable to limit wastage by adopting a 'group and save' policy. The patient's blood group is determined and the serum screened for atypical antibodies. Provided the screen is negative, blood is not routinely crossmatched.

Table 43.3 **Possible guidelines for blood ordering in a few common operations**

Protocols vary between hospitals and should be based on previous blood usage and local transfusion laboratory practice

Procedure	Recommendation[1]
Cholecystectomy	Group and save
Colectomy/hemicolectomy	2
Breast biopsy	Group and save
Heart valve replacement	8
Resection of abdominal aortic aneurysm	8
Abdominal hysterectomy	Group and save
Total hip replacement	3
Transurethral resection of prostate	Group and save

[1]Figures refer to the number of units of red cells crossmatched prior to surgery.

Most hospitals have implemented a formal surgical blood order schedule with guidelines for common operations (Table 43.3). Such guidelines are generalisations and special provision is made for unusually difficult procedures or patients who are judged to be at a higher than average risk of haemorrhage. Electronic crossmatching is very rapid and its introduction potentially reduces the number of operations for which blood is issued in advance.

Blood groups and blood testing

- The blood group antigens exist on the surface of the red cell membrane. Blood groups are highly variable in their polymorphism and clinical significance.
- The ABO system is crucial in blood transfusion as there are naturally occurring IgM antibodies in the serum targeted against non-present ABO antigens – this necessitates the use of ABO 'compatible' blood.
- Blood donors are carefully selected and donor blood tested to exclude transmissible infections.
- Testing of donor and recipient blood for ABO and Rhesus groups, antibody screening and crossmatching are routinely performed before transfusion to ensure compatibility.
- Most incompatible blood transfusions arise from clerical errors and mistaken patient identity.

42 Clinical practice

Red cell transfusion

Two questions need to be answered before transfusion of red cells is undertaken:

1. Is it indicated?
2. If it is indicated, which red cell preparation should be used?

Some general indications for red cell transfusion are listed in Table 42.1.

Whole blood is now rarely used. Haemorrhage requires transfusion of fluids to maintain blood volume and red cells to raise the haemoglobin level. For correction of anaemia not responsive to other measures red cells stored in 'optimal additive solution' are used. There are few indications for red cells stored in plasma.

Practicalities of red cell transfusion

All those involved in the prescription and administration of blood should follow local guidelines with respect to patient identification and the checking of the compatibility and viability of the transfused units. Critical information is contained on the blood bag and the attached compatibility label (Fig 42.1). No discrepancies are permissible. Most serious adverse transfusion reactions are due to transfusion of the wrong blood to the patient (Fig 42.2). Errors can be reduced by newer technologies such as bar coding and radiofrequency chips – these generally rely on machine readable data on patient wristbands.

In shocked patients blood is transfused rapidly, the precise rate dependent on the monitoring of vital signs such as pulse, blood pressure and urine output. Transfusion for correction of anaemia is usually a more elective process. Units of red cells are typically given over 2–4 hours and a rise of around 10 g/L of

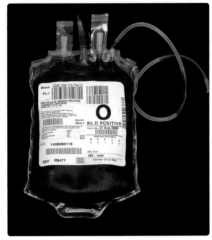

Fig 42.1 **Unit of red cells.**

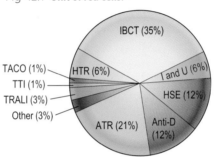

Fig 42.2 **Serious hazards of transfusion, United Kingdom 1992–2010 (data with permission of SHOT).** IBCT, incorrect blood transfused; ATR, acute transfusion reactions; HSE, handling and storage errors; I and U, inappropriate/unnecessary/delayed transfusions; HTR, haemolytic transfusion reactions; TRALI, transfusion-related acute lung injury; TACO, transfusion-associated circulation overload; TTI, transfusion-transmitted infections.

haemoglobin can be expected from each unit. Red cells are infused via specially designed sterile 'giving sets' which contain 170 μm filters. Careful monitoring is particularly important during the first 10 minutes of each unit.

Complications of red cell transfusion
Immediate
Haemolytic transfusion reactions. These potentially fatal reactions arise from the transfusion of incompatible blood (usually for ABO). Symptoms often occur within minutes and may include chest, abdominal and loin pain, vomiting, a 'burning' skin, dyspnoea and headache. Common signs are fever, tachycardia and hypotension. Renal failure and disseminated intravascular coagulation (DIC) can follow. Once a haemolytic reaction is suspected, the transfusion should be stopped and the venous access used to give crystalloid. The transfused unit should be checked

(is another patient about to get a 'wrong' unit due to a mix up?) and the blood bank informed. Initial investigations must include blood samples from the patient for a blood count and film, blood group, antibody screen and direct antiglobulin test. The blood bank will also repeat tests on the donated unit. Management of complications will require senior advice and often intensive care. The overall mortality of ABO incompatible transfusion is approximately 10%.

Non-haemolytic transfusion reactions. The majority of adverse reactions to blood are 'febrile reactions' caused by antileucocyte antibodies in the patient. Uncomplicated febrile reactions are simply managed by slowing the transfusion and giving paracetamol. Routine leucodepletion of red cells reduces such reactions. Occasionally patients develop allergic reactions with urticaria, wheezing and (rarely) anaphylaxis.

Transfusion associated circulatory overload (TACO). Care must be taken not to transfuse too rapidly, especially in elderly patients with heart disease.

Transfusion-related acute lung injury (TRALI). This is an acute syndrome occurring within 6 hours of transfusion and characterised by respiratory distress, hypoxia, bilateral pulmonary infiltrates and a fever. Donor antibodies to HLA class I and II antigens and/or granulocyte-specific antigens have been implicated in pathogenesis. Mortality is around 10%.

Delayed
Infection. Bacteria, viruses and parasites may all be transmitted via blood transfusion. Blood is screened for the relevant agents and in practice the greatest risk is of bacterial contamination. To help reduce the chance of transmission of the abnormal prion associated with variant Creutzfeldt–Jakob disease (vCJD) red cell donations are leucodepleted and plasma is increasingly imported from countries with no bovine spongiform encephalopathy (BSE). The significance of transmission of infection from blood can depend on the status of the recipient. Thus, cytomegalovirus (CMV) is of little relevance in healthy adults but potentially life-threatening in a patient receiving an allogeneic stem cell transplant or in a low birthweight premature infant.

Table 42.1 **Major indications for red cell transfusion**
To replace blood loss
Trauma
Surgery
Other haemorrhage (e.g. gastrointestinal bleed)
To correct anaemia
Marrow failure (e.g. aplastic anaemia, leukaemia)
Haemoglobinopathies (e.g. thalassaemia, sickle cell disease)
Chronic disorders (e.g. renal failure, malignancy)
Severe haemolysis (e.g. haemolytic disease of the newborn)

The final decision to transfuse requires consideration of the patient's age, clinical state, and haemoglobin concentration.

Delayed transfusion reactions. These occur approximately 5–10 days after transfusion and are caused by a previously undetected antibody being boosted by transfusion of incompatible cells. Characteristic features include fever, jaundice and a falling haemoglobin. They are only rarely fatal.

Iron overload. A unit of blood contains around 250 mg of iron. Iron is only lost from the body in small amounts and repeated transfusion can lead to accumulation and toxic effects identical to those seen in haemochromatosis. Where repeated transfusion is predictable in a younger person (e.g. in thalassaemia), chelation of iron limits overload and prolongs life.

Massive blood transfusion

Massive transfusion is defined as replacement of the patient's whole blood volume by stored allogeneic blood in less than 24 hours. There have been recent changes in practice driven by the military experience of trauma with increased early use of plasma and platelets. Problems can still arise in part due to the inevitable deficiencies of stored blood. Shortage of clotting factors and platelets in transfused blood may exacerbate haemorrhage. It is important to monitor haemostasis by checking the basic coagulation screen and replacing components accordingly. Metabolic disturbances are less common but include hyperkalaemia, hypocalcaemia, acidosis and citrate toxicity. Rapid transfusion can cause hypothermia; this can be minimised by carefully controlled blood warming.

Alternatives to allogeneic blood transfusion

Use of the patient's own blood for transfusion rather than allogeneic blood minimises the risk of infection. Selected patients awaiting elective surgery can 'pre-deposit' blood in the weeks prior to the operation. An alternative approach, now more favoured, is to use specially designed equipment to 'salvage' blood lost during surgery and reinfuse it back into the patient. Other strategies to reduce blood transfusion include the active treatment of anaemia, strict application of transfusion triggers, anaesthetic measures or drugs (e.g. tranexamic acid) to reduce blood loss and biological agents such as erythropoietin. Questions remain regarding optimal transfusion practice and there is a need for more randomized controlled trials. Possible future developments include manufactured haemoglobin solutions and platelet substitutes.

Transfusion of platelets and granulocytes

Platelet transfusion

This is used to treat or prevent haemorrhage in patients with significant thrombocytopenia. It is more useful where platelets are low due to underproduction (i.e. marrow failure) or dilution than where thrombocytopenia is due to immune destruction as in immune thrombocytopenia (ITP). Platelets are collected either from routine blood donations or from a single donor by plasmapheresis. They should ideally be matched with the patient for ABO and Rhesus. The standard dose for an adult is either a single plasmapheresis donation or 4–6 pooled standard donations. Where repeated platelet transfusions are given, patients can become sensitised against class I HLA antigens absorbed onto the platelet surface with the result that they derive a lower increment in platelet count than would be predicted ('platelet refractoriness'). In these cases, platelet donors matched with the recipient's HLA class I type can be selected. Platelet transfusion can cause non-haemolytic reactions and can transmit infection as for red cells.

Granulocyte (neutrophil) transfusion

Granulocyte transfusion is infrequently used in neutropenia and the indications are uncertain.

Transfusion of plasma and plasma products

A wide range of plasma products is available for therapeutic use:

- *Fresh frozen plasma (FFP)*. Plasma is collected from whole blood or derived from plasmapheresis prior to rapid freezing. FFP contains the full range of coagulation factors and indications for use are shown in Table 42.2. The normal dose in an

Table 42.2 Possible indications for use of fresh frozen plasma

Disseminated intravascular coagulation (DIC)
Severe liver disease (e.g. prior to liver biopsy)
Coagulopathy of massive blood transfusion
Replacement therapy of some rare congenital factor deficiencies
Bleeding in haemorrhagic disease of newborn/ malabsorption vitamin K
Thrombotic thrombocytopenic purpura (with plasma exchange)
Depletion of coagulation factors following thrombolysis

adult is one litre. FFP can transmit infection and cause immunological reactions – it is not suitable for volume expansion alone.

- *Cryoprecipitate*. This is prepared from FFP by slow thawing and separation of the resultant precipitate. It is rich in fibrinogen and may be useful in the treatment of DIC and management of massive blood transfusion.
- Factor VIII and IX concentrate. See pages 72–73.
- *Albumin*. This is produced by fractionation of pooled plasma. Solutions for clinical use include human albumin 4.5/5%, human albumin 20% and plasma protein fraction (PPF). Albumin solutions are used for the treatment of severe hypoproteinaemia, particularly when associated with a low plasma volume. Concentrated solutions can help produce a diuresis in hypoalbuminaemia (e.g. in hepatic cirrhosis).
- *Immunoglobulins*. These can be 'specific' and used in passive prophylaxis against a range of infections (e.g. varicella zoster, tetanus) or to prevent haemolytic disease of the newborn (anti-Rhesus D). 'Non-specific' immunoglobulins are used for passive prophylaxis against hepatitis A, treatment of hypogammaglobulinaemia and in selected autoimmune disorders (e.g. ITP).

Blood transfusion – clinical practice

- Before red cell transfusion is undertaken the indication should be confirmed and the optimal red cell preparation selected.
- Red cell transfusion can cause both immediate complications (e.g. haemolytic transfusion reaction) and delayed complications (e.g. infection, iron overload).
- Platelet transfusion may be helpful in the management of thrombocytopenia.
- A wide range of plasma products is available for transfusion. Selection of the appropriate product requires an understanding of the therapeutic benefit and possible side-effects.
- There are alternatives to allogeneic blood transfusion (e.g. erythropoietin) which should be considered in selected patients.

43 The immunosuppressed patient

Many patients with blood disorders are immunosuppressed. Patients with aggressive haematological malignancies such as leukaemia and non-Hodgkin's lymphoma have their immune function initially compromised by the disease and then further depressed by chemotherapy. Others have more subtle deficiencies. Patients with 'benign' diseases such as immune thrombocytopenia (ITP) and hereditary spherocytosis who have had splenectomy performed are also at increased risk of infection.

An increased susceptibility to infection can arise from multiple factors (Table 43.1). Neutropenia and neutrophil dysfunction are probably the most important causes of infectious complications in patients with leukaemia. Unlike many other forms of immunosuppression, neutropenia is easy to quantify – the risk of infection rises appreciably at counts below 0.5×10^9/L and is greatest where the count is below 0.1. Lymphopenia and lymphocyte dysfunction are seen in lymphoid malignancy and after chemo- and radiotherapy. Defects in humoral immunity are particularly seen in patients with chronic lymphoid malignancies and in myeloma. The likelihood of infection is related to the severity of hypogammaglobulinaemia.

Other common immunosuppressive factors are the loss of mucosal or skin integrity due to damage from disease or treatment, and the presence of indwelling venous catheters.

Types of infection

Bacteria
Bacterial infections in neutropenic patients are often caused by the spread of commensal flora to previously sterile sites. Fatal septicaemia can result from Gram-negative bacilli such as *Pseudomonas aeruginosa*, *E. coli*, *Klebsiella* spp. and *Enterobacter* spp. Gram-positive cocci currently cause the majority of documented bacteraemias. The skin pathogen *Staphylococcus epidermidis* often colonises indwelling venous catheters. The use of broad-spectrum antibiotics can lead to the emergence of toxin-producing *Clostridium difficile* in the stools. Methicillin-resistant *Staph. aureus* (MRSA) and bacteria producing extended-spectrum beta-lactamases (ESBLs) leading to antibiotic resistance are becoming increasingly problematic in hospitals.

Table 43.1 **Possible factors predisposing to infection in haematology patients**
Cellular defects
■ Neutropenia and neutrophil dysfunction
■ Lymphopenia and lymphocyte dysfunction
Humoral defects
■ Reduced antibody production
Anatomic defects
■ Reduced mucosal barriers (e.g. mucositis)
■ Indwelling venous catheters
Splenectomy (see p. 10)

Fig 43.1 **Skin infection caused by *Streptococcus faecalis* in a neutropenic patient.**

Bacterial infection in neutropenic patients may be overt – for instance a chest infection with a productive cough or the presence of infected skin lesions (Fig 43.1). However, bacterial sepsis can equally present with non-specific malaise and a pyrexia. In the latter case extensive cultures including blood, nose, throat, stool and urine are indicated.

Fungi
The incidence of invasive fungal infections is increasing and they are a major cause of morbidity and mortality in patients with haematological malignancy.

The most widespread fungal pathogen is *Candida*. Oral and colonic carriage of the organism is common in healthy people. Invasive *Candida* infection is most likely in neutropenic patients with indwelling catheters and severe mucositis. Disseminated candidiasis usually presents with a persistent fever and no diagnostic clinical features. Possible organ involvement includes the kidney, lung, heart and liver. Cutaneous emboli may lead to a nodular skin eruption while exudative retinal lesions can be seen through the ophthalmoscope. *Candida* spp. are grown from blood cultures in only 20% of patients with invasive candidiasis. The addition of candida PCR significantly improves detection rates.

Aspergillus species, particularly *Aspergillus fumigatus*, are potentially

Fig 43.2 **Aspergillosis complicating prolonged neutropenia.**

deadly fungal pathogens. Infection is usually via the inhalation of airborne spores and is mainly pulmonary. A chest X-ray may show pneumonia and cavitation (Fig 43.2) but it is an insensitive diagnostic method. Other infected sites can include the paranasal sinuses, skin, central nervous system and eye. Even in disseminated disease, blood and sputum cultures are rarely positive. Thirty per cent of cases of invasive aspergillosis remain undiagnosed and untreated at death. Strategies for earlier diagnosis include regular galactomannan antigen testing, aspergillus PCR, and CT scanning of the chest.

Pneumocystis jiroveci (previously *Pneumocystis carinii*) is a fungus which causes a potentially fatal bilateral pneumonia in patients with depressed cell-mediated immunity. In haematological practice it mostly affects patients receiving intensive chemotherapy regimens or stem cell transplantation and patients infected with the HIV virus. Bronchoalveolar lavage is useful in diagnosis.

Viruses
Most viral infection in immunosuppressed patients is caused by reactivation of latent organisms. Patients with deficient cell-mediated immunity (e.g. acute lymphoblastic leukaemia (ALL), stem cell transplantation, chronic lymphocytic leukaemia) are particularly susceptible. Important pathogens include herpes simplex, varicella zoster and cytomegalovirus (CMV). Clinical manifestations range from relatively trivial mouth ulcers attributable to herpes simplex through herpes zoster

Fig 43.3 **Herpes zoster following allogeneic stem cell transplantation.**

(shingles) (Fig 43.3) with the risk of dissemination to the potentially fatal CMV pneumonitis which complicates allogeneic stem cell transplantation. Measles can be a fatal illness in children with ALL. There may be no specific diagnostic features of viral infection and it must be considered as a possible cause of a febrile illness in the immunosuppressed patient. PCR-based diagnosis may allow earlier therapy of CMV infection after allogeneic stem cell transplantation.

Prevention of infection in the immunosuppressed patient

Neutropenia

General measures include the isolation of the patient, laminar airflow rooms, strict hygiene and avoidance of possible contaminants (e.g. uncooked food). Simple precautions such as hand washing by staff are crucial in reducing infection rates.

Antimicrobial prophylaxis may reduce the incidence of infection but there are well-defined adverse effects. For instance, quinolone antibiotic prophylaxis reduces the number of bacterial infections in patients with chemotherapy and transplant-induced neutropenia but this must be balanced against the side-effects of the drug and the potential emergence and dissemination of antimicrobial-resistant organisms. Increased use of antimicrobial agents increases the vulnerability of patients to nosocomial infections (e.g. *Clostridium difficile*) and community-acquired infections. Prophylaxis also complicates the treatment of a subsequent episode of febrile neutropenia. It appears that the best way to exploit the benefits of prophylaxis is to restrict its use to patients at highest risk such as those with a previous history of neutropenic fever. Similar considerations apply to the use of prophylaxis against fungal infections.

Table 43.2 **Groups of antibiotics used in the empirical treatment of infection in neutropenia**

Group	Examples
Antipseudomonal penicillins	Azlocillin, piperacillin
Aminoglycosides	Gentamicin, amikacin
Cephalosporins	Ceftazidime
Quinolones	Ciprofloxacin
Carbapenems	Meropenem, imipenem
Glycopeptides	Teicoplanin, vancomycin

Depressed cell-mediated immunity and hypogammaglobulinaemia

Impaired cell-mediated immunity leads to an increased risk of *Pneumocystis jiroveci* (*carinii*) pneumonia and viral infections. Standard prophylaxis against *Pneumocystis* is oral co-trimoxazole or nebulised pentamidine where this is not tolerated. Aciclovir is effective in reducing the incidence of viral infections. The more toxic drug ganciclovir can be used after stem cell transplantation to give additional protection against CMV. Patients with low-grade lymphoproliferative disorders and myeloma can have significant hypogammaglobulinaemia and suffer recurrent infection. Regular infusions of immunoglobulin may be helpful in these cases.

Post-splenectomy

See page 10.

Treatment of infection

The pyrexial neutropenic patient

A common clinical problem in haematology is the management of the patient with neutropenia who becomes unwell and/or develops a pyrexia. A subgroup of very carefully defined 'low-risk' patients may require only oral broad-spectrum antibiotics but high-risk patients can rapidly succumb to bacterial infection and need prompt inpatient empirical treatment with broad-spectrum intravenous antibiotics even before the infectious pathogen is identified. Blood and other cultures are taken

prior to starting antibiotics and a chest X-ray is helpful: investigations, however, should not substantially delay treatment. A microbiological diagnosis is made in only half of these cases.

The empirical antibiotic regimens are designed to provide protection against commonly implicated organisms, particularly those causing life-threatening infection (e.g. *Pseudomonas*). Regimens are constantly changing – the major groups of drugs are summarised in Table 43.2.

Monotherapy (e.g. meropenem) may be used but in patients at highest risk a combination (e.g. piperacillin/ tazobactam and gentamicin) is usually preferred.

Persistent pyrexia or clinical deterioration on first-line antibiotics is a difficult management problem. Often the infectious agent is unknown. The usual approach is to continue investigations while making a change in the antibiotic regimen. A lack of response prompts consideration of empirical antifungal treatment. To limit drug exposure, entirely empirical therapy can be replaced by a 'pre-emptive' strategy where only patients with 'probable' fungal infection (e.g. suggested by CT of chest) are treated with antifungal agents. Growth factors (e.g. G-CSF) may be given to shorten the period of neutropenia.

Treatment of specific infections

Liposomal amphotericin B has generally been the drug of choice for treatment of established *Aspergillus* infection and in the empirical antifungal role outlined above, but voriconazole and caspofungin are reasonable alternatives. Azoles, particularly fluconazole, are commonly used in the treatment of *Candida* infection. Herpes simplex and varicella zoster infections are best treated with aciclovir. Ganciclovir or foscarnet is used for CMV infection after allogeneic stem cell transplantation. *Pneumocystis jiroveci* (*carinii*) pneumonia is effectively treated by either high-dose co-trimoxazole or pentamidine.

The immunosuppressed patient

- Many patients with blood disorders are immunosuppressed. Possible factors predisposing to infection include neutropenia, lymphopenia, reduced antibody levels and anatomical defects.

- Bacteria, fungi and viruses can all cause severe systemic infection in an immunosuppressed patient.

- Measures to prevent infection in the immunosuppressed patient include isolation of the patient, strict hygiene and selective prophylactic use of antimicrobial agents.

- Infection in a neutropenic patient generally requires empirical treatment with broad-spectrum antibiotics. Persisting fever or clinical deterioration necessitates a change in antibiotics and/or antifungal treatment.

44 Pregnancy

Haematological changes

Several haematological changes occur in normal pregnancy (Fig 44.1). Beginning in the sixth week there is an increase in plasma volume accompanied by an increase in red cell mass. The plasma volume expansion peaks at around 24 weeks when it is approximately 40% greater than in a non-pregnant woman. As the increase in red cell mass is more modest (15–25%) a *dilutional anaemia* is inevitable. In practice the haematocrit and haemoglobin level start to fall at 6–8 weeks and reach a trough at around 20 weeks. It is unusual for the haemoglobin level to fall below 100 g/L and if this happens another cause for anaemia should be sought. Negative iron balance can be regarded as routine in pregnancy and as discussed below frank iron deficiency commonly occurs.

The other major changes which may be regarded as a physiological consequence of pregnancy affect the coagulation system. There are increases in the levels of the coagulation factors VII, VIII and X and a marked increase in plasma fibrinogen. The resulting hypercoagulability is helpful in limiting the likelihood of life-threatening bleeding at delivery but it does lead to an increased risk of thromboembolism. The platelet count falls about 10% during an uncomplicated pregnancy. Later in pregnancy there may also be an increase in mean platelet volume (MPV).

Anaemia in pregnancy

There are several causes of anaemia in pregnancy. The most common scenario is an exacerbation of the usual dilutional anaemia by deficiency of iron and/or folate. Erythropoietin levels increase less than in anaemic non-pregnant women, possibly suppressed by hormonal changes.

The identification of iron deficiency relies upon normal laboratory tests (p. 25). However, even in women with no overt clinical deficiency there is a progressive fall in serum iron through pregnancy. Routine dietary supplementation with modest amounts of iron (e.g. ferrous sulphate 200 mg daily) leads to a significant increase in haemoglobin level at term compared with women receiving no supplements. Parenteral iron is contraindicated in the first trimester.

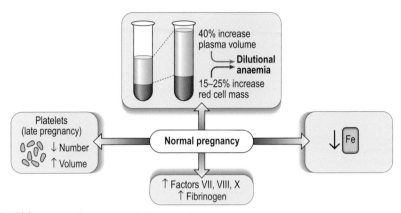

Fig 44.1 **Common haematological changes in normal pregnancy.**

The other major type of anaemia in pregnancy is megaloblastic anaemia. This usually results from deficiency of folate. As for iron, folate requirements are increased during pregnancy and the diet is frequently inadequate to meet this demand. Megaloblastic anaemia most often presents as a macrocytic anaemia in the third trimester or postpartum. It is normal practice to give folate supplements in pregnancy. The amount of folate routinely administered orally should be large enough to avoid megaloblastic anaemia but not so large as to risk masking pernicious anaemia with vitamin B_{12} deficiency which does occasionally occur in pregnancy. Folate deficiency in pregnancy has been linked with an increased incidence of neural tube defects in the fetus and recommendations for planned pregnancies are the use of folate supplements (400 µg daily) prior to conception and then particularly in the first 12 weeks. Larger doses of folate are recommended where women are at high risk of conceiving a child with a neural tube defect (e.g. previously affected pregnancy). There is no justification for the prescription of multi-ingredient vitamin preparations in pregnancy but a combined iron and folate tablet of adequate dosage may be prescribed.

It should be remembered that not all anaemia in pregnancy is caused by deficiency states. Other blood disorders may present in pregnancy and chronic blood diseases such as sickle cell anaemia can be especially difficult to manage at this time.

Thrombocytopenia in pregnancy

After anaemia, thrombocytopenia is the most common haematological disorder in pregnancy, occurring in 6–10% of all pregnant women. A few women have an obvious systemic disorder such as pre-eclampsia; disseminated intravascular coagulation (DIC) in pregnancy is further discussed below. However, the majority of women are systemically well with an apparently normal pregnancy. In these cases thrombocytopenia can be divided into two categories, with differing clinical implications for the mother and fetus.

Incidental (gestational) thrombocytopenia

Incidental thrombocytopenia is the most common cause of thrombocytopenia in pregnancy accounting for around 75% of cases. Thrombocytopenia is mild to moderate (70–150×10^9/L) and the woman is otherwise well. There is no past history suggesting a cause for the low platelet count and particularly no history of immune thrombocytopenia (ITP). The disorder is not associated with maternal haemorrhage or fetal or neonatal thrombocytopenia. As there is no diagnostic test it is often difficult to distinguish gestational thrombocytopenia from mild ITP until a non-pregnancy platelet count is available.

ITP in pregnancy

The management of pregnancy in a woman with known chronic ITP can be problematic as severe thrombocytopenia may be a threat to the mother and there is also a risk of the child becoming thrombocytopenic. The latter complication arises as the causative IgG antiplatelet autoantibody in the mother freely crosses the placenta and can target fetal platelets. Fortunately, the majority of babies escape – severe thrombocytopenia (less than 50×10^9/L) occurs in around 10% of neonates and mortality

Abruptio placentae
Amniotic fluid embolism
Septic abortion and intrauterine infection
Retained dead fetus
Hydatiform mole
Placenta accreta
Pre-eclampsia and eclampsia

Fig 44.2 **Causes of DIC in pregnancy.**

Table 44.1 General guidelines for the management of acute obstetric haemorrhage

- Secure venous access and insert a central line to measure central venous pressure (CVP)
- Seek additional (preferably senior) medical help
- Collect samples for urgent blood count, crossmatching and coagulation screen; liaise with haematology laboratory
- Restore blood volume – may have to use unmatched blood of patient's ABO and Rh group (preferred to group O Rh negative)
- Address source of bleeding
- Blood product replacement as necessary

from intracranial bleeding in those affected is less than 1%. All management decisions must thus acknowledge that fetal thrombocytopenia is uncommon and fetal mortality very rare. In this context, aggressive treatment of all mothers with ITP with corticosteroids and/or intravenous immunoglobulin and routine delivery by caesarean section are not justified. The fetal platelet count is not routinely measured. A conservative approach with normal delivery and an immediate neonatal cord blood platelet count is gaining support. If the baby's count is low or falling, intravenous immunoglobulin can be given. In more severe thrombocytopenia, transcranial ultrasound can be performed to exclude intracranial haemorrhage. Because of its low incidence of side-effects, intravenous immunoglobulin is probably the treatment of choice for severe maternal thrombocytopenia.

Coagulation abnormalities in pregnancy

Thromboembolism and anticoagulant therapy

Pulmonary embolism (PE) remains a major cause of maternal death. Approximately half of fatal PEs occur antepartum and half postpartum, the majority of the latter in the first 2 weeks of the puerperium. About 70% of women who develop venous thromboembolism in pregnancy and the puerperium have major risk factors. These include increasing age, caesarean section, obesity, previous thrombotic problems and familial thrombophilia. Hereditary thrombophilia (see p. 78) has also been linked with recurrent fetal loss, intrauterine growth restriction, pre-eclampsia and placental abruption.

Both the anticoagulants commonly used in clinical practice, heparin and warfarin, require special consideration in pregnancy.

- *Heparin.* Neither unfractionated standard heparin nor low molecular weight heparin (LMWH) cross the placenta. LMWH is widely used and is both safe and effective in the prevention and treatment of venous thromboembolism in pregnancy, with significant bleeding, usually from primary obstetric causes, in less than 2% of cases. Anti-factor X_a levels can be monitored but the optimal therapeutic range is unclear.
- *Warfarin.* Warfarin is not significantly secreted in breast milk and treatment is safe during lactation. However, it readily crosses the placenta and is a known teratogen, producing a specific warfarin embryopathy at around 6–12 weeks (approximately 5% incidence). Thus, heparin should be substituted for warfarin in the first trimester. There may be a risk of fetal haemorrhage secondary to warfarin throughout pregnancy, particularly if anticoagulant control is poor, and the risk to mother and fetus becomes unacceptable in the antepartum period. It should therefore be discontinued at 36 weeks and heparin substituted until after

delivery. Current practice is to avoid use of oral anticoagulants in pregnancy wherever possible. There is currently no place for the newer oral anticoagulants (i.e. direct thrombin and anti-X_a inhibitors) due to concerns regarding toxicity.

DIC in pregnancy

DIC is associated with a wide variety of situations in pregnancy (Fig 44.2). The chief characteristics and pathogenesis of DIC are discussed on page 76. In pregnancy, DIC may manifest as a chronic compensated state or as life-threatening haemorrhage. The latter is a frightening medical emergency and there should be a planned regimen of management with input from an obstetrician, haematologist, physician, anaesthetist and nurse (Table 44.1). It is imperative that the source of bleeding is identified and addressed as soon as possible. It is often shock which triggers DIC with a resultant increase in bleeding.

HELLP syndrome

HELLP is an acronym for microangiopathic haemolysis (H), elevated liver enzymes (EL) and low platelets (LP). The syndrome complicates less than 1% of all pregnancies but develops in 10% of women with pre-eclampsia. Both disorders generally remit within several days after delivery and delivery of the fetus is therefore central to management.

Pregnancy

- Normal pregnancy is accompanied by a modest dilutional anaemia.
- Deficiency of iron and/or folate frequently exacerbates the normal dilutional anaemia.
- Thrombocytopenia is most often 'incidental' and of little significance. Immune thrombocytopenia (ITP) may require treatment but a normal delivery is usual and severe neonatal thrombocytopenia is rare.
- There is a hypercoagulable state in pregnancy and pulmonary embolism remains a major cause of maternal death. Low molecular weight heparin is generally the preferred anticoagulant for treatment or prevention of thrombosis.
- Disseminated intravascular coagulation (DIC) can complicate pregnancy and cause life-threatening haemorrhage.

45 Paediatric haematology

Many of the blood disorders encountered in children have been discussed in the preceding pages. For instance, acute lymphoblastic leukaemia is the most common leukaemia of childhood, haemophilia is usually diagnosed in infancy and the haemoglobinopathies are a significant cause of ill health in children worldwide. Chronic and severe diseases of the blood pose particular problems in childhood and usually are best managed by a paediatrician with a special interest in haematology or in a combined paediatric/haematology clinic. The child's growth and development, and educational needs often require special attention. In this section we discuss some haematological disorders encountered in paediatric practice which are not addressed elsewhere.

Normal values

It is important to appreciate that the normal ranges for many haematological tests vary with age. Table 45.1 illustrates reference values for the total white cell count (WCC) and the differential count in children. More detailed listings of normal ranges of laboratory tests in childhood can be found in specialised paediatric haematology texts.

Neonatal disorders

Haemolytic disease of the newborn

Haemolytic disease of the newborn (HDN) is a disease of the fetus and newborn child. The haemolysis is caused by maternal IgG antibodies traversing the placenta and attaching to fetal red cells which are destroyed in the child's reticuloendothelial system. The antibodies are directed against a fetal red cell antigen not shared by the mother. Incompatibility for one of a large number of different red cell blood group systems can cause HDN but most cases of clinically significant disease affect a Rhesus (Rh)D-positive child where the mother is RhD negative. Sensitisation of the mother (i.e. the formation of anti-D) occurs following the haemorrhage of fetal red cells into the maternal circulation. This usually occurs at parturition following a normal pregnancy but may also arise earlier in pregnancy or following abortion. ABO incompatibility between mother and fetus gives some protection against sensitisation to RhD as fetal red cells are quickly destroyed by the mother's naturally occurring anti-A or anti-B antibodies. Unfortunately, in most cases baby and mother are ABO compatible. With the considerable success of prophylaxis

Table 45.1 **Normal white cell counts in children** ($\times 10^9$/L)			
Age	**White cell count**	**Neutrophils**	**Lymphocytes**
Birth (full term)	18 ± 8	5–13	3–10
Day 3	15 ± 8	3–5	2–8
1 month	12 ± 7	3–9	3–16
2–6 months	12 ± 6	1.5–9	4–10
2–6 years	10 ± 5	1.5–8	6–9
6–12 years	9 ± 4	2–8	1–5

Note: Normal haemoglobin values in childhood are shown on page 22, Table 1. The normal platelet count is the same in children and adults (150–400 × 10^9/L).

against HDN due to RhD incompatibility (see below), the most common cause of the disorder is the formation of immune antibodies against ABO; most cases are associated with only mild haemolysis.

Diagnosis

Severe HDN can result in intrauterine death. In the newborn child the presentation is entirely dependent on the degree of haemolysis but common features include anaemia, jaundice, oedema and hepatosplenomegaly. High levels of circulating unconjugated bilirubin may lead to high frequency deafness or deposition in the basal ganglia with spasticity and other neurological symptoms and signs ('kernicterus'). Further investigation of the anaemia reveals features typical of haemolysis (Fig 45.1) with a positive direct antiglobulin test (DAT). In HDN due to RhD incompatibility the baby is RhD positive and the mother RhD negative with a high level of anti-D.

Management

Management of HDN is complex, requiring close liaison between the haematology laboratory and obstetrician. In RhD alloimmunisation, if maternal anti-D levels are high and paternal testing indicates RhD heterozygosity, the fetal Rh genotype can be determined non-invasively by applying PCR technology to a maternal blood sample. Another advance is velocimetry of the fetal middle cerebral artery during an affected pregnancy. High peak systolic velocities predict severe fetal anaemia and allow the selective use of more invasive techniques such as fetal blood sampling and intrauterine transfusion. Newborns may experience ongoing anaemia and require exchange transfusion. Later anaemia may respond to erythropoietin therapy. With optimal management, a healthy child is the outcome in more than 90% of cases.

RhD prophylaxis in RhD-negative mothers

The breakthrough in the prevention of HDN has been the introduction of prophylaxis (Fig 45.2). A dose of Rh anti-D immunoglobulin (Ig) is given to all

Fig 45.1 **Peripheral blood film in a newborn child with severe HDN.** Note the numerous nucleated red cells and polychromasia.

RhD-negative mothers who deliver a RhD-positive infant. A larger than average feto-maternal haemorrhage necessitates a greater dose of anti-D Ig. It is most likely that anti-D administration prevents HDN by a negative modulation of the primary immune response rather than by simple removal of fetal RhD-positive cells. General recommendations for Rh prophylaxis are shown in Table 45.2. As some women undoubtedly become sensitised earlier in a normal pregnancy, routine antenatal prophylaxis is widely recommended.

Anaemia of prematurity

The haemoglobin concentration falls after birth in all babies but in premature infants it falls faster and to a lower level. At 1–3 months of age haemoglobin concentrations of less than 70 g/L are common and in babies born at less than 32 weeks gestation this anaemia is often associated with inadequate adaptive responses including tachycardia, tachypnoea and apnoeic attacks. The anaemia is due in part to shortened red cell lifespan and the effects of rapid growth but the fundamental problem appears to be a poor erythropoietin response. Erythropoietin levels are highest in premature infants with the most severe anaemia and hypoxia but even in these cases levels are inadequate compared to those achieved in anaemic adults. Recombinant erythropoietin is of benefit in some infants.

Polycythaemia in the neonate

Polycythaemia in the neonate is most simply defined as a packed cell volume (PCV) exceeding 0.65. Causes include

Table 45.2 Recommendations for Rh prophylaxis[1]

Table 45.2 Recommendations for Rh prophylaxis[1]

Rh prophylaxis after delivery

Anti-D (usually 500 IU) is given within 72 hours in RhD-negative mothers where the infant is RhD positive (or group undetermined). If there is a large feto-maternal haemorrhage (assessed in a Kleihauer test) additional anti-D is given

Rh prophylaxis and abortions

In RhD-negative mothers anti-D is given after all therapeutic abortions and after spontaneous or threatened abortions later than 12–13 weeks' gestation and in selected cases of threatened abortion before 12 weeks (usual dose 250 IU before 20 weeks and 500 IU after 20 weeks)

Rh prophylaxis during pregnancy

Anti-D is given after possible sensitising events in RhD-negative women. These include: amniocentesis, chorionic villus sampling, abdominal trauma, external cephalic version, antepartum haemorrhage, ectopic pregnancy (usual dose of anti-D is 250 IU before 20 weeks and 500 IU after 20 weeks). Anti-D (500 IU) should be given to non-sensitised RhD-negative mothers at 28 and 34 weeks

[1]*United Kingdom guidelines.*

Table 45.3 Some causes of thrombocytopenia in the neonate

- DIC in various severe systemic disorders
- Intrauterine infection (e.g. rubella, cytomegalovirus)
- Platelet antibodies:
  - autoimmune (maternal ITP)
  - alloimmune
  - drugs
- Hereditary/congenital disorders:
  - Wiskott–Aldrich syndrome
  - thrombocytopenia with absent radii (TAR) syndrome
- Post exchange transfusion
- Neonatal leukaemia
- Giant haemangioma

placental transfusion (e.g. delayed clamping of the cord), intrauterine hypoxia, endocrine disorders (e.g. maternal diabetes) and genetic disorders (e.g. trisomy 21). Polycythaemia is often well tolerated but if severe it may cause hyperviscosity with congestive heart failure, respiratory distress, neurological disturbances and even gangrene. Partial exchange transfusion using a crystalloid solution to reduce the haematocrit is indicated where a high PCV is associated with symptoms and signs of hyperviscosity.

Thrombocytopenia in the neonate

Some causes of thrombocytopenia in neonates are listed in Table 45.3. In practice the major divide is between seriously ill infants where the low platelet count is caused by disseminated intravascular coagulation (DIC), and relatively well infants where thrombocytopenia is most often of immune aetiology or occurs secondary to a specific inherited syndrome.

Immune thrombocytopenia (ITP) may be seen in infants born to mothers with ITP where there is passive transfer of IgG across the placenta. Alloimmune thrombocytopenia arises where the healthy mother becomes sensitised against a fetal platelet antigen in a manner analogous to HDN; the platelet antigen HPA-1a is most commonly implicated.

Iron deficiency in infancy

Iron deficiency has already been discussed (p. 24) but some aetiological factors in infancy are unique to this period of life. Blood loss may still be the major cause of deficiency but other factors worthy of consideration are decreased total body iron at birth (e.g. prematurity, feto-maternal haemorrhage, twins), the impact of growth with increased demands for iron, and dietary inadequacy (e.g. excessive dependence on unsupplemented cow's milk).

Red cell aplasia in childhood and adolescence

Pure red cell aplasia (PRCA) is characterised by anaemia, reticulocytopenia and reduced or absent erythroid precursor cells in the bone marrow. There are many causes of PCRA including infection (e.g. parvovirus B19), connective tissue

disorders, and malignancies (e.g. thymoma). However, two types of PCRA are unique to childhood: Diamond–Blackfan anaemia and transient erythroblastopenia.

Diamond–Blackfan anaemia

This is a rare heterogeneous disorder caused by defects in structured ribosomal proteins. The majority of cases are sporadic but various patterns of inheritance have been documented. An anaemia with the features of red cell aplasia usually presents within the first 12 months of life. This runs a chronic course and can be combined with developmental abnormalities. There is an increased risk of haematological malignancy and other cancers. Beyond blood transfusion, therapeutic options include corticosteroids, ciclosporin and allogeneic stem cell transplantation.

Transient erythroblastopenia of childhood

This is a transient form of red cell aplasia of probable immune origin which must be distinguished from Diamond–Blackfan anaemia. It generally affects older children (1–4 years) and may be diagnosed simultaneously in siblings or in seasonal clusters. In over half of cases there is a previous viral illness. The normocytic anaemia may be accompanied by mild neutropenia. Full recovery within 4–8 weeks is the rule.

Congenital dyserythropoietic anaemias (CDAs)

This is a group of rare inherited anaemias. There are various subtypes but common features include ineffective erythropoiesis and multi-nucleated erythroblasts. The white cell and platelet counts are normal. Anaemia is usually first diagnosed in infancy or childhood. It may be of normocytic or macrocytic type. Transfusion is required in more severe cases.

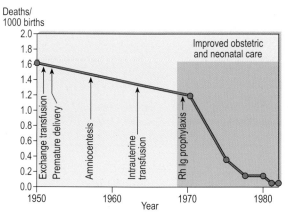

Fig 45.2 **Perinatal deaths/1000 births caused by HDN.** (From Derrick Tovey, LA 1992 Haemolytic disease of the newborn and its prevention. In: Contreras, M (ed) ABC of Transfusion. BMJ Publishing.)

> *Paediatric haematology*
>
> - Chronic and severe blood disorders in children are usually best managed by a paediatrician with a special interest in haematology or in a combined paediatric/haematology clinic.
>
> - In haemolytic disease of the newborn (HDN), haemolysis is caused by maternal IgG antibodies crossing the placenta and attaching to fetal red cells. Most clinically significant cases affect a RhD-positive fetus or newborn child where the mother is RhD negative.
>
> - RhD prophylaxis has much reduced the incidence of severe HDN.
>
> - Prematurity is associated with a particular type of anaemia.
>
> - In pure red cell aplasia in children it is important to distinguish between Diamond–Blackfan anaemia and the more benign transient erythroblastopenia of childhood.

46 Haematology in the elderly

Average life expectancy is increasing. Elderly people (>65 years) are likely to make up more than 20% of the world's population by 2050. This effect is particularly marked in the developed world where in some countries the population over 65 years already outnumbers those below 20 years. An ageing population has implications for the practice of clinical haematology. There are significant age-related changes in haematopoiesis and haemostasis. Many blood diseases, especially malignant disorders, are more common in older people. The management of blood diseases in the elderly is often complicated by frailty, comorbidity and a need for extra care in the hospital and community.

Haematopoiesis and ageing

There is an age-associated decline in haematopoietic stem cells and haematopoietic cell function. The reasons for this are unclear and much of our knowledge is derived from studies of mouse models rather than humans. It is probable that this decline arises from a combination of accumulated genetic and epigenetic changes, alterations in the marrow microenvironment and systemic effects such as inflammation. Practical consequences of these biological changes include reduced immune function, an increased incidence of cancer, and a lesser tolerance of haematopoietic stress (e.g. chemotherapy). Stem cells from older donors are less efficient at reconstituting haematopoiesis in transplant recipients.

Anaemia

Anaemia is a common clinical problem in the elderly. The prevalence rises rapidly after 50 years and approaches 20% in people aged over 80 years. In general, one third of cases will have an identifiable nutritional deficiency (iron, vitamin B_{12} or folate) (Fig 46.1). Where iron deficiency is the cause of anaemia it is often secondary to gastrointestinal blood loss, and underlying bowel pathology (e.g. colonic carcinoma) should be excluded. Another third of cases have the anaemia of chronic disease. These patients have an obvious chronic inflammatory condition (see p. 36) and will often have a measurable acute phase response (e.g. elevated C-reactive protein). In the final third of elderly patents, there is no clear cause for the anaemia (sometimes termed 'anaemia unexplained'). This entity is a diagnosis of exclusion and has been the focus of much recent interest. A few cases may be explained by myelodysplastic syndrome or other rarer causes of anaemia but it is probably

mainly due to a combination of age-related suppression of erythroid colony formation, insensitivity to erythropoietin and impaired iron utilisation.

Whatever its aetiology, anaemia in the elderly is a relevant finding. It is associated with reduced physical and cognitive functioning, an increased chance of falls, an aggravation of comorbidity such as cardiac and neurological disease, and reduced survival. A low haemoglobin level should not be readily dismissed as part of 'normal ageing'.

Where the anaemia has an explained cause (e.g. iron deficiency), treatment is specific for that disorder. Erythropoeitin may be used in chronic renal failure. Blood transfusion is needed in only a minority of cases (e.g. for the symptomatic anaemia of myelodysplastic syndrome), and in the very elderly and frail must be undertaken cautiously to avoid fluid overload and the exacerbation of cardiac failure. The treatment of unexplained anaemia in the elderly remains controversial with no clear guidelines.

Thrombosis and anticoagulation

Old age is a relatively hypercoagulable state. Ageing leads to increased plasma levels of fibrinogen and various clotting factors and delayed fibrinolysis. The incidence of both arterial and venous thrombosis increases with age (Fig 46.2). Advanced age is not in itself a contraindication to the use of anticoagulant therapy – older patients may derive the greatest benefit – but there are

particular considerations. Patients over 60 years usually require lower doses of vitamin K antagonists to maintain a therapeutic range than younger patients. Some studies have suggested an increased risk of adverse events such as bleeding in older patients on anticoagulants. It is not clear whether this is related to age alone or the presence of comorbidity. It is sensible to monitor elderly patients more frequently. It is likely that the newer oral anticoagulants (see p. 102) will also have to be used cautiously in this group of patients.

Haemophilia and other inherited bleeding disorders

Haemophilia is not generally thought of as a disease of the elderly. Recent changes in management such as the prophylactic use of coagulation factors have focused on children and young adults. However, at least in the West, regular coagulation factor replacement means that life expectancy is now

Fig 46.1 **Causes of anaemia in the elderly.**

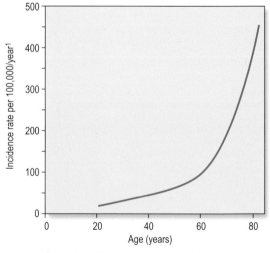

^{1} New episodes of venous thromboembolism

Fig 46.2 **The incidence of venous thrombosis increases exponentially with age.**

approaching that of the whole male population. This means that older patients increasingly present with both the clinical problems of haemophilia (e.g. joint arthropathy and pain, blood-borne infections) and age-related illnesses such as cancer and cardiovascular disease. The treatment of such comorbidities routinely involves invasive practical procedures and drugs which further derange haemostasis, and patients will often need intensive coagulation factor replacement to counter the increased risk of bleeding. The same considerations apply to other inherited bleeding disorders.

Haematological malignancy and chemotherapy

Haematological malignancy can occur at any age but most types are more common in the elderly. The median age at diagnosis for all blood neoplasms combined is around 70 years (Fig 46.3). There is a male excess except for over 80 years when more women are diagnosed. This may be because of greater female life expectancy. Some haematological malignancies in the elderly are diagnosed incidentally, are indolent, and require little or no intervention. Examples are described in other sections and include monoclonal gammopathy of undetermined significance (MGUS), monoclonal B-cell lymphocytosis and early stage chronic lymphocytic leukaemia. Other neoplasms are aggressive and will reduce quality of life and shorten life expectancy in the absence of effective treatment.

Older patients tolerate chemotherapy less well than younger patients and they are less likely to be cured of their malignancy (Table 46.1). Changes in pharmacodynamics account for part of this reduced effectiveness and increased toxicity. Reducing the dose of chemotherapy drugs to minimise side-effects will reduce cure rates. Other factors leading to poorer outcomes in the elderly are increased comorbidity and adverse disease characteristics. For example, elderly patients with acute myeloid leukaemia have a higher incidence of poor risk cytogenetic changes compared with younger patients. They also have an increased number of significant chemotherapy side-effects including more profound myelosuppression, neurotoxicity and cardiotoxicity.

Fig 46.3 **Median ages of presentation of haematological malignancies.**

In the very elderly (>80 years), it may be judged that intensive chemotherapy is contraindicated. This might also apply to younger patients with very significant comorbidity. Where chemotherapy is undertaken, this should follow a careful assessment of the benefit and risk to the individual patient. A formal geriatric assessment should be considered in patients 70 years and older. This can identify potential reversible conditions which might exacerbate the complications of treatment including anaemia, depression, poor nutrition and a lack of available care and social support. Other practical steps to reduce the complications of chemotherapy are dose adjustment for renal dysfunction (based on the glomerular filtration rate), the prophylactic use of growth factors (e.g. granulocyte colony-stimulating factor (G-CSF)) to shorten the period of myelosuppression and the selection of drug regimens with relatively low toxicity. An example of the latter is the avoidance of anthracycline drugs in patients with cardiac failure. Targeted therapies (e.g. imatinib in chronic myeloid leukaemia) are particularly attractive in the elderly

Table 46.1 **Guidelines for the management of chemotherapy in older cancer patients**
Geriatric assessment for patients over 70 years
Adjust doses to individual GFR in patients over 65 years
Prophylactic use of G-CSF in patients over 65 years receiving regimens comparable to CHOP[1]
Maintenance of haemoglobin level around 120 g/L
Use of drugs with low toxicity where feasible

GFR: glomerular filtration rate; G-CSF: granulocyte colony-stimulating factor.
[1]*See page 61.*

as they potentially combine high levels of efficacy with fewer side-effects than conventional chemotherapy.

Population studies show lower survival rates for older people with all types of haematological malignancy. This group of patients is generally under-represented in formal clinical trials of chemotherapy. Many are excluded because of multiple comorbidities. Where older patients are entered into such trials the results must be interpreted cautiously as the selective nature of trial entry means that the results may not be applicable to the whole elderly population.

Haematology in the elderly

- An ageing population has implications for the practice of clinical haematology. Many blood disorders (e.g. malignant diseases) are commoner in the elderly.

- There are significant age-related changes in haematopoiesis and haemostasis.

- Anaemia is a common clinical problem in the elderly; in a third of cases there is no clear cause.

- Old age is a relatively hypercoagulable state.

- Older people tolerate chemotherapy less well than younger people and are less likely to be cured of their haematological malignancy.

47 Palliative care in haematological malignancy

The World Health Organization defines palliative care as 'an approach that improves the quality of life of patients and their families facing the problems associated with life-threatening illness, through the prevention and relief of suffering by means of early identification and impeccable assessment and treatment of pain and other problems, physical, psychosocial and spiritual'. As the modern specialty of palliative medicine was born in the hospice movement, there has been a tendency to regard it as an end-of-life intervention, an option only when disease-modifying cancer treatments have been exhausted. It is more correctly viewed as being entirely complementary to ongoing anti-tumour treatment – for instance, a patient with myeloma presenting with refractory bone pain is likely to benefit from expert symptom control early in their illness (Fig 47.1). Good palliative care requires a multidisciplinary team approach with staff expert in communication and control of symptoms and with the organisational skills to coordinate care. Patients commonly derive palliative care input from diverse sources (Fig 47.2). There is not space here to comprehensively review all aspects of palliative care but a number of applications with particular relevance to patients with haematological malignancy will be discussed.

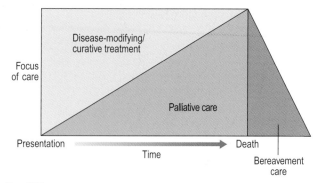

Fig 47.1 **Current model of cancer management.**

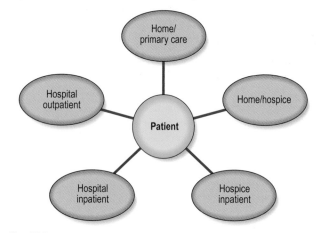

Fig 47.2 **Schematic view of a patient's access to palliative care services.**

Palliative chemotherapy and radiotherapy

Chemotherapy and radiotherapy are primarily employed as disease-modifying treatments but they may also be used in a palliative context to relieve symptoms and improve quality of life. Any side-effects of such treatment must be carefully weighed against the likely symptom control. Chemotherapy may thus be used to limit the degree of troublesome lymphadenopathy in advanced lymphoma or to reduce the systemic upset from a high malignant cell burden in end-stage leukaemia. Similarly, attenuated radiotherapy can give local relief from tumour infiltration in lymphoma and can reduce pain from myeloma bone lesions (Fig 47.3). Surgical interventions are used more sparingly but lymphomatous pleural effusions can be drained and the severe pain of myelomatous spinal disease can be ameliorated by the operation of vertebroplasty where the vertebrae are reinforced with a cement-like substance.

Management of cancer pain

Pain is a common symptom of cancer, particularly in patients with advanced or refractory disease. The means are available to give the great majority of patients good quality pain relief but, in practice, this goal may be compromised by the time, skill and commitment required of the medical team. Before initiating therapy, it is important to fully assess the severity (pain scales are available) and nature of the pain – visceral pain is often described as a dull ache, somatic pain may be sharp and postural, while neuropathic pain can be 'burning' or 'numbing'.

Pharmacological therapy is the mainstay of pain management in patients with haematological malignancy. Patients experiencing mild pain on no analgesia may be commenced on an oral non-opiate agent (e.g. paracetamol, nonsteroidal anti-inflammatory drug (NSAID)) but more severe pain is likely to require an opiate analgesic given at an appropriate dose and interval, possibly in combination with a specific co-analgesic dependent on the nature of the pain. There is no one optimal opiate dose and the correct dose must be achieved by proactive titration so that the patient is pain free without unacceptable toxicity. For most patients with chronic cancer pain, the oral route is preferable but parenteral, transdermal and rectal preparations are also widely employed. Pain prevention must be complemented by management of drug side-effects – patients on opiates will generally need laxatives and antiemetics. Particular care is necessary when analgesics are changed. This requires an understanding of their relative strengths and durations of action.

Opiates may be combined with co-analgesics to maximise their effect. Examples in haematological practice include the use of corticosteroids (usually dexamethasone) to tackle symptoms of raised intracranial pressure or nerve infiltration secondary to lymphoma and the prescription of NSAIDs and bisphosphonates to optimise control of bone pain in myeloma. Tricyclic antidepressants can be a useful adjunct in neuropathic pain.

Control of non-pain symptoms

Fatigue. In the haematology clinic, many patients with leukaemia, lymphoma and myeloma complain of demoralising fatigue. This is usually of multifactorial aetiology with a mixture of physiological and psychosocial factors, the latter including anxiety and sleep disruption. Anaemia is the most common reversible physical cause and regular administration

Fig 47.3 **The need for palliative care in a patient with myeloma.** An MRI scan of the spine in a patient with myeloma showing vertebral collapse. Back pain is a common symptom in this disease.

Fig 47.4 **A syringe driver used to give continuous drug infusions.**

of subcutaneous erythropoietin improves haemoglobin levels and quality of life in selected patients with myeloma, lymphoma and other cancers.

Nausea and vomiting. These symptoms are common, both due to tumour infiltration and as a side-effect of chemotherapy and analgesics. It is crucial to identify the cause. A centrally acting antiemetic drug (e.g. ondansetron) is indicated for drug-induced nausea whereas a pro-kinetic agent (e.g. metoclopramide) is more appropriate for gastric stasis or functional bowel obstruction. In more difficult cases, it is important to combine antiemetics logically and to consider alternative routes of administration.

Anorexia and cachexia. Patients with loss of appetite and weight loss need expert dietary assessment and advice. Oral corticosteroids can improve appetite and lead to weight gain. Poor nutrition may be exacerbated by drug-induced mucositis, painful neutropenic mouth ulcers and oral infections such as candida and herpes simplex. This can be minimised by good mouth care and early recognition of infections.

Dyspnoea. Lymphoma can cause dyspnoea because of bulky mediastinal lymphadenopathy or lung infiltration. Patients with advanced leukaemia more commonly develop the symptom during fulminant respiratory infections or after

bleeds into the lung parenchyma. Once correctable causes of dyspnoea have been excluded, other options include the selective administration of oxygen, opiates and sedation to minimise the subjective sensation of breathlessness.

Care at of the end of life. In patients with advanced disease and refractory symptoms in the final days of life, sedation may be used in the form of continuous drug infusions via portable syringe drivers (Fig 47.4). Strict criteria must be used for patient selection and fully informed consent must be obtained from the patient (where possible) and their family. Such measures should only be resorted to after consultation with the palliative care team.

Psychosocial oncology

It is important (but not always easy) to distinguish the inevitable emotional upset following a diagnosis of a life-threatening disease such as leukaemia from a more severe disturbance that meets the criteria for a mental disorder. In practice, there is a need for a multidisciplinary strategy with the involvement of specialist haematology/oncology nurses, psychologists, psychiatrists and social workers. High quality communication between the patient and their physician and other members of the caring team is crucial to blunt the

distress caused by setbacks and the toxicity of treatment. Psychotherapeutic approaches may be on an individual or group basis and have been shown to diminish any sense of isolation and to boost optimism. The provision of good quality information, exploiting the internet and other new technologies, is complementary to this process. Where there is significant anxiety and depression – and correctable causes have been excluded – anxiolytics and antidepressants can be beneficial. Support must also be given to the patient's family, particularly at the time of bereavement.

Complementary therapy

Patients may turn to complementary and alternative medicine. Staff specialising in traditional cancer medicine may be ignorant of and even threatened by such modalities. However, they should not hesitate to advise against any unorthodox intervention which is likely to lead to harm. There is some evidence for the use of hypnosis in pain relief, for acupuncture in the management of drug-induced nausea and vomiting, and for massage and meditation techniques in decreasing distress and improving sense of well-being. Centres specialising in the treatment of haematological malignancy are increasingly offering these therapies to their patients.

Palliative care in haematological malignancy

- Palliative care is designed to improve the quality of life of patients and their families – it is complementary to ongoing anti-cancer treatment.
- Optimal provision of palliative care requires a multidisciplinary team with specialist skills.
- Good communication is a vital therapeutic tool.
- Chemotherapy and radiotherapy may be used to palliate symptoms.
- Pain is a common symptom of haematological malignancy and is often poorly treated. Patients with advanced disease may require an actively titrated opiate analgesic and an appropriate co-analgesic.
- Normal emotional distress following the diagnosis of a haematological cancer must be distinguished from mental disorders requiring specific treatment.

48 Systemic disease

Clinical haematologists spend a considerable part of their time investigating blood abnormalities in patients with diseases of other organ systems. Some of the more common diagnostic challenges are discussed here.

Renal disease

Diseases of the kidney are associated with a remarkably wide range of possible haematological abnormalities (Table 48.1).

Anaemia is almost inevitable in chronic renal failure. The pathogenesis is complex but impaired erythropoietin production is the principal cause. Other possible contributory factors include the release of inhibitors of erythropoiesis, mild haemolysis and iron deficiency. The anaemia of renal failure is typically normocytic and normochromic. A characteristic finding in the blood film is the presence of *burr cells* (Fig 48.1). The best treatment of anaemia is resolution of the underlying renal problem (e.g. by transplantation), but where this is not feasible, recombinant erythropoietin is the treatment of choice. Intermittent bolus administration generally leads to a marked improvement in anaemia and transfusion independence. A failure of the anaemia to respond to erythropoietin should prompt a search for other aetiologies such as iron deficiency.

Paradoxically, some forms of renal disease can lead to increased red cell production and clinical polycythaemia (see Table 48.1). This arises either from inappropriate secretion of erythropoietin by a kidney tumour or from local renal hypoxia promoting erythropoietin release from normal cells. Polycythaemia can be the presenting feature of renal carcinoma and rapid identification of the malignancy may allow curative surgical treatment. Benign diseases such as polycystic disease and hydronephrosis probably cause polycythaemia by inducing renal ischaemia. The polycythaemia of renal disease is not an appropriate physiological response and patients with high haematocrits can derive benefit from regular venesection.

Chronic renal failure is also associated with a large number of possible platelet and coagulation abnormalities. The increased risk of bleeding in these patients is generally caused by the complex interaction of abnormalities shown in Table 48.1. Anaemia tends to

Table 48.1   Haematological changes in renal disease

	Abnormality	Clinical association
Red cells	Anaemia	Chronic renal failure
	Polycythaemia	Renal carcinoma, cystic disease, hydronephrosis, parenchymal disease, Bartter's syndrome, renal transplantation
	Burr cells	Renal failure
Haemostasis	Abnormal platelet function	Renal failure
	Thrombocytopenia	
	Disordered coagulation[1]	

[1]The complex coagulation abnormalities of renal failure usually lead to a bleeding tendency but nephrotic syndrome is associated with an increased incidence of thrombosis.

Fig 48.1   **Burr cells in the blood in renal failure.**

worsen bleeding by interfering with the normal interaction between platelets and vascular endothelium.

Liver disease and alcohol

Significant liver disease is associated with haemostatic problems (see p. 77) and red cell abnormalities including macrocytosis and target cells. Excessive alcohol consumption commonly causes macrocytosis and thrombocytopenia.

Malignancy

Anaemia is seen in around half of patients with non-haematological malignant tumours. The anaemia of chronic disease is the most common aetiology (p. 36) but other causes include chemotherapy, blood loss, haemolysis and marrow infiltration. Invasion of the bone marrow by solid tumours can result in a pancytopenia and a characteristic leucoerythroblastic blood picture with circulating nucleated red cells and myelocytes (Fig 48.2a). Clumps of malignant cells may be seen in a bone marrow aspirate but a bone marrow trephine is a more reliable way of demonstrating solid malignancy (Fig 48.2b).

Malignancy can be associated both with a hypercoagulable state and a bleeding tendency. The presence of hypercoagulability was first suggested by the increased incidence of deep vein thrombosis and pulmonary embolism seen in cancer patients. The mechanism is thought to be activation of the normal clotting system with low-grade intravascular coagulation and secondary fibrinolysis. In the laboratory, common findings are elevated levels of clotting factors and a shortened prothrombin time and activated partial thromboplastin time. It is presumed that cancer cells secrete thromboplastin which initiates clot formation. Treatment of venous thrombosis in malignancy is difficult, as anticoagulant control is often poor. Low molecular weight heparin is generally preferred to warfarin.

Disseminated intravascular coagulation (DIC) can complicate malignancy. It may be an acute haemorrhagic state but is more often a chronic low-grade disorder with no bleeding. It is particularly likely to accompany carcinomas of the prostate, stomach, colon, breast, ovary, lung, gallbladder and melanoma. DIC is further discussed on page 76.

Connective tissue disorders

Systemic disorders such as rheumatoid arthritis, systemic lupus erythematosus (SLE) and mixed connective tissue disease often lead to abnormal blood counts. In practice the most common finding, particularly in rheumatoid arthritis, is the anaemia of chronic disease. Immune thrombocytopenia is more often seen in SLE and this heterogeneous disorder may also be complicated by the presence of the lupus anticoagulant (p. 79). Neutropenia can arise in several connective tissue disorders; the triad of long-standing rheumatoid arthritis, splenomegaly and neutropenia is termed Felty syndrome. There may be a small increased risk of haematological malignancy in patients with rheumatoid arthritis. In Sjögren's syndrome there is a substantially increased risk of non-Hodgkin's lymphoma.

Fig 48.2 **Patient with prostatic carcinoma and invasion of the bone marrow. (a)** Leucoerythroblastic blood picture: note the nucleated red cell and myelocyte. **(b)** Bone marrow trephine specimen showing replacement of normal haematopoiesis by carcinoma.

Infections

Infections are probably the most common cause of abnormal blood counts in a typical haematology laboratory. Different infections are associated with different abnormalities but it is possible to make some generalisations.

Bacterial infections commonly cause a neutrophil leucocytosis. The neutrophils are classically 'left-shifted' (i.e. reduced nuclear segmentation) with increased cytoplasmic granulation (toxic granulation). Very severe bacterial infections such as disseminated tuberculosis can induce a leukaemoid reaction with immature myeloid cells appearing in the blood.

Viral infections most commonly cause a transient lymphocytosis with reactive changes in the cells. Two types of viral infection merit more detailed description: infectious mononucleosis and HIV infection.

Infectious mononucleosis

Infectious mononucleosis (or glandular fever) is a disorder caused by the Epstein–Barr virus (EBV). It predominantly affects adolescents and young adults. Clinical features often include malaise, fever, pharyngitis, lymphadenopathy, splenomegaly and hepatitis. There is a small risk of splenic rupture. The haematological hallmark of the disease is the presence of numerous atypical lymphocytes in the blood (Fig 48.3). These lymphocytes are mainly activated T-cells produced as an immunological response to EBV-infected B-lymphocytes. Other possible blood changes are neutropenia, thrombocytopenia and a cold-type autoimmune haemolytic anaemia. The differential diagnosis is essentially other viral diseases, but where the blood abnormalities are severe the disease may be confused with acute lymphoblastic leukaemia. The diagnosis is supported by positive Paul–Bunnel or Monospot tests which rely on the detection of heterophile antibodies that appear in the serum. If these tests are negative and there remains clinical suspicion of the disorder then EBV-specific serodiagnostic tests should be performed. Treatment of infectious mononucleosis is essentially symptomatic, although corticosteroids can be helpful in unusually difficult cases.

HIV infection

Progressive HIV infection has many possible haematological consequences (Table 48.2). These result from a combination of a direct effect of the virus, opportunistic infection and side-effects from the drugs used in treatment. The blood changes are often similar to those seen in other viral infections but a chronic decline in the lymphocyte count is a particular feature. Examination of the bone marrow often reveals non-specific features such as changes in cellularity, fibrosis, trilineage myelodysplasia, increased plasma cells and prominent haemophagocytosis. The presence of granulomas can signify infection by atypical mycobacteria or other opportunistic pathogens. In clinical practice the major haematological problems associated with HIV infection are immune thrombocytopenia (ITP) and lymphomas. The latter are typically aggressive B-cell malignancies with extranodal involvement.

Fig 48.3 **Atypical lymphocyte in infectious mononucleosis.**

Table 48.2 **Possible haematological changes in HIV infection**	
Blood	Lymphopenia
	Anaemia
	Neutropenia
	Thrombocytopenia
	Atypical lymphocyte morphology
	Anisopoikilocytosis
	Macrocytosis[1]
Bone marrow	Variable changes in cellularity
	Dysplasia
	Increased plasma cells
	Increased fibrosis
	Haemophagocytosis
	Opportunistic infection (e.g. granulomas)
	Lymphoid aggregates
	Lymphoma
Other	Positive direct antiglobulin test (DAT)
	Lupus anticoagulant

[1]*Particularly in patients receiving the drug zidovudine.*

Systemic disease

- Renal disease can cause anaemia, polycythaemia and abnormalities in platelets and coagulation.

- Malignancy often causes anaemia. Invasion of the bone marrow by solid tumour is a cause of a leucoerythroblastic blood picture.

- Bacterial and viral infections are common causes of abnormal blood counts.

- Infectious mononucleosis is a disease caused by the Epstein–Barr virus. Numerous atypical lymphocytes are seen in the blood.

- The many possible blood changes of HIV infection result from a combination of a direct viral effect, opportunistic infection and drugs used in treatment.

49 The developing world

The term 'developing world' is used to describe the majority of tropical countries which are 'hot, humid and poor'. An alternative term is the 'less economically sound' nations, as these countries are often advanced in human and cultural resources. Haematological practice is different to that in most developed countries. Genetic diseases such as the haemoglobinopathies and red cell enzymopathies are frequent in many tropical regions. Deficiency anaemia and haemolytic anaemia are often secondary to infections such as ancylostomiasis (hookworm) and malaria. Medical treatment regarded as routine in the developed countries is commonly unavailable. For instance, only about 20% of the world's haemophiliac population has access to factor VIII replacement therapy.

With the ever-increasing availability of 'exotic' holidays and regular foreign travel within immigrant populations, doctors in the developed world are seeing more tropical diseases. In the patient with unexplained symptoms such as malaise and fever, or signs such as splenomegaly, a history of travel should not be overlooked.

Malaria

Malaria is a protozoal disease, the infectious agent being *Plasmodium falciparum, P. vivax, P. ovale* or *P. malariae*. Mortality from the disease has fallen over the last decade but it remains a serious health risk throughout the tropics and subtropics where insecticide resistance of anopheline mosquitoes and multiple drug resistance of malarial parasites make control and treatment challenging. According to the World Health Organization, there were 216 million cases of malaria and an estimated 655 000 deaths in 2010. Most deaths occur in children living in Africa where the disease accounts for 20% of all childhood mortality.

Pathogenesis

The life cycle of the malaria parasite is illustrated in Figure 49.1. When taking a meal of blood an infected mosquito initiates human infection by the inoculation of malarial sporozoites. These rapidly pass to the liver where they enter hepatocytes and divide. After several days, enormously increased numbers of parasites (merozoites) depart the liver and invade red cells. Here the merozoites develop via ring forms and trophozoites into schizonts. Rupture of the schizont releases 12–20 merozoites back into the blood, thus perpetuating the cycle. The duration of the blood cycle varies between malarial species, explaining the different periodicity of fever in each type. A further mosquito becomes infected when it feeds on blood containing gametocytes, the sexual form of the parasite.

Diagnosis

Although malarial parasites may be detected in normal blood films, their identification is generally easier in Leishmann or Giemsa stain at a higher pH. A thick film is best for detection and a thin film for determination of the species. Prolonged inspection of the film is sometimes necessary to spot malarial parasites as there can be a low level of parasitaemia. Where malaria is suspected on clinical grounds repeated samples may be needed to make or exclude the diagnosis. *P. falciparum* is often associated with higher parasite counts. Paradoxically,

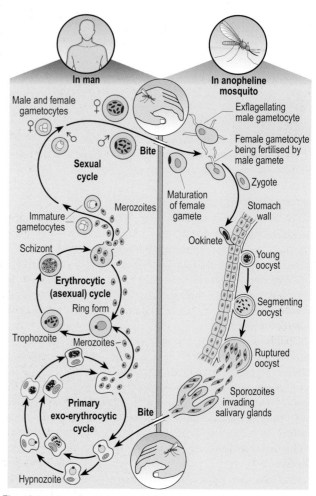

Fig 49.1 **Life cycle of the malarial parasite.**

some very ill patients with malaria initially have no detectable parasites in the blood as there is sequestration of parasite-laden red cells in the tissues. It is beyond the scope of this book to make a detailed comparison of the four species but some typical appearances are shown in Figure 49.2. Supplementary methods of parasite detection include antigen and antibody detection and DNA-based techniques.

Clinical features

Malaria has a different clinical presentation in non-immune and immune patients.

Non-immune patient

The interval between the mosquito bite and the onset of symptoms is typically 1–2 weeks. Common symptoms are rigors, sweats, headache, vomiting, diarrhoea and muscle pains. *P. vivax* and *P. ovale* are classically associated with bouts of fever on alternate days and *P. malariae* on every third day. Possible clinical signs include a rising temperature, tachycardia, herpes labialis, jaundice, dehydration and splenomegaly. *P. falciparum* infection is the most dangerous form of malaria. The onset can be insidious and the fever has no particular pattern. Life-threatening complications such as cerebral malaria (with development of coma), acute renal failure and blackwater fever (rapid intravascular haemolysis), can suddenly develop in a patient previously not particularly ill. Children are particularly at risk of a sudden demise.

Fig 49.2 **Malarial parasites in the blood. (a)** Ring-forms in *P. falciparum* malaria. **(b)** Schizonts in *P. ovale* malaria. **(c)** Gametocytes in *P. vivax* malaria.

Endemic malaria

In indigenous populations, malaria presents variably depending on the degree of endemicity, the age of the patient and the development of immunity. Thus in hyperendemic areas where there are seasonal variations, adults develop considerable immunity, malaria causing only short episodes of fever and a palpable spleen. In holoendemic areas there is infection through the year and usually the disease manifests as a transient low parasitaemia with no symptoms. In hypoendemic areas, epidemics occur and the disease resembles that in the non-immune. *Tropical splenomegaly syndrome* is the development of massive splenomegaly in adults in hyperendemic areas. The patient has a low parasitaemia with an exaggerated immune response and very high levels of IgM.

Treatment and prophylaxis

Ill patients should be rested and rehydrated. A rational choice of drug treatment requires knowledge of both the clinical syndrome and the likelihood of drug resistance. The mainstay of treatment of severe malaria is quinine. This is given intravenously. The dosage must be carefully calculated to avoid undertreatment or toxicity. Recent trials have suggested that artesunate, a derivative of the plant compound artemisin, is both easier to give and more effective than quinine in severe malaria. Its use in Africa may be limited by its cost. Specialist advice should be sought in difficult cases.

Chemoprophylaxis is advised for non-immune travellers entering malarial areas. Specific recommendations depend on the risk of exposure to malaria, the extent of drug resistance, the efficacy of drugs, drug side-effects and patient-related criteria (e.g. pregnancy, renal impairment). Drugs used include chloroquine, proguanil, mefloquine and doxycycline. Where there is doubt, expert advice should be sought. Simple preventative measures such as protective clothes, mosquito nets and insect repellent creams also help reduce the risk of infection. The recently discovered red cell surface receptor which allows *P. falciparum* to invade may provide a target for a future vaccine.

Visceral leishmaniasis (kala-azar)

This protozoal disease is transmitted by sandflies and caused by the organism *Leishmania donovani*. It is a cause of massive splenomegaly. The organism may be detected in a blood film within monocytes or neutrophils but bone marrow aspiration is more sensitive.

Other parasitic diseases detectable in the blood

These include the following:

- *Filariasis*. Microfilariae are released into the blood during an acute attack of disease. As the organisms are motile, examination of a wet preparation is useful.
- *Babesiosis*. This tick-borne disease only occasionally affects humans. Trophozoites which resemble small ring-forms of *P. falciparum* can be found in red cells.
- *Trypanosomiasis*. The parasites are extracellular and motile.

Iron deficiency in hookworm infection

Hookworms infect approximately a billion people worldwide. They are a major cause of gastrointestinal blood loss and iron deficiency anaemia in tropical regions. Worms attach to the upper small intestine and remove blood from the host; the daily loss can be as great as 250 mL. Management of anaemic patients should include both treatment of worms with an effective anthelminthic agent and oral iron supplements to replenish stores.

Endemic Burkitt's lymphoma

Endemic Burkitt's lymphoma is an aggressive B-lymphoblastic lymphoma which is found particularly in African children. In areas where malaria is holoendemic it is the most common childhood cancer. The disease is associated with Epstein–Barr virus (EBV) infection and the chromosomal rearrangement t(8;14). The classic clinical presentation is with a massive tumour of the jaw or other extranodal disease. Cure rates exceeding 90% are possible with combination chemotherapy.

> ### The developing world
>
> - The incidence of many haematological disorders and the availability of treatment is different in the developing world and developed countries.
> - Malaria is a protozoal disease transmitted to humans by anopheline mosquitoes. It is a major health problem in tropical and subtropical regions.
> - Laboratory diagnosis of malaria depends on the identification of parasites in thick and thin blood films.
> - Optimum drug treatment of established malaria and the best choice of prophylaxis require expert knowledge of clinical syndromes and possible drug resistance.
> - Hookworm infection is a major cause of iron deficiency in tropical areas.

50 Molecular biology

Molecular techniques now play a central role in the diagnosis and management of blood disorders, particularly haematological malignancies. This is a rapidly changing field and the following is a summary of some of the most commonly used and newest technologies and applications.

Selected techniques used in the analysis of DNA

Polymerase chain reaction (PCR)

The object of PCR is to amplify a preselected sequence of DNA many times over. This amplification greatly facilitates subsequent analysis of the DNA sequence for point mutations and polymorphisms, and often allows direct analysis of the product by gel electrophoresis without the use of probes.

The method can only be briefly described here. Essentially two specific oligonucleotide primers are added to the DNA. These have sequences matching the regions flanking the region of interest. A DNA polymerase is added and the mixture heated, causing the DNA to dissociate into two single strands. Following cooling the single strands bind to the oligonucleotides which are in excess. The oligonucleotide then acts as a primer for DNA polymerase and is extended to form a new double-stranded molecule. With each repeat of the cycle the amount of DNA is doubled. Generally about 30 cycles are used and amplification of approximately 10^6 can be achieved.

Fluorescence in situ hybridisation (FISH)

FISH describes the hybridisation of specific DNA or RNA sequences in situ to cellular targets attached to microscope slides. The most popular probes are chromosome-specific DNA sequences which generate a brilliant signal in both metaphase and interphase nuclei. The technique is particularly useful in the demonstration of chromosomal monosomies or trisomies but chromosome translocations (Fig 50.1), deletions and amplification of specific genes can also be detected. The results of FISH may be further improved by image processing.

Comparative genomic hybridisation

This technique is designed to detect regions in the genome which are undergoing quantitative changes. Different tumours show distinct genomic hybridisation patterns of gains and losses. The method is especially useful in the analysis of leukaemias.

Microarrays/gene profiling

Microarray technology allows the simultaneous profiling of tens of thousands of genes thus painting a molecular portrait of a tumour cell. Several methods are available for analysis of a large number of RNA transcripts. These include complementary DNA microarrays, oligonucleotide microarrays and serial analysis of gene expression (SAGE). The most commonly used 'platforms' are the two microarray technologies in which each experiment reveals the expression levels of over 20 000 genes. cDNA fragments and oligonucleotides can be spotted onto glass slides. The DNA arrayed on the slide is generally referred to as the 'probe' and the cDNA or cRNA derived from the sample is referred to as the 'target'. The

Fig 50.1 **Use of FISH in a case of chronic myeloid leukaemia (CML).** Probes for *BCR* and *ABL* are used – juxtaposition of the two probes (giving a yellow signal as in cell lower right) indicates the *BCR–ABL* rearrangement seen in Ph+ CML.

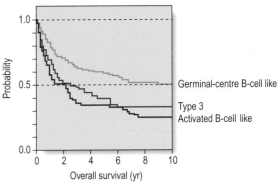

Fig 50.2 **Subgroups of diffuse large B-cell non-Hodgkin's lymphoma (DLBCL) according to gene expression profiles.** In the top panel each column represents a single DLBCL and each row a single gene. Red areas indicate increased expression and green areas reduced expression. Survival after chemotherapy is different in the three groups. (Reprinted with permission from Margalit O et al 2005 Micro-array based gene expression profiling of hematologic malignancies: basic concepts and clinical applications. Blood Reviews 19: 226.)

complex gene expression data generated requires powerful statistical analysis. Microarrays are enhancing our understanding of haematological malignancy (see below and Fig 50.2).

Fig 50.3 **Whole genome sequencing for detection of mutations in chronic lymphocytic leukaemia.** For each tumour genome, copy number (solid lines), density of mutations per 5-Mb window (bars) and protein-coding mutations (dots) are shown. The shaded rectangle indicates the location of the 13q14 deletion present in three of the four cases. Chromosome numbers are listed below the four profiles. (Reprinted by permission from Macmillan Publishers Ltd: Puente XS et al 2011, Whole genome sequencing identifies recurrent mutations in chronic lymphocytic leukaemia. Nature 475: 101–105.)

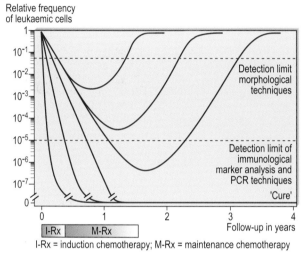

I-Rx = induction chemotherapy; M-Rx = maintenance chemotherapy

Fig 50.4 **The detection of minimal residual disease.** The greater sensitivity of PCR and immunological marker analysis compared with traditional morphological techniques in the detection of residual leukaemic cells can be seen. (Reproduced with permission of JJM van Dongen, Department of Immunology, Erasmus University, Rotterdam, and Medicultura International B.V.)

Next-generation sequencing

Massively parallel sequencing (also termed next- or second-generation sequencing) results in the simultaneous generation of millions of short DNA sequences. In studies of haematological malignancy, it is important to sequence both the tumour cells and normal tissue (e.g. skin) from the patient to identify relevant acquired (somatic) mutations. In whole genomic sequencing (Fig 50.3), the object is to sequence the entire genome. More specific next-generation techniques include exome and transcriptome sequencing.

Application of molecular biology in haematology

Carrier detection and antenatal detection in genetic disorders

Molecular techniques are crucial in antenatal diagnosis and genetic counselling in genetic disorders of the blood. For instance, PCR technology to detect DNA point mutations or deletions in chorionic villus samples, enabling first trimester testing for thalassaemia. Extraction of fetal cells or DNA from maternal blood may allow less invasive prenatal diagnosis.

Haematological malignancy
Diagnosis and classification

Leukaemias and lymphomas were originally diagnosed and classified on the basis of their morphological appearance. As is discussed in the disease sections, optimum management of these disorders now requires the supplementation of traditional clinical and morphological information with detail of immunophenotypic, karyotypic and molecular characteristics. Molecular analysis allows the confirmation of specific disease markers (e.g. *BCR-ABL* in chronic myeloid leukaemia) and also reveals key prognostic information (e.g. Ig gene mutation in chronic lymphocytic leukaemia). Microarray-based gene expression and next-generation sequencing studies, described above, provide novel insights into the biology of leukaemia, lymphoma and myeloma. Simplification of this expensive research technology is likely to permit its eventual use in the hospital laboratory.

Minimal residual disease

Traditional definitions of remission in leukaemia have relied on crude morphological criteria. Many patients in remission subsequently relapse, implying the existence of occult neoplastic cells undetectable by normal morphological or cytogenetic methods – so-called *minimal residual disease* (MRD) (Fig 50.4). Reliable detection of MRD potentially allows improved management with escalation of therapy for patients with persistent disease and the avoidance of excessive treatment in patients showing a good response to previous intervention. Detection of MRD relies upon the presence of disease markers that can be targeted (e.g. *PML-RAR* α in acute promyelocytic leukaemia). In childhood and adolescent ALL the tandem application of flow cytometry and PCR can be used to study MRD in almost all patients and this information is being employed in clinical trials. In CML quantitative PCR assay of *BCR-ABL* transcripts is routinely used to direct management. Very low levels of *BCR-ABL* mRNA predict a good clinical outcome.

Stem cell transplantation

Molecular techniques can be used both to monitor MRD post-transplant and to improve the level of HLA matching between unrelated donors and recipients.

Molecular biology

- Molecular biology techniques routinely used in haematology include the polymerase chain reaction (PCR), fluorescence in situ hybridisation (FISH) and comparative genomic hybridisation.

- Molecular techniques play a key role in carrier detection and antenatal detection in genetic disorders such as thalassaemia and haemophilia.

- In haematological malignancy, molecular techniques refine diagnosis and classification, and improve detection of minimal residual disease (MRD) after therapy.

- Recent developments include microarray-based gene expression profiling and whole genome sequencing of haematological malignancies.

51 Potential advances in treatment

This section addresses some potential advances in the treatment of blood disorders only briefly alluded to in the coverage of specific diseases. Inevitably any such listing of advances is subjective. Most clinicians would expect an expanding role for the targeting of the microenvironment in haematological malignancy, the wider use of new oral anticoagulant agents, and the introduction of gene therapy for single-gene disorders such as haemophilia and thalassaemia.

Targeting the microenvironment in haematological malignancy

The tumour microenvironment is currently thought to play a crucial role in cancer biology. A better understanding of the complex interactions between tumour and non-malignant cells is likely to translate into better characterization of tumour pathophysiology and novel approaches to therapy. In haematological malignancy, follicular lymphoma (see also p. 61) provides an excellent model for the study of the microenvironment. This disease accounts for approximately a quarter of all cases of non-Hodgkin's lymphoma. Modern treatment with a combination of chemotherapy agents and the anti-CD20 monoclonal antibody rituximab has improved overall survival but cure is elusive. Better therapeutic strategies are needed. Technologies such as immunocytochemistry, functional cytotoxicity assays and 3-D confocal imaging have improved our understanding of the role of the microenvironment in this disease and offered the prospect of new treatments which tip the balance against the tumour cells. The various interactions are complex (Fig 51.1) but it is clear that CD8+ cytotoxic lymphocytes play an active role and have the potential to be employed in the treatment of follicular lymphoma. Most simplistically, a higher content of T-cells appears to confer a better prognosis while pro-tumour macrophages may worsen the outlook. Follicular lymphoma cells can manipulate the microenvironment to their own advantage. Stimulation of CD4+ T-cell cytokine release promotes tumour cell growth and survival. The tumour cells also employ mechanisms to block entry of cytotoxic T-cells into the tumour site and to inhibit recruitment and trafficking of previously healthy T-cells. The challenge is to find ways of supplementing current immunotherapy regimens (e.g. rituximab and chemotherapy) by tipping the balance in the tumour microenvironment towards enhanced T-cell anti-tumour activity and away from immunosuppression. Possible agents include immunomodulating drugs such as lenalidomide. Such considerations may also apply in other haematological malignancies. For instance, encouraging clinical results have been obtained in chronic lymphocytic leukaemia following the targeting of the tumour cells with genetically modified autologous T-cells.

New oral anticoagulant drugs

Anticoagulant drugs are used both in the treatment and prevention of thromboembolic disease (see pp. 80–81). Conventional heparin and warfarin were discovered over 60 years ago while low

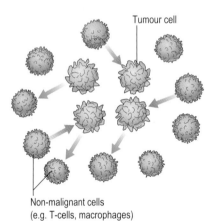

Fig 51.1 **A schematic view of the microenvironment in follicular lymphoma.** Cytotoxic CD8+ lymphocytes exert anti-tumour effects (red arrows) while tumour cells seek self-preservation (green arrows) by stimulating CD4+ T-cells to secrete favourable cytokines, inhibiting cytotoxic T-cells, and erecting a 'tumour barrier'.

molecular weight heparin is a more recent addition. All of these drugs have disadvantages, none fulfilling all the criteria for an 'ideal' anticoagulant, namely a high efficacy to safety index, a predictable dose response with no need for laboratory monitoring, administration by parenteral and oral routes, a rapid onset of action, a safe antidote, freedom from non-anticoagulant side-effects and minimal interaction with other drugs. Any new agent must aspire to meet as many of these requirements as possible without being prohibitively expensive. Attempts to develop better anticoagulants have focused on specific steps or enzymes in the coagulation pathway. Agents under evaluation include inhibitors of the factor VIIIc/tissue factor pathway, factor Xa inhibitors, activated protein C and soluble thrombomodulin and direct thrombin inhibitors (Fig 51.2).

Direct thrombin inhibitors and direct factor X_a inhibitors are now entering clinical practice and their use is likely to change the current practice of anticoagulation. *Dabigatran etexilate* is a prodrug. It is rapidly absorbed and converted in the liver to the active form dabigatran which acts as a direct thrombin inhibitor binding both free and clot-bound thrombin. The drug is administered orally and no therapeutic monitoring (i.e. laboratory testing of drug levels or activity) is required. *Rivaroxaban* is a direct inhibitor activated X (factor X_a) and is also given orally without the need for routine monitoring. *Apixaban* and *edoxaban* are other oral factor X_a inhibitors under

	Coagulation pathway	Possible anticoagulant
Initiation	Tissue factor / VIIa	Tissue factor pathway inhibitors
Thrombin generation	IX X IXa, VIIIa Xa, Va II	Protein C pathway (e.g. activated protein C) Xa inhibitors (e.g. rivaroxaban)
Thrombin activity	Thrombin Fibrin	Thrombin inhibitors (e.g. dabigatran)

Fig 51.2 **Possible new anticoagulants.** See text for discussion.

development. The indications for all these agents are gradually increasing as they are tested in clinical trials. There are still questions regarding long-term safety. Also, there are no specific antidotes to reverse the anticoagulant effects. Fortunately, the drugs have a short half-life and the bleeding risk is relatively low.

Gene therapy

Gene therapy is potentially a very powerful therapeutic tool applicable to a wide range of diseases including several blood disorders. After years of failure, there have been recent successes in the treatment of infants with immunodeficiency and in selected patients with malignancy. The basis of the technique is the insertion of a new functional gene into a cell (Fig 51.3). The gene is introduced into the target cell by use of a 'vector'. Disabled viruses are commonly used as vectors because they can undertake tasks necessary for successful gene transfer such as binding to the target cell and delivering the viral genome to the nucleus for transcription. Non-viral vectors based on plasmid DNA produced in bacteria and combined with lipids are also used. The optimum vector and delivery method is likely to vary depending on the disease under treatment. Early protocols mainly involved an ex vivo approach where the gene was inserted into cells taken from the patient. However, more recently the vector is normally given directly to the patient (in vivo approach). The problems have been numerous and have included difficulties in characterising and accessing the target cells, poor efficacy of gene transfer, short-lived expression of the newly introduced gene, and safety issues. The latter especially relate to viral vectors which have caused clinical symptoms of infection and induced massive immunological responses. Two children cured of their immunodeficiency by gene therapy subsequently developed leukaemia as a result of insertional mutagenesis.

As single-gene disorders, both haemophilia and thalassaemia are good candidates for cure by gene therapy. Haemophilia is a particularly attractive target disease as only a very small sustained increase in factor VIII or IX levels (1–2%) significantly reduces the bleeding tendency. A variety of methods for transferring genes for factor VIII and IX are under investigation. No single technique has emerged as being definitely superior. Animal studies with viral-derived vectors suggest that it is possible to provide sustained therapeutic levels of the clotting factors. Allowing the possibility that gene therapy for haemophilia may involve unforeseen risks, a number of carefully designed clinical studies in consenting patients are under way. In an early trial, a small number of patients with severe haemophilia B were treated using a non-pathogenic, non-integrating adeno-associated virus (AAV) as a DNA carrier. An intravenous schedule with gradually increased doses was used. Patients achieved increased factor IX levels with sustained clinical benefit, some being able to stop prophylactic factor IX treatment. In thalassaemia initial efforts at gene therapy have been directed against diseases of the β-globin gene. The therapeutic strategy involves insertion of a normally functioning γ-globin or β-globin gene into the patient's haematopoietic stem cells. At the time of writing, one patient with β-thalassaemia has been rendered transfusion independent following gene therapy but it is unclear if this was fortuitous or if this success can be reproduced in larger trials.

Gene therapy is also likely to have a role in malignant disorders. Leukaemia is essentially a genetic disease and, in theory, gene therapy could eventually be used to correct the abnormality in the malignant cell and cure the patient with minimal side-effects. Alternatively, gene therapy might be used to augment the patient's own immune response against malignant cells.

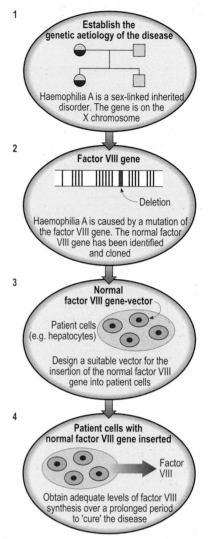

Fig 51.3 **The essential steps necessary for successful gene therapy in haemophilia A.**

Potential advances in treatment

- The tumour microenvironment plays a crucial role in some haematological malignancies (e.g. follicular lymphoma). It is likely to be increasingly targeted.

- New anticoagulant agents are under active development. Oral thrombin and factor Xa inhibitors potentially give safe anticoagulation without laboratory monitoring.

- The enormous promise of gene therapy is likely to be soon translated into clinical benefits. There is a real prospect of successful treatment of haemophilia.

52 Venepuncture and venous access

Obtaining a sample of venous blood from a patient is the most commonly performed practical procedure in haematology. The technique is apparently straightforward but poorly performed venepuncture can both upset the patient and compromise the quality of the sample. Gaining venous access for the delivery of fluids, blood or drugs is also fundamental to good haematological practice. This section is an overview of venepuncture and venous cannulation. These skills are best learnt by practice with expert supervision.

Taking a venous blood specimen (venepuncture)

The patient should be the correct patient – check their identity! Most serious haemolytic transfusion reactions arise from careless identification of patients and incorrect form labelling. Patients should sit or lie comfortably in such a way that no serious injury could result from a faint. The operator washes his hands and wears plastic gloves – insist on gloves that fit properly. The procedure is explained to the patient and the necessary consent obtained. The presence of a little transient pain when the needle is inserted should be acknowledged but not exaggerated.

Under normal circumstances blood is most easily taken from a vein in the antecubital fossa; the median cubital vein is preferred (Figs 52.1 and 52.2). It is considerate to ask whether the patient is left- or right-handed and then to choose the non-dominant arm. A tourniquet is applied well proximal to the site. This should cause distension of the veins but not discomfort. Gentle palpation is the best method of identifying a vein and checking its patency. If a suitable vein proves elusive it may help to gently tap the area or to warm the arm in water. The skin over the chosen vein is thoroughly cleaned with antiseptic solution. Usually a 21- or 22-gauge needle is used but a smaller size (e.g. 23) can be used where the veins are fragile, or in children. The syringe should be adequate for the sample – where larger blood samples necessitate more than one syringe a 'butterfly needle' may be preferred to a conventional venepuncture needle. The needle is inserted bevel uppermost along the line of the vein at an angle of around 20°. There is a distinctive 'give' as the vein is entered. Blood is aspirated into the syringe slowly to avoid haemolysis. The tourniquet is released and the needle withdrawn after a dry swab has been held to the site. Pressure should be applied by the patient or an assistant with the arm held straight or slightly elevated. The needle is removed from the syringe – not resheathed – and placed directly into a sharps container. The specimen is expelled gently from the syringe into the relevant bottles. Mixing with anticoagulant is best achieved by gently inverting the bottle several times – violent shaking will damage the sample. An adhesive plaster can be applied to the venepuncture site (check for allergy) when bleeding has stopped.

The above describes the procedure for a conventional needle and syringe. Increasingly, venepuncture is performed using closed evacuated container systems where a double-ended venepuncture needle is screwed into a holder and the evacuated tube inserted into the holder following entry of the vein. Blood is automatically aspirated into the tube as the vacuum is released. It is important to understand how the system works *before* undertaking venepuncture.

Precautions

Blood should not be taken from a vein proximal to an intravenous infusion as the sample can be diluted. Neither should eczematous or infected areas be used for venepuncture. If patients are known to have a blood-transmissible infection (e.g. hepatitis B or C, HIV) or are at increased risk of such an infection this must be indicated on the specimen bottle and request form. Due care must be taken as this is sensitive information – labels stating an infective risk are generally available. In view of the possibility of needle-stick injuries, those performing venepuncture should be vaccinated against hepatitis B.

Common problems

Venepuncture is not always easy. If blood is not aspirable following perceived entry of the vein it is worth withdrawing the needle slowly with suction applied as the vein may have been transfixed. If a vein cannot be located in the antecubital fossa it is permissible to use veins at the wrist or on the dorsum of the hand. If two attempts fail a more experienced colleague

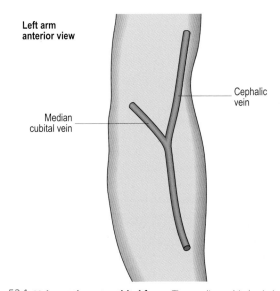

Fig 52.1 **Veins at the antecubital fossa.** The median cubital vein is preferred for routine venepuncture.

Fig 52.2 **Taking blood from a vein in the antecubital fossa.**

should be sought. As a last resort a sample can be taken from the femoral vein. The operator must be familiar with the anatomy of the femoral region as the vein lies close to the femoral artery and nerve.

Children

In babies and infants a blood sample is often more easily obtained from a stab wound made with a lancet (capillary blood). The usual site is the heel, although fingers and ear-lobes can be used. Venepuncture may also be from scalp veins.

Fig 52.3 **A large gauge plastic cannula.**

Venous access

Peripheral venous cannulation

Almost all haematology patients admitted to hospital require a drip to infuse fluids, blood products or drugs. Before inserting a cannula into a vein, an appropriate giving set should be prepared in accordance with instructions and the bag or bottle containing the infusion fluid inverted and hung on the drip stand. The set should be properly primed and all bubbles excluded. The operator must wash hands and wear gloves. It is vital to ensure that the patient is comfortable and fully understands the procedure and that necessary consent is obtained. The choice of cannula depends both on the quality of the veins and the duration and type of infusion. For short-term infusions or small veins a winged metal cannula (butterfly needle) is often suitable. In other circumstances a larger gauge plastic cannula is used (Fig 52.3). In adults, 18–20-gauge catheters provide good flow rates without too much discomfort for the patient.

The best site is the non-dominant forearm or the dorsum of the hand. The antecubital fossa is best avoided as it is uncomfortable to have the elbow immobilised. A tourniquet is applied and the skin cleaned as for venepuncture. The skin at the site may be stretched slightly to immobilise the vein. The cannula assembly (metal needle and surrounding plastic cannula) is introduced through the skin and into the vein. Once blood enters the cannula chamber or is easily drawn into a syringe, the tourniquet is released and the metal needle withdrawn from the plastic cannula which may be advanced further into the vein. The pre-prepared giving set is attached to the cannula and fluid allowed to enter the vein while the insertion site is carefully inspected for possible extravasation. The needle is promptly disposed of in a sharps receptacle. To minimise the chance of the drip being infected or dislodged the site is

protected with a sterile dressing and the cannula secured with a bandage or adhesive tape.

The most common problem is failure to locate a vein in the favoured sites. A more experienced operator may be successful. Where problems persist in experienced hands, other veins such as those in the region of the ankle or the subclavian, jugular or saphenous veins may be cannulated. Regular inspection of the drip site and careful hygiene will minimise the chance of infection. Where there is local inflammation or an otherwise unexplained bacteraemia, the cannula should be removed and another site used.

Central venous cannulation

Insertion of wide-lumen silicon rubber catheters (generally referred to as Hickman catheters) is routinely undertaken in clinical haematology where recurrent intravenous access is required. Examples include:

- patients with haematological malignancy receiving intensive chemotherapy
- patients with thalassaemia having regular blood transfusions
- children with haemophilia A on prophylactic factor VIII treatment.

The catheter is normally inserted into the subclavian vein and the location of the distal tip checked on X-ray (Fig 52.4). The proximal end of the catheter can be tunnelled under the skin with an exit

Fig 52.4 **Chest X-ray showing a central venous catheter in situ.**

site on the anterior chest wall. A catheter cuff within the tunnel promotes the formation of fibrous tissue which helps secure the device. The procedure is usually performed in the operating theatre by a surgeon or anaesthetist. Once in place the catheter may be used for several months. Strict aseptic technique is necessary as infection with coagulase-negative staphylococci is the most common complication.

> **Intravenous administration of cytotoxic drugs (chemotherapy) should only be undertaken following appropriate training in the use of these agents.**

> ### Venepuncture and venous access
>
> - Obtaining a venous blood sample (venepuncture) is a commonly performed practical procedure in haematology; poor technique can upset the patient and ruin the sample.
> - In babies and infants, capillary blood sampling is often easier than venepuncture.
> - Peripheral venous cannulation is commonly performed to infuse fluids, blood products and drugs.
> - Where there is serious difficulty in locating a vein for venepuncture or cannulation, more experienced help should be sought.
> - For recurrent venous access, insertion of an indwelling central venous catheter can be helpful.

53 Bone marrow aspiration and trephine biopsy

The indications for performing bone marrow aspiration and trephine biopsy procedures have previously been discussed (p. 19). In this section the practical aspects of obtaining these samples are outlined. More detailed accounts can be found in books of practical procedures, but ultimately the only way to perfect techniques is to practise under expert supervision.

Although the anterior iliac crest is occasionally preferred, most operators get the best specimens from the posterior iliac crest. The sternum is now rarely used. This is, in part, due to the small risk of causing catastrophic damage to the mediastinum, but mainly because it is not possible to obtain a trephine biopsy. Only the posterior iliac crest approach is described here.

Bone marrow aspiration

As for all procedures the sequence of events should be explained to the patient, reassurance given and consent obtained. A degree of discomfort should be acknowledged but it should be emphasised that this is transitory. In most adults, local analgesia is adequate but sedation is considered where patients are unusually anxious. A general anaesthetic is the norm in children. A clean, no touch technique is mandatory and operators should wear gloves. Stringent asepsis is needed in immunosuppressed cases.

The patient lies in the left or right lateral position and the skin over the posterior iliac crest is cleaned with antiseptic prior to screening with sterile drapes. The crucial next stage is to properly identify the bony landmarks (Fig 53.1). This is straightforward in most patients but can be problematic in obese subjects. If there are real difficulties in locating the posterior iliac crest then the anterior crest or the sternum may be considered or the procedure may be performed under CT guidance. A local anaesthetic is infiltrated into the skin and then down to the periosteum. Before use it should be checked that the marrow aspirate needle stylet is easily withdrawn and the guard is removed (this is only required for sternal aspirates). The needle (Fig 53.2) is inserted through the skin and subcutaneous tissues at the site of local anaesthetic infiltration until the periosteum is encountered. It is pushed through the periosteum with a deliberate screwing motion (alternating clockwise and anticlockwise) – a 'give' is felt as the marrow cavity is entered. The stylet is withdrawn and a syringe attached to the needle (Fig 53.3). Approximately 0.5 mL of marrow is aspirated into the syringe. The patient should be warned that this stage often causes pain but that it is momentary.

Fig 53.1 **Anatomy of the posterior iliac crest.** Possible sites for marrow sampling are indicated in red.

Fig 53.2 **Bone marrow aspirate needle.**

Marrow aspirate smears must be made promptly at the bedside before the marrow clots. If a larger volume is needed for tests such as cytogenetics and immunophenotyping, it is best to use a second syringe as large samples dilute the marrow with peripheral blood and reduce the quality of the morphological preparations. If it proves difficult or impossible to aspirate marrow it is worth replacing the stylet and carefully advancing or retracting the needle a short distance before repeating aspiration. It is important to remember that a 'dry tap' can result from marrow pathology (particularly fibrosis or solid malignancy) and is not always caused by poor technique.

Once the aspirate needle is withdrawn, firm pressure is applied to the site for a few minutes and then a sterile dressing or plaster used as protection. The patient lies on his back for 15 minutes to ensure a period of recuperation and that further light pressure is

Fig 53.3 **Aspiration of bone marrow from the posterior iliac crest.**

applied to the puncture site. Outpatients should probably be observed for at least an hour before being allowed home (more if sedated). Troublesome haemorrhage from the site is rare but it is sensible to correct a severe coagulation defect before undertaking the procedure. Thrombocytopenia alone is generally not a problem.

Patients often ask how quickly the 'results' will be available. Aspirate slides can be processed for microscopy (see

Table 53.1 **Ancillary tests which may be performed on bone marrow aspirate samples**

- Cytochemistry
- Cytogenetics
- Immunophenotyping
- Molecular studies
- Microbiological culture
- Cell culture studies
- Drug resistance studies

Fig 53.4 **Bone marrow trephine needle.**

p. 19) within a few hours but most ancillary tests (Table 53.1) take longer.

Bone marrow trephine biopsy

In practice the trephine procedure is usually performed immediately following the aspirate at the same site. It is helpful to enlarge the aspiration puncture site slightly with a scalpel blade. There is sometimes more prolonged discomfort than in the aspirate procedure and sedation is indicated in anxious adults, and a general anaesthetic is necessary in children. A number of different disposable needles are available – the Jamshidi type is illustrated in Figure 53.4. Smaller needles are available for paediatric use.

It is important to ensure that the device is complete and that the stylet can be easily withdrawn. The trephine needle is inserted in a similar fashion to the aspirate needle through the periosteum and approximately 0.5 cm into the cortex (Fig 53.5a) – when properly inserted the needle should easily support its own weight. The stylet is removed prior to advancing the needle 2–3 cm using the same oscillatory movement. The needle is aimed towards the anterior iliac crest. The method for breaking off the biopsy varies with the needle used. Some have devices designed to grip the biopsy and ensure its retention. The needle is then withdrawn taking care not to catch the skin and lose the biopsy in subcutaneous tissue. A special blunt probe is provided to push the biopsy out of the needle. The probe is inserted (with great care to avoid injury to the operator) at the sharp end of the needle so as not to traumatise the sample.

If the aspirate is a 'dry tap' it is worthwhile gently dabbing the trephine biopsy onto a glass slide before putting it into histological fixative. This 'touch preparation' is not useful for subtle morphological diagnosis but can permit rapid identification of malignant infiltration. It usually takes several days to process the trephine biopsy. Aftercare is the same as for the aspirate, although as it is a slightly more invasive procedure the patient also having a trephine may require a longer period of recuperation. Nevertheless, trephine biopsies are routinely performed in the outpatient clinic.

Bone marrow harvesting

Bone marrow can be harvested from a patient (for autologous stem cell transplantation) or from a donor (for allogeneic stem cell transplantation). The procedure is performed under a general anaesthetic, the marrow being collected from the iliac crests using multiple punctures with specialised harvest needles. Normally, approximately 1 litre is harvested from an adult in under an hour. Donors are hospitalised for around 48 hours. Serious side-effects are rare but some short-lived discomfort over the aspiration sites is common. The procedure is now undertaken less often

(a)

(b)

Fig 53.5 **Obtaining a trephine biopsy from the posterior iliac crest. (a)** Insertion of the needle. **(b)** CT guidance is useful in obese patients.

as peripheral blood stem cells are more commonly used than bone marrow in both autologous and allogeneic transplants (see page 56).

> ### Bone marrow aspiration and trephine biopsy
>
> - The optimal site for both bone marrow aspiration and trephine biopsy procedures is the posterior iliac crest.
>
> - Local analgesia is often adequate but nervous adults require sedation and children normally require a general anaesthetic.
>
> - Marrow aspiration smears may be stained for microscopy immediately after the procedure whereas trephine biopsies are processed over several days.
>
> - Serious side-effects from posterior iliac crest aspiration and trephine biopsy are very rare. Occasionally there can be excessive haemorrhage or local infection at the site.
>
> - Bone marrow can be harvested from the iliac crests in patients (for autologous stem cell transplantation) or healthy donors (for allogeneic stem cell transplantation).

Appendices

Appendix I: Reference ranges in normal adults

These figures are for guidance only. 'Normal' reference ranges vary in different populations and in different laboratories. Patient results should always be compared with local reference ranges.

Blood count

Haemoglobin	Male 130–180 g/L	Female 115–165 g/L
Packed cell volume	Male 0.40–0.52	Female 0.37–0.47
Red cell count	Male $4.5–5.9 \times 10^{12}$/L	Female $3.8–5.2 \times 10^{12}$/L
MCV	80–96 fl	
MCH	27–32 pg	
MCHC	315–345 g/L	
Reticulocytes	$50–100 \times 10^9$/L (0.5–2.5%)	
White cell count	$4.0–12.0 \times 10^9$/L	
Neutrophils	$2.00–7.50 \times 10^9$/L	
Lymphocytes	$1.50–4.00 \times 10^9$/L	
Monocytes	$0.20–1.00 \times 10^9$/L	
Eosinophils	$0.02–0.40 \times 10^9$/L	
Basophils	$0.02–0.20 \times 10^9$/L	
Platelet count	$150–400 \times 10^9$/L	

MCV, mean corpuscular volume; MCH, mean corpuscular haemoglobin; MCHC, mean corpuscular haemoglobin concentration.

Acute phase response

ESR[1]	Male 0–5 mm/h	Female 0–7 mm/h
Plasma viscosity	1.50–1.72 mPa·s (25°C)	
C-reactive protein	0–10 mg/L	

[1]*Higher levels (up to 15 mm/h) may be seen in the elderly.*
ESR, erythrocyte sedimentation rate.

Other

Ferritin	Male 21–300 µg/L	Female 15–150 µg/L
Serum iron	13–32 µmol/L	
TIBC	45–70 µmol/L	
Transferrin	1.2–2.0 g/L	
Serum vitamin B_{12}	160–760 ng/L	
Serum folate	3–20 µg/L	
Red cell folate	160–640 µg/L	

TIBC, total iron binding capacity.

Appendix II: Selected immunophenotypic (cell surface) markers

Cluster differentiation (CD) designation	Normal reactivity/Comments
CD2	T-lymphocytes
CD3	T-lymphocytes
CD4	Helper/inducer T-lymphocytes
CD5	T-lymphocytes, B-lymphocyte subset (expressed in B-CLL)
CD7	T-lymphocytes
CD8	Cytotoxic/suppressor T-lymphocytes
CD10	Precursor B-lymphocytes (expressed in common ALL)
CD11c	Monocytes, granulocytes, NK cells, activated T-lymphocytes, hairy cells
CD13	Monocytes, granulocytes (expressed in AML)
CD14	Monocytes
CD19	B-lymphocytes
CD20	B-lymphocytes (except pre-B)
CD22	B-lymphocytes
CD33	Monocytes, myeloid cells (expressed in AML)
CD34	Haematopoietic stem cells
CD36	Platelets, monocytes (platelet GP IIIa)
CD38	Plasma cells, some lymphocytes
CD41	Platelets (GP IIb)
CD42a/b	Platelets (GP Ib)
CD45	Leucocytes
CD55	Broad (decay accelerating factor[1])
CD56	NK cells
CD57	NK cells
CD59	Broad (membrane inhibitor of reactive lysis[1])
CD61	Platelets (GP IIIa)
CD68	Macrophages, neutrophils
CD75	B-lymphocytes
CD79	B-lymphocytes
CD103	Hairy cells
CD114	Granulocytes, monocytes
CD117 (expressed in AML)	Mast cells, plasma cells, expressed in AML

[1]Deficient in paroxysmal nocturnal haemoglobinuria.
CLL, chronic lymphocytic leukaemia; ALL, acute lymphoblastic leukaemia; NK, natural killer; AML, acute myeloid leukaemia; GP, glycoprotein.

Appendix III: International prognostic index (IPI) for non-Hodgkin's lymphoma (NHL)

The IPI was initially designed for predicting the outcome of diffuse large B-cell lymphoma (see non-Hodgkin's lymphoma section for further discussion of IPI). However, it has been shown to also have validity in other types of NHL. Patients in the higher risk groups have poor outcomes with conventional chemotherapy regimens.

Pretreatment criteria	Score 0	Score 1
Age (years)[1]	60 or under	Over 60
Stage (Ann Arbor)	I or II	III or IV
Number of extranodal sites of disease	1 or less	Greater than 1
Performance status (ECOG/WHO scale[2])	0 or 1	2 or greater
Serum lactate dehydrogenase (LDH)	Low or normal	High
These five scores are added to define the risk group as follows:		
Low	0 or 1	
Low intermediate	2	
High intermediate	3	
High	4 or 5	

[1]An age-adjusted model for patients less than 60 years is also available.
[2]The ECOG/WHO performance status scale is defined as follows: (0) able to carry out all normal activities without restriction; (1) restricted in physically strenuous activity but ambulatory and able to carry out light work; (2) ambulatory and capable of all self-care but unable to carry out any work; up and about more than 50% of waking hours; (3) capable of only limited self-care; confined to bed or chair for more than 50% of waking hours; (4) completely disabled; cannot undertake any self-care; totally confined to bed or chair; (5) dead.

Case histories

These case histories and the attached questions are designed to illustrate themes discussed in the main text. They are in no particular order. For Case 1, there is an obvious clue in one of the anaemia sections to help you get started. For the subsequent cases, you will have to dig a little deeper into the book for the answers. Relevant page numbers are shown is square brackets next to each case number. Where not appended, the normal ranges for the laboratory test results are listed in Appendix I.

Good luck!

Case 1 [pp. 24–25]

A 53-year-old Caucasian man attends his primary care practitioner complaining of gradually increasing fatigue and shortness of breath on exertion. He has also noted a few kilograms weight loss but there are no other symptoms. His doctor decides to check a *full blood count*, the results of which are summarised:

Haemoglobin	75 g/L
MCV	69 fl
MCH	24 pg
White cell count	9.2×10^9/L
Platelet count	460×10^9/L

1. What type of anaemia is this?
2. What is the most likely cause in this man? What simple blood investigation would confirm this?
3. If you confirm the anaemia aetiology you suspect, are further investigations necessary?

Notes to Case 1
1. This is a microcytic hypochromic anaemia.
2. The most likely cause in a Caucasian man of this age is *iron deficiency*. Measurement of serum ferritin is a simple test to confirm the diagnosis. It is usually reliable. A low level always indicates iron deficiency but a normal level does not guarantee normal stores as ferritin is increased in chronic inflammation and liver disease. The result here was 7 µg/L. This low level confirms the presence of iron deficiency. This may also be the cause of the slight thrombocytosis.
3. A cause for iron deficiency must always be sought. In this man, it is

vital to exclude gastrointestinal bleeding despite the lack of gastrointestinal symptoms. Clinical examination should include rectal examination. A colonoscopy revealed a large bowel carcinoma which was successfully resected.

Case 2 [pp. 28–29]

A 15-year-old girl presents to her primary care practitioner. According to her parents, she is constantly pale and tired. They have also noticed occasions when her eyes are a little yellow. She eats a normal diet and there is nothing else of note in the remainder of the history. The mother has had life-long similar symptoms but these have been only mild and never investigated. She thinks other members of her family might also be affected. The doctor decides to check a *full blood count* as he suspects anaemia:

Haemoglobin	94 g/L
MCV	92 fl
MCH	31 pg
White cell count	8.3×10^9/L
Platelet count	301×10^9/L

1. What type of anaemia is this?
2. The mother and other family members have similar symptoms so this might be an inherited form of anaemia. Do you know of any causes of inherited anaemia?
3. What further simple blood tests can be performed in the haematology laboratory to help elucidate the cause of the anaemia in this girl?

Notes to Case 2
1. This is a normocytic normochromic anaemia.
2. Inherited causes of anaemia include the haemoglobinopathies (e.g. thalassaemias, sickle cell syndromes), disorders of the red cell membrane (e.g. hereditary spherocytosis) and abnormalities of red cell metabolism (e.g. glucose-6-phosphate dehydrogenase deficiency). A thorough family history is very important in the diagnosis of these disorders. In them all, the anaemia is at least in part due to haemolysis. The patient's history of intermittent jaundice also supports a diagnosis of haemolytic anaemia.

3. Simple blood tests to clarify the cause of the anaemia should include a reticulocyte count and inspection of a blood film. Her reticulocyte count was raised at 9% and the blood film revealed large numbers of spherocytes (see p. 28, Fig. 14.2). A diagnosis of *hereditary spherocytosis* was made and was later also confirmed in the mother. In the Haemolytic anaemia II section, you should be able to find an acquired form of haemolytic anaemia which is also a cause of spherocytes in the blood film.

Case 3 [pp. 40–41]

A previously well 26-year-old man presents to the accident and emergency department of his local hospital with a 24 hour history of spontaneous bruising and bleeding from his gums. He has also felt unusually tired for the last few weeks. On examination he is pale with numerous small bruises and a scattered petechial rash. The accident and emergency doctor suspects that this might be a blood disorder and he takes blood samples for a *full blood count* and some *tests of coagulation*:

Haemoglobin	84 g/L
MCV	95 fl
MCH	31 pg
White cell count	25.4×10^9/L
Platelet count	62×10^9/L
Prothrombin time	22 seconds (9–12)
Activated partial thromboplastin time	58 seconds (26–36)
Fibrinogen level	1.1 g/L (1.7–4.5)

The automated haematology analyser does not generate a white cell differential count but the biomedical scientist in the haematology laboratory has inspected a blood film and reports that the white cell count is increased because of numerous leukaemic blast cells with marked cytoplasmic granularity. An urgent request for specialist clinical haematology advice is made.

1. What is the most likely diagnosis?
2. How urgent is the treatment of this blood disorder?

Notes to Case 3

1. The combination of the symptoms, the blood count, the coagulation test results and the appearance of the leukaemic blast cells strongly suggest that this is *acute myeloid leukaemia with t (15;17) (q22;q12) (M3:M3v)*. This subtype of the disease is also known as acute promyelocytic leukaemia. It is associated with a high incidence of disseminated intravascular coagulation and a high risk of spontaneous bleeding into vital organs. The blood film is shown on page 40 as Figure 20.2b.

2. Very urgent. Immediate treatment with the differentiating agent all-trans retinoic acid (ATRA) reduces the risk of early death from bleeding. Tests to make a more definitive diagnosis (e.g. molecular testing to detect the genetic abnormality) should not delay the initiation of this treatment where there is clinical suspicion of the disorder.

Case 4 [pp. 46–47]

A 72-year-old woman has a full blood count checked as part of the routine monitoring of her diabetes. She is feeling very well and wonders whether her doctor really needs to take these blood samples. The *full blood count* is surprisingly abnormal, as follows:

Haemoglobin	121 g/L
MCV	88 fl
MCH	30 pg
White cell count	30.4×10^9/L
Neutrophils	2.4
Lymphocytes	21.5
Monocytes	0.8
Eosinophils	0.2
Basophils	0.1
Platelet count	262×10^9/L

Inspection of the blood film reveals the increased lymphocytes to resemble normal lymphocytes but they are perhaps a little larger. Numerous 'smear cells' are noted. Flow cytometry of the cells confirms a diagnosis of *chronic lymphocytic leukaemia*. The blood film is illustrated in the chronic lymphocytic leukaemia section (Fig. 23.2). Subsequent examination of the patient is normal with no palpable lymphadenopathy or hepatosplenomegaly.

1. What is the stage of the disease?
2. What is your treatment plan for this lady?

Notes to Case 4

1. The lack of symptoms, absence of palpable lymphadenopathy and the normal haemoglobin level and platelet count are consistent with stage A disease.

2. This is an entirely incidental diagnosis of early stage chronic lymphocytic leukaemia in an elderly person. The prognosis is very good and there is no immediate need for treatment. The patient can be reassured and periodically followed up in the haematology outpatient clinic.

Case 5 [pp. 72–73]

A 10-month-old male infant is brought to the accident and emergency department by his very anxious parents. They report that he has had more bruising than his older siblings and that over the previous 2 days he has developed swelling of the left knee which he is now reluctant to bend. There is no history of trauma and he has been otherwise well with normal development. There is no family history of a similar problem. On examination, the baby is irritable. He is confirmed to have multiple small ecchymoses and a swollen left knee. The doctor decides to check a full blood count and some first-line coagulation tests. The blood count is normal but the *coagulation screen* is abnormal as follows:

Prothrombin time	11 seconds (9–12)
Activated partial thromboplastin time	82 seconds (26–36)
Fibrinogen level	3.1 g/L (1.7–4.5)

1. Suggest a possible diagnosis.
2. What further blood test would you request to confirm this diagnosis?

Notes to Case 5

1. The presence of multiple bruises and joint swelling in a baby raises the possibility of non-accidental injury. It is important to remember that a bleeding disorder can lead to a very similar presentation. In this case, the combination of the symptoms and the very prolonged activated partial thromboplastin time (APTT) is very suggestive of *haemophilia*. The lack of a family history does not rule out this diagnosis as up to 30% of all new cases of haemophilia are due to recent sporadic mutations.

Symptoms may only become apparent after 6 months when the baby begins to crawl.

2. The most common form of haemophilia is haemophilia A which is characterised by a deficiency of factor VIII. A factor VIII assay was performed and this revealed a very low level (1 unit/dL) of the coagulation factor consistent with severe disease.

Case 6 [pp. 68–69]

A 62-year-old woman is admitted to hospital with a chest infection. She has no history of any blood disorder and a normal blood count. Her infection is treated with intravenous antibiotics. She is also prescribed a daily subcutaneous dose of low molecular weight heparin as prophylaxis against thromboembolism. After a week in hospital she is feeling much better with improvement in her pneumonia but the medical team notice that her platelet count is starting to fall. By day 10 of her admission it is 65×10^9/L. She has no symptoms of bleeding. On the following day, she develops a swollen left lower leg.

1. What is the most likely cause of the thrombocytopenia?
2. What is the most likely cause of the leg swelling?

Notes to Case 6

1. This patient's 'isolated thrombocytopenia' (her haemoglobin level and white cell count were normal) occurred following her admission to hospital. A diagnosis of immune thrombocytopenia (ITP) is possible but the timing is suspicious of some other cause. She is not obviously ill enough for the low platelet count to be a sign of disseminated intravascular coagulation (DIC) but it would be sensible to check first-line coagulation tests. The most likely cause is a newly commenced drug and heparin is the obvious candidate. The drug chart should be carefully scrutinised to exclude other agents which might be responsible (see p. 69, Table 34.3).

2. *Heparin induced thrombocytopenia (HIT)* is a distinct syndrome characterised by the development of antibodies to platelet factor 4 and heparin. The thrombocytopenia is typically non-severe and occurs 5–10 days after starting heparin.

Unlike other drug-induced thrombocytopenias, HIT leads to an increased risk of thromboembolism. This patient had developed a deep vein thrombosis; an ultrasound of the affected leg ruled out a haematoma and confirmed this diagnosis. Heparin was discontinued and an alternative anticoagulant substituted.

Case 7 [pp. 86–87]

A 42-year-old man is diagnosed as having stage IV *diffuse large B-cell non-Hodgkin's lymphoma*. He is treated with the RCHOP chemotherapy regimen. Two weeks after the first cycle, he presents to the haematology outpatient clinic complaining of general malaise. There are no more specific symptoms. He is initially reviewed by the clinic nursing staff who report him to appear pale and unwell. He has a pyrexia, a slight tachycardia and a normal blood pressure. A blood sample is taken for investigations including a *full blood count*:

Haemoglobin	115 g/L
MCV	83 fl
MCH	31 pg
White cell count	0.8×10^9/L
Neutrophils	0.1
Lymphocytes	0.6
Monocytes	0.1
Platelet count	132×10^9/L

1. You are asked for your opinion? What diagnosis do you suspect?
2. What is your management plan?

Notes to Case 7
1. This man has severe neutropenia following chemotherapy. His malaise and pyrexia are very likely due to *neutropenic sepsis*. It is common for the symptoms of infection in these patients to be vague with no localisation.
2. Suspected neutropenic sepsis is a medical emergency. A significant delay in the empirical administration of intravenous broad-spectrum antibiotics leads to increased mortality. He should have blood and other relevant cultures performed prior to starting antibiotics but investigations should never significantly delay antibiotic treatment. The antibiotics can be commenced in the clinic before transfer to the haematology ward. The empirical antibiotic regimens

are designed to provide protection against commonly implicated organisms (see p. 87, Table 43.2).

Case 8 [pp. 58–59]

A previously well 32-year-old man presents to his primary care practitioner complaining of a 12 week history of malaise, anorexia, weight loss and drenching night sweats. It is calculated that he has lost 15% of his normal body weight. He has also found a lump in his left neck which the doctor identifies as a 3 cm enlarged non-tender cervical lymph node. On more general examination, he has similar enlarged nodes in the axillary and inguinal regions but nothing else. He is urgently referred to the local hospital where a cervical lymph node biopsy confirms the suspected diagnosis of *classical Hodgkin's lymphoma* (nodular sclerosing histological subtype). A blood count reveals moderate anaemia and an eosinophilia. A CT scan of the neck, chest and abdomen confirms the enlarged cervical, axillary and inguinal nodes and also shows significant mediastinal and intra-abdominal lymphadenopathy. The liver and spleen are normal. Bone marrow examination is also normal.

1. What is the stage of this man's Hodgkin's lymphoma?
2. Suggest a treatment plan.
3. What is the prognosis?

Notes to Case 8
1. He has lymph node involvement above and below the diaphragm but no evidence of disease outside nodal areas (e.g. liver, bone marrow). He has night sweats and significant weight loss. This is stage IIIB disease (see p. 59, Fig. 29.3).
2. Stage IIIB disease is 'advanced stage disease'. He should receive a full course of chemotherapy with the possible addition of radiotherapy for bulky disease. The ABVD regimen is most commonly used. 'Alternating' or 'hybrid' regimens containing a larger number of drugs are under investigation. The role of PET scanning in staging and assessment of response to treatment is also under review.
3. In younger patients, the prognosis of Hodgkin's lymphoma is generally good with cure rates of 80% achievable even in advanced disease. With such high cure rates, the

potential long-term side-effects of chemotherapy (e.g. increased risk of second malignancy, sterility, cardiac disease, lung damage, endocrine dysfunction) should be fully acknowledged.

Case 9 [pp. 78–79]

A 27-year-old woman presents to the hospital accident and emergency department complaining of a day's history of a swollen right lower leg. This developed shortly after a long flight. An ultrasound scan of the leg confirms a deep vein thrombosis. The patient tells the doctor that she has a strong family history of venous thrombosis and that she has previously tested positive as being *heterozygous for the factor V Leiden mutation*. This is confirmed in her hospital notes – other thrombophilia tests were normal. She is otherwise entirely well and has had no previous episode of thrombosis.

1. What is the increased risk of venous thrombosis in people with the factor V Leiden mutation?
2. Was it the correct decision to screen her for this mutation?
3. How will the presence of heterozygosity for the factor V Leiden mutation alter the immediate clinical management?

Notes to Case 9
1. Heterozygosity for the factor V Leiden mutation gives a 4–8-fold increase in risk for venous thrombosis. This is a relatively small risk and thrombosis often only occurs where there are coexistent risk factors (e.g. prolonged immobility). Homozygosity carries a much greater venous thrombotic risk, around 50–100-fold.
2. We must presume that she was screened because one or more of her relatives tested positive for the factor V Leiden mutation and/or other thrombophilia abnormalities after an episode of venous thrombosis. Testing strategies for thrombophilia are controversial but there is generally no indication for case finding of asymptomatic relatives with low risk thrombophilia (such as factor V Leiden heterozygosity). Her testing was very likely unnecessary.
3. Patients with heritable thrombophilia should have a deep vein thrombosis treated with

heparin and warfarin as in patients without heritable thrombophilia. Thus, the presence of the factor V mutation does not affect her immediate management. The precise role of thrombophilia testing in clinical decision making remains nuclear.

Case 10 [pp. 52–53]

A 25-year-old man presents to his primary care practitioner with a 6 week history of increasing fatigue and shortness of breath on exertion. He has also noticed an intermittent sore throat and that he has been bruising more easily than usual. He has been previously well and is on no medication. On examination, he appears pale and there are a few small ecchymoses. His doctor suspects anaemia and decides to perform a *full blood count*:

Haemoglobin	64 g/L
MCV	94 fl
MCH	30 pg
Reticulocyte count	0.1%
White cell count	0.9×10^9/L
Neutrophils	0.1
Lymphocytes	0.7
Monocytes	0.1
Platelet count	9×10^9/L

On receipt of the blood count result, the doctor makes an urgent referral to the local hospital haematology department. Here, the blood count is repeated and the result confirmed. There are no abnormal cells in the blood film. A bone marrow aspirate and trephine procedure is performed. This shows a grossly hypocellular bone marrow appearance with no abnormal cells.

1. How could you describe the abnormal blood count in one word?
2. What is the likely diagnosis?
3. What is the severity of this disorder?
4. Suggest a treatment plan.

Notes to Case 10
1. *Pancytopenia*. There is reduction in haemoglobin level, white cell count and platelet count.
2. The marked hypocellularity of the bone marrow is consistent with *aplastic anaemia*. There are no abnormal cells to suggest infiltration by leukaemia or another malignant disorder. Possible causes of secondary aplastic anaemia such as

drugs and viral infections must be excluded (p. 52, Tables 26.1 and 26.2). This man had idiopathic aplastic anaemia.
3. The blood results are consistent with *very severe aplastic anaemia* (p. 53, Table 26.4).
4. In a young fit person with very severe aplastic anaemia, the best definitive therapy is likely to be an allogeneic stem cell transplant from an HLA-matched sibling or unrelated donor. In the meantime, he will need judicious use of red cell and platelet transfusions to manage symptoms arising from anaemia and thrombocytopenia. If he develops a systemic infection, he will need prompt broad-spectrum antibiotic treatment in view of his severe neutropenia.

Case 11 [pp. 64–65]

A 74-year-old man presents to his primary care practitioner complaining of a week's history of cough and increased dyspnoea. His medical records reveal that he is a smoker and that he has a history of chronic lung disease. The doctor's initial diagnosis of a chest infection is confirmed by a chest X-ray and he prescribes a course of oral antibiotics. As the patient has also complained of more longstanding fatigue he decides to check some blood tests including a *full blood count*:

Haemoglobin	196 g/L
Packed cell volume (haematocrit)	0.54
MCV	95 fl
MCH	31 pg
White cell count	9.8×10^9/L
Platelet count	182×10^9/L

In view of this abnormal result, the patient is referred to the haematology department at the local hospital. More investigations are performed including the following:

Oxygen saturation 89% (95–100)
Serum erythropoietin level 28 mU/mL (2–20)

1. What is the abnormality in the blood count?
2. What is the most likely cause of this abnormality?
3. What is the best treatment of the blood abnormality?

Notes to Case 11
1. *Polycythaemia*. This is indicated by the significantly raised haemoglobin

level and packed cell volume (also known as the haematocrit).
2. This is *secondary polycythaemia* caused by the hypoxia of chronic lung disease. The clinical history, low oxygen saturation and raised erythropoietin level are all supportive of this diagnosis. In this patient, further investigations for the cause of polycythaemia, such as screening for the *JAK2* mutation and bone marrow examination, are unnecessary (p. 64, Fig. 32.2).
3. The management of secondary polycythaemia is essentially that of the underlying cause. This man's polycythaemia is likely to improve if he stops smoking and if his respiratory function can be improved. The role of venesection in this situation is not well defined. It may be helpful where the haematocrit is very high (e.g. greater than 0.55).

Case 12 [pp. 50–51, 84–85]

A 62-year-old woman with *myelodysplastic syndrome* receives regular blood (red cell) transfusions to improve her haemoglobin level and relieve symptoms of anaemia. She has received these without problems every 3–4 weeks for the previous 6 months. On this occasion, the nurses on the hospital haematology day unit inform the duty doctor that the patient has become suddenly unwell only a few minutes after the start of the transfusion of the first unit of red cells. She is complaining of chest and loin pain and has become acutely short of breath. Her clinical observations, normal before the start of the transfusion, now show pyrexia, tachycardia and hypotension. The doctor is alarmed.

1. What diagnosis should he suspect?
2. What immediate action should he take?

Notes to Case 12
1. The doctor should strongly suspect a potentially fatal *haemolytic transfusion reaction*. The acute onset of the symptoms within minutes of starting the red cell transfusion and the changes in temperature, pulse and blood pressure are all highly suggestive of this.
2. He should immediately stop the transfusion and maintain the venous access with crystalloid. The transfused unit should be checked

(is another patient about to get a 'wrong' unit due to a mix-up?) and the blood bank informed. Urgent measures to resuscitate the patient should be undertaken as necessary. If an ABO incompatible transfusion is confirmed, or even suspected, senior medical advice should be quickly sought to ensure proper investigation, to guide the management of complications (e.g. renal failure, disseminated intravascular coagulation) and to establish the need for intensive care input.

Case 13 [pp. 62–63]

A previously well 59-year-old man presents with a 3 month history of persistent increasingly severe back and rib pain. He also complains of loss of energy. There is nothing diagnostic on examination although he appears pale and unwell. The doctor decides to arrange some investigations including blood tests. These show the patient to have a moderate normocytic normochromic anaemia with a blood film reported as 'rouleaux formation'. The biochemical tests reveal mild renal failure and hypercalcaemia.

1. This man has a haematological malignancy. What is the likely diagnosis?
2. Suggest further investigations to confirm the suspected diagnosis.
3. Suggest a treatment plan.

Notes to Case 13

1. The combination of chronic severe back and rib pain, normocytic normochromic anaemia, rouleaux formation in the blood film, renal failure and hypercalcaemia is highly suggestive of *myeloma*.
2. Vital tests to establish the diagnosis of myeloma include serum and urine electrophoresis to detect a monoclonal protein and bone marrow examination (aspirate and trephine biopsy) to assess the number of clonal plasma cells. The degree of bone disease can be determined with a combination of traditional X-rays ('skeletal survey') and MRI scanning.
3. The above tests confirmed myeloma with numerous bony lesions in the ribs and spine. In a younger fitter patient such as this man, induction chemotherapy (see p. 63) is generally followed by stem cell harvesting and intensification of

treatment with high dose melphalan and autologous stem cell transplantation. He should also receive bisphosphonate therapy.

Case 14 [pp. 34–35]

A 25-year-old man with *sickle cell anaemia (Hb SS)* presents to the casualty department of his local hospital with a 24 hour history of increasing back and shoulder pain unresponsive to oral analgesics. He has had numerous episodes of similar pain in the past, some of which have led to admission to hospital. He is clearly in distress with severe pain but the doctor can elicit no other symptoms. His medication includes a folate supplement, penicillin and hydroxycarbamide. His *full blood count* is as follows:

Haemoglobin	72 g/L
MCV	90 fl
MCH	32 pg
White cell count	9.8×10^9/L
Platelet count	365×10^9/L

1. Why does the patient not have more obvious symptoms from his significant anaemia?
2. Explain the aetiology of his pain.
3. How would you manage his symptoms?
4. What is the mechanism of action of hydroxycarbamide in this disease?

Notes to Case 14

1. When anaemia is chronic as in sickle cell disease the symptoms are often less pronounced than when anaemia of similar severity (i.e. similar haemoglobin level) develops acutely. Also, because HbS releases oxygen more readily than HbA, the symptoms of anaemia are often surprisingly mild.
2. He has a vaso-occlusive crisis. This is caused by polymerisation of deoxygenated HbS leading to inflexible sickle cells becoming lodged in small vessels. This in turn leads to oxygen deprivation of tissues and avascular necrosis of the bone marrow. Over 90% of hospital admissions for patients with sickle cell disease are for a painful crisis.
3. Management should include rest, warmth, intravenous fluids, opiate analgesia and reassurance. Patients who are ill should be referred urgently for more specialist care.
4. Hydroxycarbamide can reduce the severity of the disease by increasing

the level of fetal haemoglobin in red cells.

Case 15 [pp. 76–77]

A 55-year-old woman is admitted to hospital with a chest infection. Despite prompt antibiotic treatment she deteriorates and develops the symptoms and signs of severe sepsis. She is transferred to the intensive care unit. Here it is noted that she has oozing of blood from her cannulation sites. The medical team request a *full blood count* and *coagulation tests*:

Haemoglobin	102 g/L
MCV	81 fl
MCH	30 pg
White cell count	9.2×10^9/L
Platelet count	31×10^9/L
Prothrombin time	26 seconds (9–12)
Activated partial thromboplastin time	58 seconds (26–36)
Fibrinogen level	0.8 g/L (1.7–4.5)
Fibrin degradation products (FDPs)	Increased

1. What is the likely cause of the patient's bleeding?
2. How should this acquired bleeding disorder be managed?

Notes to Case 15

1. The combination of thrombocytopenia, prolonged prothrombin time (PT) and activated partial thromboplastin time (APTT), reduced fibrinogen level and increased fibrin degradation products (or D-dimers) in a very ill patient with widespread bleeding is characteristic of *disseminated intravascular coagulation (DIC)*.
2. The cornerstone of management of DIC is the treatment of the underlying disorder – in this case sepsis. In addition, bleeding may be reduced by the transfusion of platelets, fresh frozen plasma (FFP – a source of coagulation factors) and cryoprecipitate (a source of fibrinogen). Careful monitoring of the bleeding symptoms and repeated blood counts and coagulation tests are vital to guide the appropriate use of these blood products. Recombinant activated protein C may be of benefit in DIC associated with sepsis and could be considered here.

Index

Page numbers ending in 'b', 'f' and 't' refer to Boxes, Figures and Tables respectively

A

AA see Aplastic anaemia (AA)
Abdomen, examination, 17
Abdominal lymph nodes, examination, 16
Abnormalities
  blood count, 15
  clotting tests, first-line, 20t
  coagulation see Coagulation disorders
  common haematological, 14t
  fibrinogen, 75
  genetic see Genetic abnormalities
  haemoglobin, 29
  lymphocytes, 9
  neutrophils, 7
  red cells
    indices, 22
    metabolism, 29
  splenic, 10–11
  stomach and ileum (vitamin B_{12} deficiency), 27
ABO blood grouping, 82–83
  neonatal disorders, 84, 90
  platelet transfusion, 85
ABVD (doxorubicin, bleomycin, vinblastine, dacarbazine) chemotherapy protocol, 59
Aciclovir, 87
Acidosis, 85
Acrocyanosis, 30
Actin, 4
Actin–myosin assembly, cell membrane, 6
Activated partial thromboplastin time (APTT)
  acquired haemophilia, 77
  disseminated intravascular coagulation, 76
  haemostasis, 12–13
  and heparin, 80
  laboratory haematology, 20
  prolonged, in haemophilia, 72
  vitamin K deficiency, 77
  Von Willebrand disease, 75
  see also Prothrombin time (PT)
Activated protein C (APC), 78, 102
Activating receptors, natural killer (NK) cells, 9
Acupuncture, 95
Acute graft-versus-host disease, 56
Acute immune thrombocytopenia (ITP), 68, 68t, 69f
Acute lymphoblastic leukaemia (ALL)
  and acute myeloid leukaemia, 40
  in adults, 43
  allogeneic stem cell transplantation, 56
  in children, 43
  classification, 42
  clinical features, 42
  diagnosis, 42–43
  incidence, at different ages, 42f

lymphocytosis, 9
  management and outcome, 43
  poor prognosis, factors predicting, 43t
  subtypes, 42
Acute monocytic leukaemia, 40f
Acute myeloid leukaemia (AML)
  and acute lymphoblastic leukaemia, 40
  age of presentation and AML characteristics, 41f
  allogeneic stem cell transplantation, 56
  and aplastic anaemia, 53
  blood count and film, 40
  bone marrow aspirate and trephine, 40
  chemotherapy, 41
  chromosome deletions and additions, 38
  classification, 40
  clinical features, 40
  common genetic abnormalities, 41t
  cytochemistry, 40–41
  cytogenetics, 41
  diagnosis, 40–41
  epigenetic therapies, 55
  essential thrombocythaemia, progression from, 66
  FLT3 inhibitors, 55
  fluorescence in situ hybridisation, 38f
  immunophenotyping, 41
  management, 41
  molecular biology, 41
  monoclonal antibodies, 55
  multi-drug resistance, 54
  and myelodysplastic syndromes, 39, 50
  and myeloproliferative disorders, 39
  peripheral blood film, 39f
  platelet function disorders, 71
  polycythaemia, 65
  prognosis, 41
  smoking, 15
  stem cell transplantation, 41
  supportive care, 41
  tyrosine kinase inhibitors, 55
Acute obstetric haemorrhage, 89t
Acute phase response
  in elderly people, 92
  lack of, in essential thrombocythaemia, 66
  measurement, 20–21
Acute promyelocytic leukaemia, 40–41
Acute venous thrombosis, 79
Adaptive immune response, 9
Adeno-associated virus (AAV), 103
Adenopathy, 16
Adenosine triphosphate (ATP), 5
Adhesion molecules
  bone marrow structure, 2
  neutrophils, 6
  splenic structure, 10

Adult T-cell leukaemia lymphoma (ATLL), 39f, 49
Afibrinogenaemia, 75
Afro-Caribbean population, sickle cell anaemia, 34
Agglutination, cold (cold autoimmune haemolytic anaemia), 31f
AIHA see Autoimmune haemolytic anaemia (AIHA)
Albumin, 20, 85
Alcohol misuse, 15, 96
Aldosterone, 4
Alemtuzumab, 48, 53, 55
ALK1 (gene mutation), 71
Alkylating agents, 54
ALL see Acute lymphoblastic leukaemia (ALL)
Allergic disorders, 7, 15
Alloantibodies, 30–31
Allogeneic stem cell transplantation
  acute lymphoblastic leukaemia, 43
  adult T-cell leukaemia lymphoma, 49
  aplastic anaemia, 53
  bone marrow harvesting, 107
  chronic lymphocytic leukaemia, 47
  chronic myeloid leukaemia, 45
  defined, 56
  herpes zoster following, 87f
  myelodysplastic syndromes, 51
  non-myeloablative ('reduced intensity'), 57
  and syngeneic SCT, 56
  thalassaemias, 33
Alloimmune thrombocytopenia, 91
All-trans-retinoic acid (ATRA), 41, 55
Alpha-1-antitrypsin, acute phase response, 21
Alpha-2-macroglobulin, 20
Alteplase, 81
AML see Acute myeloid leukaemia (AML)
Anaemia
  acute lymphoblastic leukaemia, 42
  acute phase response, 20
  aetiological classification, 22–23
  aplastic see Aplastic anaemia (AA)
  blood count, 18
  of chronic disease see Anaemia of chronic disease (ACD)
  classification, 22–23, 23f
  congenital dyserythropoietic anaemias, 91
  definition, 22
  Diamond–Blackfan, 91
  dilutional, in pregnancy, 88
  in elderly people, 22–23, 92
  Fanconi's anaemia, 52
  general features, 22

haemolytic see Haemolytic anaemia
  hypersplenism, 11
  iron deficiency see Iron deficiency anaemia
  macrocytic, 22, 25, 27
  management, 23
  megaloblastic see Megaloblastic anaemia
  microcytic, 22
  morphological classification, 22
  myelodysplastic syndromes, 50
  myelofibrosis, 67
  myeloma, 62
  normochromic, 22
  normocytic, 22
  packed cell volume, 22
  pernicious, 16, 26–27, 88
  platelet function disorders, 71
  in pregnancy, 22, 88
  of prematurity, 90
  prevalence, 22
  prolymphocytic leukaemia, 48
  symptoms attributable to, 14
  T-cell large granular lymphocyte leukaemia, 48–49
  unexplained, in elderly people, 92
  see also Haemoglobin; Red cells
Anaemia of chronic disease (ACD), 36–37
Anagrelide, 66
Anaphylaxis, 25
Angiogenesis, bone marrow abnormality, 67
Angular stomatitis, 24f, 26
Ankyrin, 4
Anopheline mosquitoes, 98
Anorexia, malignant disease, 95
Antecubital fossa, veins at, 104
Anterior iliac crest, 106–107
Anthracycline, 41, 54
Anti-angiogenic agents, 55
Antibiotic treatment, 87, 87t
Antibodies
  antileucocyte, 84
  HTLV-1, 49
  immune, 82–83
  isoantibodies, 30–31
  monoclonal, 55
  naturally occurring, 82
Antibody screening, 82–83
Anti-CD33 (Mylotarg), 55
Anti-chymotrypsin, acute phase response, 21
Anticoagulation
  in elderly people, 92
  heparin, 80
  new agents, 81
  new drugs, 102–103
  in pregnancy, 89
  thrombolytic therapy, 81
  warfarin, 80–81, 80f
Anti-D immunoglobulin (Ig), 90
Antidiuretic hormone (ADH), 4
Antiemetics, 95
Antifibrinolytic agents, 70, 73
Antigen-presenting cells, 8f, 10

Antiglobulin test, 83f
Anti-helminthic agents, 99
Antileucocyte antibodies, 84
Anti-leukaemic drugs, 54
Antimetabolites, 54
Antimicrobial prophylaxis, 87
Antiphospholipid antibody
    syndrome, 79
Antithrombin (AT), 13, 79–80
Antithymocyte globulin (ATG), 51,
    53
Anti-tissue transglutaminase, 25
Aorto-gonad-mesonephros (AGM)
    region, embryo, 2
APCR (activated protein resistance
    ratio), 78–79
Apixaban, 102–103
Aplastic anaemia (AA)
    aetiology, 52
    classification, 52
    clinical features, 52
    diagnosis, 52–53
    immunosuppression, 52–53
    management, 53
    removal of cause, 53
    restoring normal
        haematopoiesis, 53
    severity measurement, 53
Apoptosis, 38, 60
Arteriovenous malformations
    (AVMs), 71
Ashkenazi Jews, factor VI
    deficiency, 75
Aspergillus fumigatus, 86–87
Aspirate, bone marrow
    acute lymphoblastic leukaemia,
        42
    acute myeloid leukaemia, 40
    advantages and disadvantages,
        19
    aplastic anaemia, 52–53
    aspiration procedure, 106–107
    chronic lymphocytic leukaemia,
        46
    examination procedure, 19
    hairy cell leukaemia, 48
    increased reticuloendothelial
        iron stores in anaemia of
        chronic disease, 37f
    iron deficiency anaemia, 25
    in megaloblastic anaemia, 26f
    needle, 106f
    pernicious anaemia, 26
    polycythaemia, 64
    systemic disease, 96
    thrombocytopenia, 69
Aspirin
    essential thrombocythaemia, 66
    platelet function disorder caused
        by, 70–71
    polycythaemia, 64–65
Asplenia syndrome, 10–11
Asplenism, 10–11, 11t
ATG see Antithymocyte globulin
    (ATG)
ATRA see All-trans-retinoic acid
    (ATRA)
Autoantibodies, 27, 30
Autoimmune haemolysis, 46
Autoimmune haemolytic anaemia
    (AIHA), 30
Autoimmune thrombocytopenia,
    46

Autologous stem cell
    transplantation, 56–57
    acute lymphoblastic leukaemia,
        41, 43
    bone marrow harvesting, 107
    Hodgkin's lymphoma, 59
    myeloma, 63
Automated haematology counters,
    18
Axillary lymphadenopathy,
    lymphoma, 60f
Axillary nodes, examination, 16
Azacitidine, 55
Azathioprine, 30
Azoles, 87

B

Babesiosis, 99
Backache, myeloma, 62
Bacterial infection, 86, 97
    see also Antibiotic treatment
Basophils, 7
B-cell lymphomas, 55, 97
BCL2 gene, non-Hodgkin's
    lymphoma, 60
BCR-ABL oncogene, 38
    chronic myeloid leukaemia,
        44–45
    molecular biology, 101
    treatments, 55
Bence Jones protein, myeloma,
    62
Bendamustine, 47, 54
Bernard–Soulier syndrome, 70
Biliary obstruction, vitamin K
    deficiency, 77
Bilirubin, 5
Biopsy
    lymph node
        Hodgkin's lymphoma, 58, 58f
        non-Hodgkin's lymphoma,
            60–61
    trephine see Trephine biopsy,
        bone marrow
Bisphosphonate, myeloma, 63, 94
Black people, neutrophil counts, 7
Blast cells
    acute lymphoblastic leukaemia,
        42
    acute myeloid leukaemia, 40
    morphology, 42f
Blast crisis, chronic myeloid
    leukaemia, 44–45
Bleeding
    disseminated intravascular
        coagulation, 76
    haemophilia A, 72–73, 72f
    intracranial see Intracranial
        bleeding
    liver disease, 77
    myeloma, 62
    thrombocytopenia, 14, 68
    tranexamic acid, 73
    Von Willebrand disease, 74–75
Bleeding time, 70–71
Bleomycin, 59
Blood
    clotting of see Clotting of blood
    lymphocytes, mature, 8f
    ordering practicalities, 83
    peripheral see Peripheral blood

    see also Blood count; Blood
        groups; Blood tests; Blood
        transfusion; Plasma; Platelet
        function disorders; Platelets
Blood count
    abnormalities, past medical
        history, 15
    acute lymphoblastic leukaemia,
        42
    acute myeloid leukaemia, 40
    aplastic anaemia, 52
    Hodgkin's lymphoma, 58–59
    iron deficiency anaemia, 25
    laboratory haematology, 18
    lymphocytes, 9, 46
    neutrophils, 6
    pernicious anaemia, 24
    report, 18–19
    Von Willebrand disease, 75
Blood films
    acute lymphoblastic leukaemia,
        42
    acute myeloid leukaemia, 39f,
        40
    anaemia of chronic disease,
        36–37
    aplastic anaemia, 52
    chronic lymphocytic leukaemia,
        46, 46f
    chronic myeloid leukaemia, 44,
        45f
    cold autoimmune haemolytic
        anaemia, cold agglutination
        in, 31f
    essential thrombocythaemia, 66f
    haemolytic disease of the
        newborn, 90f
    hereditary spherocytosis, 29
    hyposplenism, 11f
    iron deficiency, 25f
    making, 18–19
    megaloblastic anaemia, 27f
    microangiopathic haemolytic
        anaemia, 31f
    morphological terms, 19t
    myelofibrosis, 66f
    myeloma, 62f
    pernicious anaemia, 24
    sickle cell anaemia (HbSS), 34f
    thalassaemias, 33f
    thrombocytopenia, 68f–69f
    warm autoimmune haemolytic
        anaemia, 30f
Blood groups
    ABO group, 82–85, 90
    gel system, using, 82f, 83
    incompatibility, 82, 90
    tests, 82–83
    Von Willebrand disease, 75
Blood tests
    antibody screening, 83
    antiglobulin, 83f
    blood grouping, 82–83
    chronic myeloid leukaemia, 44f
    crossmatching, 83
    donor blood, 82
    prior to transfusion, 82–83
    see also Venepuncture; Venous
        access
Blood transfusion
    acute myeloid leukaemia, 41
    allogeneic, alternatives to, 85
    anaemia, 23

aplastic anaemia, 53
    complications, 84–85
    delayed complications, 84–85
    in elderly people, 92
    granulocytes, 85
    haemolytic reactions, 84
    immediate complications, 84
    incompatibility, 82
    infection, 84
    massive, 85
    myelodysplastic syndromes, 51
    non-haemolytic reactions, 84
    platelets, 71, 85
    practicalities, 85
    red cells, 84–85, 84t
    safety factors, 82
    sickle cell anaemia (HbSS), 35
    testing before, 82–83
    transfusion associated
        circulation overload, 84
    transfusion-related acute lung
        injury, 84
    see also under Platelets; Stem cell
        transplantation (SCT)
B-lymphocytes, 8–9
    antigen-stimulated mature, in
        CLL, 46
    cold autoimmune haemolytic
        anaemia, 30
    germinal-centre, in HL, 58
    splenic structure, 10
Bone disease, myeloma, 62–63
Bone marrow
    acute myeloid leukaemia
        subtypes, appearance in,
        40f
    angiogenesis, 67
    aspirate see Aspirate, bone
        marrow
    examination, 19
    failure of production, in
        thrombocytopenia, 68
    haematopoiesis, 2–3, 3f
    harvesting, 107
    normal, 2f
    prostatic carcinoma, 97f
    regulators, haematopoiesis, 2–3,
        3f
    specific conditions, effects
        Hodgkin's lymphoma, 58–59
        myelodysplastic syndromes,
            50
        myelofibrosis, 66
        myeloma, 62, 62f
    stem cell hierarchy, 2, 3f
    structure, 2
    trephine appearance, in human
        T-cell leukaemic lymphoma,
        39f
Bortezomib, 55, 63
Bovine spongiform
    encephalopathy (BSE), 84
Brentuximab, 55, 59
Bronchoalveolar lavage, 86
Bruising, acquired haemophilia,
    76f
Bullae, haemorrhagic, 76f
Burkitt's lymphoma, 42, 60–61
    endemic, 99
Burr cells, renal failure, 96
Busulfan, 54
'Butterfly needle,' venepuncture,
    104

C

Cachexia, malignant disease, 95
Cancer see Malignant disease
Candida infection, 86
Cannulation, 105
Carbon dioxide, transport, 4
Cardiac overactivity, anaemia, 22
Cardiopulmonary bypass, platelet
    function disorders, 71
Caspofungin, 87
CD4 surface marker
    HIV/AIDS, 9
    and T-lymphocytes, 8
    treatment advances, 102
CD8 surface marker, 8
CD20 antigen, 55
Cell cycle, 54
Cellulose acetate electrophoresis,
    35f
Central nervous system (CNS)
    disease
    acute lymphoblastic leukaemia,
        42
    monocytic/monoblastic
        leukaemia, 40
    non-Hodgkin's lymphoma, 60
Central venous cannulation, 105
Cerebral malaria, 98
Cervical lymph nodes,
    enlargement, 16
Chemotaxis, 6
Chemotherapy
    acute myeloid leukaemia, 41
    combination, 54, 99, 102
    consolidation, 41
    elderly people see under Elderly
        people
    general principles, 54
    high-dose, in stem cell
        transplantation, 56–57
    Hodgkin's lymphoma, 59
    immunosuppression in, 86
    induction, 41
    major classes of conventional
        drugs, 54
    multi-drug resistance, 54
    myelodysplastic syndromes, 51
    palliative, 94
    phase-specific and phase
        non-specific, 54
    and Philadelphia chromosome,
        43
    related treatments, 54–55
Children see Paediatric
    haematology
Chlorambucil, 54
    chronic lymphocytic leukaemia,
        47
    follicular lymphoma, 61
    myeloma, 63
Chloroquine, 99
Cholesterol, 4
CHOP regimen, diffuse large
    B-cell lymphoma, 61
Chromosomal abnormalities see
    Genetic abnormalities
Chromosome deletions and
    additions, leukaemia, 38
Chronic benign neutropenia, 7
Chronic graft-versus-host disease,
    56

Chronic granulomatous disease, 7
Chronic immune
    thrombocytopenia (ITP),
    68t, 69
Chronic lymphocytic leukaemia
    (CLL)
    clinical features, 46
    diagnosis, 46
    in elderly people, 46, 93
    humoral immunity defects, 86
    incidence, 38
    lymphocytosis, 9
    management, 46–47, 47f
    monoclonal antibodies, 55
    prognosis, 47t
    staging, 46
    whole genome sequencing,
        101f
Chronic myeloid leukaemia
    (CML)
    accelerated phase, 44–45
    advanced disease, 45
    allogeneic stem cell
        transplantation, 56
    chronic phase, 44–45
    clinical features, 44
    diagnosis and monitoring,
        44–45
    drug therapy, 45, 45t, 55, 93
    and essential thrombocythaemia,
        66
    fluorescence in situ
        hybridisation, 100f
    pathogenesis, 44
    Philadelphia (Ph) chromosome,
        38–39, 44, 44f
    predisposing factors, 39
    treatment, 45, 55
Chronic myelomonocytic
    leukaemia (CMML), 50
Chronic renal failure
    platelet function disorders, 71
    systemic disease, 96
Chronic thrombocytopenia, 68
Ciclosporin, 30, 53
Circulating pool, neutrophils, 6
Cirrhosis, hepatitis risk, 73
Citrate agar electrophoresis, 21
Citrate toxicity, massive blood
    transfusion, 85
Cladribine (2-CDA), 48, 49f
CLL see Chronic lymphocytic
    leukaemia (CLL)
Clostridium difficile, 86
Clotting of blood, 12
    first-line tests, 20t
    prothrombin time test, 20
Clubbing of nails, polycythaemia,
    65f
Cluster differentiation (CD), 21
CML see Chronic myeloid
    leukaemia (CML)
CMV see Cytomegalovirus
    (CMV)
Coagulation
    abnormal, symptoms
        attributable to, 14
    disorders see Coagulation
        disorders
    physiological pathways, 12–13,
        13f
    regulation of, 13
    tests, 20

Coagulation cascade
    defects, 14
    haemostasis, 12, 13t
Coagulation disorders
    acquired, 76–77
    chronic renal failure, 96
    disseminated intravascular
        coagulation see
        Disseminated intravascular
        coagulation (DIC)
    factor deficiencies, 75
    fibrinogen abnormalities, 75
    haemophilia, acquired, 76f, 77
    history taking, 14
    hypercoagulability in malignant
        disease, 96
    liver disease, 77
    in pregnancy, 89
    vitamin K deficiency, 76–77
Coagulation factors, 12
Coeliac disease, splenic atrophy,
    10–11
Cold autoimmune haemolytic
    anaemia, 30
Collagen receptors, 12
Colon carcinoma, iron deficiency
    anaemia, 24f
Colonoscopy, iron deficiency,
    25
Colony-forming units (CFUs), 2
Colony-stimulating factors (CSFs),
    3
Combination chemotherapy, 54,
    99, 102
Comparative genomic
    hybridisation, 100
Complementary therapy, 95
Complete remission (CR), acute
    myeloid leukaemia, 41
Computed tomography (CT) scan,
    59, 61
Congenital dyserythropoietic
    anaemias (CDAs), 91
Connective tissue disease, 71, 96
Coombs' test, autoimmune
    haemolytic anaemia, 30
Cords of Billroth, 10
Coronary atherosclerosis, 79
Corticosteroid treatment
    anorexia and cachexia, in
        malignancy, 95
    monocytopenia, 7
    pain relief, 94
    in pregnancy, 89
    see also Prednisolone; Steroid
        treatment
Co-trimoxazole, 87
Counselling see Genetic
    counselling
C-reactive protein (CRP), 21,
    36–37
Creutzfeldt-Jakob disease (CJD), as
    contradiction to blood
    donation, 82
Crossmatching, blood tests, 83
Cryoprecipitate
    acquired coagulation disorders,
        76–77
    transfusion, 85
Crystalloid solution, 84, 91
CT scans see Computed
    tomography (CT) scan
Cultures, cell, 2

Cyanmethemoglobin method,
    automated haematology
    counters, 18
Cyanotic congenital heart disease,
    65f
Cyclical neutropenia, 7
Cyclooxygenase-1 (COX-1), 70–71
Cyclophosphamide, 54
    acute lymphoblastic leukaemia,
        43
    aplastic anaemia, 53
    chronic lymphocytic leukaemia,
        47
    diffuse large B-cell lymphoma, 61
    follicular lymphoma, 61
    myeloma, 63
Cytochemistry, 40–42
Cytogenetics, 41, 43
Cytokines, 6, 10, 66
Cytomegalovirus (CMV)
    pneumonitis, 87
    red cell transfusion
        complications, 84
    thrombocytopenia, 68
Cytopenia, supportive care, 55
Cytoplasm, platelets, 12
Cytosine arabinoside, 54
    acute lymphoblastic leukaemia,
        43
    acute myeloid leukaemia, 41
Cytoskeleton, 4
Cytotoxic drugs
    major classes, 54
    side-effects, 54
    see also Chemotherapy

D

Dabigatran etexilate, 102–103
Dacarbazine, 59
Dactylitis, sickle cell anaemia, 34f
Dasatinib, 45, 55
Daunorubicin, 54
    acute lymphoblastic leukaemia,
        43
    acute myeloid leukaemia, 41
DDAVP (desmopressin) see
    Desmopressin (DDAVP)
Decitabine, 55
Deep vein thrombosis (DVT), 78,
    89
Desferrioxamine, subcutaneous, 32
Dendritic cells, follicular, 10
Desmopressin (DDAVP)
    haemophilia, 73
    platelet function disorders,
        70–71
    Von Willebrand disease, 75
Developing world, diseases
    affecting, 7, 22, 98–99
Dexamethasone, 63, 94
Dialysis, 71
Diamond–Blackfan anaemia, 91
DIC see Disseminated
    intravascular coagulation
    (DIC)
Diet
    malabsorption see
        Malabsorption
    vitamin B12 deficiency see
        Vitamin B12 deficiency
    and vitamin K deficiency, 77

Differential white cell count, 18

Differentiating agents, 55

Diffuse large B-cell lymphoma (DLBCL), 61, 100f

Direct antiglobulin test (DAT), 30, 90

Disseminated intravascular coagulation (DIC)
  acute myeloid leukaemia, 40
  bleeding, 76
  diagnosis and management, 76
  fibrinogen, quantitation, 20
  haemolytic transfusion reactions, 84
  haemorrhagic bullae and gangrene, 76f
  malignant disease, 96
  pathophysiology, 76f
  in pregnancy, 88–89
  protein C and S deficiencies, 78–79
  thrombocytopenia in neonate, 91
  and thrombophilia, 78

DNA analysis techniques, 83, 100–101

DNA synthesis, megaloblastic anaemia, 24

Donor blood, 82

Donor lymphocyte infusions (DLIs), 57

Doxorubicin, 54
  diffuse large B-cell lymphoma, 61
  Hodgkin's lymphoma, 59

Doxycycline, malaria, 99

Drug history, 15, 69

Drug-induced conditions
  aplastic anaemia, 52t
  glucose-6-phosphate dehydrogenase (G6PD) deficiency, 29
  nausea and vomiting, 95
  platelet function disorders, 70–71
  thrombocytopenia, 69

Drug treatment
  anticoagulant therapy see Anticoagulation
  side-effects see Side-effects
  specific conditions
    chronic myeloid leukaemia, 45, 45t, 93
    leukaemia, 54
    malaria, 99
    myeloma, 63, 94
    nausea and vomiting, 95
    polycythaemia, 64–65
    syringe drivers, continuous infusions, 95
  see also Chemotherapy; Treatment of conditions; specific drugs

'Dry tap,' bone marrow aspiration, 106

Dyes, blood film, 18–19

Dysfibrinogenaemia, 75, 79

Dyskeratosis congenita, 52

Dyspnoea, 22, 95

E

Edoxaban, 102–103

Ehlers–Danlos syndrome, 71

Elderly people
  anaemia, 22–23, 92
  anticoagulation, 92
  chronic lymphocytic leukaemia in, 46, 93
  essential thrombocythaemia, 66
  haematopoiesis, 92
  haemophilia and other inherited blood disorders, 77, 92–93
  iron deficiency, 24, 92
  malignant disease, 92–93, 93t
    chemotherapy contraindications, 41, 43, 93
    chronic lymphocytic leukaemia, 46
    prolymphocytic leukaemia, 48
    thrombosis, 92, 92f
    vitamin K supplementation, 92

Electrical impedance, cell counting and sizing, 18

Electronic crossmatching, 83

Electron microscopy, 48f

Electrophoresis, 21
  cellulose acetate, 35f
  electrophoretic strip, myeloma, 62f
  sickle cell anaemia, 34, 35f
  thalassaemias, 33f

Embden–Meyerhof pathway, 5, 29

Endemic Burkitt's lymphoma, 99

Endemic malaria, 99

End of life care, 95

Endoglin (gene mutation), 71

Endoscopy, iron deficiency, 25

Endothelial cell barrier, 12

Enterobacter spp., 86

Eosinophils, 7

Epigenetics, 38–39, 55

Epipodophyllotoxins, 54

Epstein–Barr virus (EBV)
  endemic Burkitt's lymphoma, 99
  Hodgkin's lymphoma, 58
  mononucleosis, 97
  non-Hodgkin's lymphoma, 60

Erythrocyte sedimentation rate (ESR)
  acute phase response, measurement, 20
  anaemia of chronic disease, 36–37
  myeloma, 62

Erythropoiesis, 22–23, 64

Erythropoietin, 4, 55
  anaemia of chronic disease, 37
  myelodysplastic syndromes, 51
  myeloma, 63
  in pregnancy, 88
  radioimmunoassay, estimation by, 64
  renal failure, in elderly, 92

Escherichia coli (E. coli), 31, 86

ESR see Erythrocyte sedimentation rate (ESR)

Essential thrombocythaemia (ET)
  clinical features, 66
  diagnosis, 66
  management, 66
  polycythaemia, 64
  splenic atrophy, 10–11
  systemic enquiry, 15

Ethnic origin
  disorder type, 16
  factor VI deficiency, 75

neutrophil counts, black people, 7
  sickle cell anaemia, 34

Ethylene diamine tetra-acetic acid (EDTA), 18, 21

Etoposide, 54

Examination
  blood films, 18–19
  bone marrow, 19
  of patient, 16–17

Exsanguination, 12

Extended spectrum beta-lactamases (ESBLs), 86

Extracorporeal photochemotherapy, adult T-cell leukaemia lymphoma, 49

Extrinsic pathway, platelets, 12–13, 13f

Eyes, sickle cell anaemia, 34

F

FAB (French–American–British) classification, 39
  acute lymphoblastic leukaemia, 42
  acute myeloid leukaemia, 40
  myelodysplastic syndromes, 50

Factor II, 12

Factor V
  activated partial thromboplastin time, 20
  coagulation disorders, deficiencies in, 75
  platelets, 12–13
  prothrombin time test, 20

Factor Va, 12

Factor V Leiden (FVR506Q), familial thrombophilia, 78

Factor VII
  platelets, 12–13
  pregnancy, increase in, 88
  prothrombin time test, 20

Factor VIIa, 12–13
  factor VI deficiency, 75
  platelet function disorders, 70

Factor VIII
  activated partial thromboplastin time, 20
  C assay, 75
  haemophilia, 72–73, 73f
    clinical severity of haemophilia A and factor VIII level, 14, 72t
    see also Haemophilia A
  platelets, 12–13
  pregnancy, increase in, 88

Factor VIIIa, 12–13

Factor VIIIc/tissue factor pathway inhibitors, 102

Factor IX
  activated partial thromboplastin time, 20
  haemophilia B, 73
  platelets, 12–13

Factor X
  activated partial thromboplastin time, 20
  platelets, 12–13
  pregnancy, increase in, 88
  prothrombin time test, 20

Factor Xa, 12

Factor XI
  activated partial thromboplastin time, 20
  coagulation disorders, deficiencies in, 75
  platelets, 12–13

Factor XII
  activated partial thromboplastin time, 20
  coagulation disorders, deficiencies in, 75
  platelets, 12–13

Factor XIII, 12–13, 75

Familial thrombophilia, 78–79

Family history, 15
  haemophilia, 72

Fanconi's anaemia, 52

Fatigue, in malignant disease, 94–95

Felty syndrome, 96

Fetus, sites of blood production in, 2f

Fibrinogen, plasma
  abnormalities, 75
  acute phase response, 21
  pregnancy, increase in, 88
  quantitation, 20

Fibrinolysis/fibrinolytic system, 13

Fibroblasts, Hodgkin's lymphoma, 58

Filariasis, 99

Flow cytometry
  acute myeloid leukaemia, 41
  haematopoiesis, 2
  laboratory haematology, 21
  platelet function disorders, 70

FLT3 inhibitors, acute myeloid leukaemia, 55

Fluconazole, 87

Fludarabine, 54
  chronic lymphocytic leukaemia, 47
  follicular lymphoma, 61
  myeloma, 63
  prolymphocytic leukaemia, 48

Fluorescence in situ hybridisation (FISH), 38f, 100

Folate deficiency
  megaloblastic anaemia, 26–27
  in pregnancy, 88

Follicular lymphoma, 61, 102, 102f

Fondaparinux, 80

French-American-British classification see FAB (French–American–British) classification

Fresh frozen plasma (FFP)
  acquired coagulation disorders, 76–77
  indications for use, 85t

Full blood count (FBC), 18

Functional assay, vWF antigen, 75

Functional cytotoxicity assays, 102

Fungal infection, 86–87

G

Gaisbock's syndrome, 64–65

Gametocytes, 98

Ganciclovir, 87

Gangrene, 76f

G-CSF *see* Granulocyte colony-stimulating factor (G-CSF)
Gel technology, blood grouping, 82f, 83
Gene profiling, 100
General anaesthesia, bone marrow aspiration in children, 106
General examination, 16
Gene therapy
　haemophilia A, 73
　sickle cell anaemia (HbSS), 35
　treatment advances, 103
Genetic abnormalities
　17p deletions, in CLL, 47
　adult T-cell leukaemia lymphoma, 48
　antenatal detection, 101
　aplastic anaemia, 52
　β-chain gene, in sickle cell syndromes, 34–35
　carrier detection, 101
　haemophilia A, 72
　leukaemia, 38–39, 41t
　　acute lymphoblastic leukaemia, 42, 43t
　　acute myeloid leukaemia, 41
　　adult T-cell leukaemia lymphoma, 49
　　chronic myeloid leukaemia, 44–45
　myelodysplastic syndromes, 50
　myeloma, 62–63
　non-Hodgkin's lymphoma, 60
　Philadelphia chromosome *see* Philadelphia (Ph) chromosome
　platelet function disorders, 71
　polycythaemia, 64
　in tropical regions, 98
　see also Cytogenetics; Epigenetics
Genetic counselling
　haemophilia A, 73
　sickle cell syndromes, 35
　thrombophilia, 79
　Von Willebrand disease, 75
Genitourinary complications, sickle cell anaemia, 34
Gentamicin, 87
Germ cells, prechemotherapy storage, 54
Gestational thrombocytopenia, 88
Giemsa stain, 18–19, 98
Glanzmann's thrombasthenia, 70
Globin chains, 5
Glossitis
　iron deficiency, 24f
　pernicious anaemia, 26, 27f
Glucose-6-phosphate dehydrogenase (G6PD) deficiency, 29
Glycoprotein (GP) la/IIa complex, 12
Glycoprotein (GP) lb/IX/V complex, 12, 70
Glycoprotein (GP) llb/IIIa complex, 12, 70
Gonadal failure, chemotherapy treatment, 54
Gout, 64, 65f
Graft-versus-host disease (GVHD), 56, 57f
Graft-versus-leukaemia (GVL) effects, 57

Graft-versus-tumour (GVT) effects, 57
Gram-negative bacilli, 86
Granulocyte colony-stimulating factor (G-CSF), 93
　chemotherapy and related treatments, 55
　stem cell transplantation, 56–57
Granulocytes
　blood transfusion, 85
　defined, 6
　Hodgkin's lymphoma, 58
　see also Basophils; Eosinophils; Neutrophils
Growth factors
　aplastic anaemia, 53
　and bone marrow, 2–3
　haematopoietic growth factor therapy, 55
　neutropenia, 87

H

Haem, protoporphyrin of, 5
Haemarthroses (bleeding into joints), 14
Haematoma, haemophilia, 72
Haematopoiesis
　and ageing, 92
　aplastic anaemia, restoring in, 53
　bone marrow, 2–3, 3f
　myelodysplastic syndromes, abnormalities in, 50
　splenic structure, 10
Haematopoietic growth factor therapy, 55
Haematopoietic stem cells (HSCs), 2
Haematoxylin and eosin (H&E) stain, 19
Haemoglobin
　abnormalities, 29
　blood count, 18
　cellulose acetate electrophoresis, to separate, 35f
　high concentration in polycythaemia, 64
　low concentration *see* Anaemia
　molecule, essential elements, 5f
　normal concentrations, 22, 22t
　transport, 5
Haemoglobinaemia, 30
Haemoglobin molecule (HbA), 5
Haemoglobinopathies
　in children, 15–16
　electrophoresis, 21
　see also specific conditions, such as thalassaemia
Haemoglobinuria, 30
Haemolysis
　autoimmune, 46
　autoimmune haemolytic anaemia, 30
　chronic lymphocytic leukaemia, 46–47
　general features, 28–29
Haemolytic anaemia
　acquired disorders, 30–31
　autoimmune, 30
　classification, 28t
　diagnosis, 28–29
　general features and inherited disorders, 28–29

　isoimmune, 30–31
　microangiopathic, 31, 31f
　and sickle cell anaemia, 34
Haemolytic disease of the newborn (HDN), 90, 90f
　blood group incompatibility, 82, 90
Haemolytic transfusion reactions, 84
Haemolytic uraemic syndrome (HUS), 31
Haemophilia
　acquired, 76f, 77
　in children, 15
　on demand treatment, 72–73
　in elderly people, 77, 92–93
　gene therapy, 103
　joint examination, 16
　see also Haemophilia A; Haemophilia B
Haemophilia A
　access to therapy, 98
　bleeding, 72–73, 72f
　carrier state and genetic counselling, 73
　clinical features, 72
　clinical severity and factor VIII level, 14, 72t
　diagnosis, 72
　treatment complications, 72
Haemophilia B, 73, 103
Haemophilia centres, 72
Haemophilus influenzae, 11
Haemorrhage
　acute obstetric, 89t
　coagulation disorders, 14
　fibrinogen abnormalities, 75
　thrombocytopenia, 14, 68
　see also Bleeding
Haemorrhagic bullae, 76f
Haemosiderin, 28
Haemosiderinuria, 31f
Haemostasis, 12–13
　complexity, 20
　primary tests, 75
Hairy cell leukaemia (HCL), 48, 55
Ham test, paroxysmal nocturnal haemoglobinuria, 31
Haptoglobins, 21, 28
Hb-Bart hydrops syndrome, 32
HbH disease, 32
HDN *see* Haemolytic disease of the newborn (HDN)
Helicobacter pylori, 60, 68
HELLP syndrome (haemolysis, elevated liver enzymes and low platelets), 89
'Helper' cells, 8
Henoch–Schönlein purpura, 71
Heparin
　acute venous thrombosis, 79
　cardiopulmonary bypass, 71
　low molecular weight (LMW), 79–80, 89, 102
　in pregnancy, 89
　unfractionated, 80, 89
Heparin-induced thrombocytopenia (HIT), 69
Hepatitis
　aplastic anaemia, 52
　as contradiction to blood donation, 82

　haemophilia, 72–73
　marginal zone lymphoma, 60
　thrombocytopenia, 68
　venepuncture precautions, 104
Hepatobiliary complications, sickle cell anaemia, 34
Hepatocellular cancer, 73
Hepatomegaly, 67
Hereditary elliptocytosis, 29
Hereditary haemorrhagic telangiectasia (HHT), 71
Hereditary pyropoikilocytosis, 29
Hereditary spherocytosis, 28f, 29, 86
Hereditary thrombophilia, 89
Herpes simplex, 87
Herpes zoster, 87f
Hexose monophosphate shunt (pentose phosphate pathway), 5
Hickman catheters, 105
History taking
　common haematological abnormalities, 14t
　presenting complaint, 14
　systemic enquiry, 15
　thrombophilia, 78
　Von Willebrand disease, 74–75
HIV/AIDS
　CD4 count, 9
　as contradiction to blood donation, 82
　haemophilia, 72–73
　and Hodgkin's lymphoma, 58
　immunosuppression, 86
　systemic disease, 97
　thrombocytopenia, 68
Hodgkin's lymphoma (HL)
　advanced stage disease, 59
　aetiology, 58
　age distribution, 58
　classical, 58
　classification, 58
　clinical presentation, 58
　diagnosis, 58
　early stage disease, 59
　late effects of treatment, 59
　lymphocyte predominant nodular, 58
　management, 59
　monoclonal antibodies, 55
　prognosis, 59
　spleen, absent, 11
　staging, 58–59, 59f
Hormone replacement therapy (HRT), 79
Howell–Jolly bodies, 10–11
HPA-1a (platelet antigen), 69
HTLV-1 antibodies, adult T-cell leukaemia lymphoma, 49
Human leucocyte antigens (HLA), 8
　platelet transfusion, 85
　stem cell transplantation, 56
Humoral immunity, 8
　defects, 86
Hydronephrosis, 60
Hydroxycarbamide
　essential thrombocythaemia, 66
　myelofibrosis, 67
　polycythaemia, 64–65
　sickle cell anaemia (HbSS), 35
Hypercoagulability, in malignant disease, 96

Hyperdiploid mutations, myeloma, 62–63
Hypereosinophilic syndrome, 7
Hyperhomocysteinaemia, 27
Hyperkalaemia, 85
Hypersensitivity reactions, 7
Hypersplenism, 11
Hyperviscosity syndrome, 21, 63–64
Hypervolaemia, 11
Hypnosis, 95
Hypocalcaemia, 85
Hypocellular myelodysplastic syndrome, 52–53
Hypochromia, 22
Hypofibrinogenaemia, 75
Hypogammaglobulinaemia, 46, 87
  chronic lymphocytic leukaemia, 47
  immunosuppression, 87
Hyposplenism, 10–11, 11f, 11t
Hypothermia, 71, 85
Hypoxia-inducible factor (HIF), 4

I

Ibrutinib, 47
Idarubicin, 54
Idiopathic aplastic anaemia, 52
Idiopathic erythrocytosis, 65
Idiopathic venous thrombosis, 81
Ileum abnormalities, vitamin B$_{12}$ deficiency, 27
Imaging
  computed tomography (CT) scan, 59, 61
  magnetic resonance imaging, 59, 61
  positron emission tomography (PET) scans, 59, 61
Imatinib
  chronic myeloid leukaemia, 45, 55, 93
  hypereosinophilic syndrome, 7
Immune antibodies, 82–83
Immune neutropenia, 7
Immune thrombocytopenia (ITP), 68–69, 68t, 69f
  chronic lymphocytic leukaemia, 47
  haematopoietic growth factor therapy, 55
  and HIV/AIDS, 97
  paediatric haematology, 91
  in pregnancy, 88–89
  systemic disease, 96
  see also Thrombocytopenia
Immunochemistry, 102
Immunodeficiency, in chronic lymphocytic leukaemia, 46
Immunoglobulins
  acute phase response, 20
  basic structure, 9f
  and B-lymphocytes, 9
  intravenous, 30, 89
  thrombocytopenia, 69
  transfusion, 85, 87
Immunological tolerance, natural, 9
Immunophenotyping
  acute lymphoblastic leukaemia, 42

acute myeloid leukaemia, 41
  flow cytometry, 21
  non-Hodgkin's lymphoma, 61
Immunosuppression
  allogeneic stem cell transplantation, 56
    see also Allogeneic stem cell transplantation
  antibiotic treatment, 87, 87t
  aplastic anaemia, 52–53
  bone marrow aspiration, 106
  and chemotherapy, 86
  chronic lymphocytic leukaemia, 46f
  depressed cell-mediated immunity, 87
  infection types, 86–87
  neutropenia, 87, 87t
  prevention of infection, 87
  treatment of infection, 87
  see also Infection
Infection
  and anaemia of chronic disease, 36f
  aplastic anaemia, 52
  bacterial, 86, 97
  blood transfusion, 84
  chronic lymphocytic leukaemia, 47
  fungal, 86–87
  history taking, 14
  HIV/AIDS, 97
  hookworm, 99
  immunosuppression, 86–87
  lymphadenopathy secondary to, 16
  lymphocytosis, 9
  mononucleosis, 97, 97f
  neutropenia, 7
  parasitic, 7, 98–99
  prevention, 87
  red cell transfusion complications, 84
  systemic disease, 97
  systemic enquiry, 15
  treatment, 87
  viral see Viral infection
Infertility, chemotherapy treatment, 54
Inflammation, systemic enquiry, 15
Inguinal nodes, examination, 16
Inherited blood disorders
  connective tissue disease, 71
  in elderly people, 92–93
  examples, 15t
  familial thrombophilia, 78
  haemolytic anaemia, 29
  platelet function, 70–71
  sickle cell syndromes, 34f
  vascular purpuras, 71
  see also Genetic abnormalities; Haemophilia
Inhibitory receptors, 9
Interference phase microscopy, splenic function quantitation, 11
Interferon alfa, 55
  essential thrombocythaemia, 66
  hairy cell leukaemia, 48
  polycythaemia, 64–65
Interleukin 5, eosinophils, 7
International normalised ratio (INR), 20, 80–81

International prognostic index (IPI), 61
International Prognostic Scoring System for Primary MDS (IPSS), 50–51, 51t
International sensitivity index (ISI), 81
Intracranial bleeding
  haemophilia A, 72
  thrombocytopenia, 68
Intrinsic factor (IF), megaloblastic anaemia, 24–25
Intrinsic pathway, platelets, 12–13, 13f
Iron
  definition/role, 24
  malabsorption, 24–25
  normal cycle, 24f
  oral, failure to respond to, 25t
  overload, 85
  reuse of, 5
Iron chelation therapy
  aplastic anaemia, 53
  myelodysplastic syndromes, 51
  thalassaemias, 33
Iron deficiency
  anaemia see Iron deficiency anaemia
  characteristics, 24
  correction, 25
  in elderly people, 24, 92
  erythropoiesis, 64
  hookworm infection, 99
  identification in pregnancy, 88
  in infancy, 91
  unexplained, 16
Iron deficiency anaemia
  and anaemia of chronic disease, 37t
  causes, 24–25
  clinical features, 24–25
  confirmatory tests, 25
  diagnosis, 25
  investigation of underlying cause, 25
  management, 25
Isoantibodies, 30–31
Isoimmune haemolytic anaemia, 30–31

J

Janus kinase 2 (JAK2) gene mutations
  essential thrombocythaemia, 66
  myelofibrosis, 67
  polycythaemia, 64
Janus kinase 2 (JAK2) inhibitors
  myelofibrosis, 67
  myeloproliferative disorders, 55
  polycythaemia, 65
Joints
  bleeding into, 14
  examination, 16
  haemophilia, effects on, 72

K

Kaolin cephalin clotting time (KCCT), 20
Kidney enlargement, 17

see also Renal disease; Renal failure
Klebsiella spp., 86
Knee damage, haemophilia A, 72f

L

Laboratory haematology
  blood and bone marrow, 18–19
  blood films see Blood films
  coagulation and acute phase response, 20–21
Lactate dehydrogenase (LDH), 61
Leishmania donovani, 99
Leishmann stain, 98
Lenalidomide, 55
  myelofibrosis, 67
  myeloma, 63
Leucocytosis, 6–7, 7t, 97
Leucopenia
  hypersplenism, 11
  myelodysplastic syndromes, 50
  symptoms attributable to, 14
Leukaemia
  acute lymphoblastic see Acute lymphoblastic leukaemia (ALL)
  acute monocytic, 40f
  acute myeloid see Acute myeloid leukaemia (AML)
  adult T-cell leukaemia lymphoma, 39f, 49
  aetiology, 38–39
  annual causes of death, 38f
  anti-leukaemic drugs, 54
  blood count, 18
  chronic lymphocytic see Chronic lymphocytic leukaemia (CLL)
  chronic myeloid see Chronic myeloid leukaemia (CML)
  classification, 39
  definition, 38
  dyspnoea in, 95
  gene therapy, 103
  genetic abnormalities, 38–39
  hairy cell, 48
  history taking, 14
  immunophenotype, cells, 21
  immunosuppression, 86
  incidence, 38
  minimal residual disease, 21
  predisposing factors, 39
  prolymphocytic, 48
  social history, 15
  T-cell large granular lymphocyte, 48–49
Leukapheresis, peripheral blood stem cells harvested by, 56, 57f
Leukocytes, listed, 6
  see also White cell count (WBC)
Light microscopy, spleen, 11f
Light scattering, cell counting and sizing, 18
Lipid bilayer, red cells, 4
Liver disease
  and alcohol, 96
  coagulation disorders, 20, 77
  hepatitis see Hepatitis
  protein C and S deficiencies, 78–79

sickle cell anaemia, 34
and thrombophilia, 78
Liver function tests, 53
Local anaesthesia, bone marrow
aspiration, 106
Low molecular weight (LMW)
heparin, 79–80, 89, 102
Lumps, examination, 16
Lymph, location of lymphocytes
in, 8
Lymphadenopathy
chronic lymphocytic leukaemia,
46
defined, 16
history taking, 14
Hodgkin's lymphoma, 48f
infection, 16
massive cervical, 16f
mediastinal, in HL, 48f
non-Hodgkin's lymphoma, 60
Lymph nodes
biopsy, 58, 58f, 60–61
examination, 16–17
location of lymphocytes in, 8
neck, 17f
Lymphocyte predominant nodular
Hodgkin's lymphoma, 58
Lymphocytes, 8–9
atypical, infectious
mononucleosis, 97f
B-lymphocytes see
B-lymphocytes
changes in disease, 9
count, 9, 46
depletion, 56
donor lymphocyte infusions,
57
dysfunction, 86
hairy cell leukaemia, 48f
Hodgkin's lymphoma, 58
mature, in blood, 8f
mononucleosis, infectious, 97
natural killer (NK) cells, 9
T-lymphocytes see
T-lymphocytes
see also Chronic lymphocytic
leukaemia (CLL)
Lymphocytosis
chronic lymphocytic leukaemia,
46, 93
common causes, 9t
infection, 9
Lymphoid follicles, splenic
structure, 10
Lymphoid organs, 8–9
Lymphoma
axillary lymphadenopathy, 60f
B-cell, 55, 97
Burkitt's see Burkitt's lymphoma
diffuse large B-cell, 61, 100f
dyspnoea in, 95
follicular, 61, 102, 102f
and HIV/AIDS, 97
Hodgkin's lymphoma see
Hodgkin's lymphoma (HL)
mantle cell, 61
marginal zone, 61
mucosa-associated lymphoid
type, 61
non-Hodgkin's see Non-
Hodgkin's lymphoma
pain management, 94
peripheral T-cell, 61

poorly differentiated large cell,
46
T-cell leukaemic see Adult T-cell
leukaemia lymphoma
Lymphopenia, 86

M

Macrocytic anaemias, 22, 25, 27
Macrocytosis, alcohol misuse, 15,
96
Macrophages, 7, 10
Magnetic resonance imaging
(MRI), 59, 61
Malabsorption
folate, 27
iron, 24–25
vitamin K, 77
Malaria, 98–99
history taking, 15
removal of malarial parasites, 10
Malignant disease
chemotherapy see
Chemotherapy
colon cancer, 24f
current management model, 94f
in elderly people see under
Elderly people
end of life care, 95
hypercoagulability in, 96
lymphocytosis, 9
median ages of presentation, 93f
microarrays/gene profiling, 100
microenvironment, targeting,
102
minimal residual disease, 21, 101
molecular biology applications,
101
non-pain symptoms, control,
94–95
pain management, 14, 94
palliative treatment see Palliative
treatment
prostatic carcinoma, bone
marrow invasion, 97f
psychosocial oncology, 95
rectal, 16
renal carcinoma, 96
secondary, mediastinal
irradiation, 59
staging
chronic lymphocytic
leukaemia, 46
Hodgkin's lymphoma, 58–59,
59f
myeloma, 62–63
non-Hodgkin's lymphoma,
60–61
stem cell transplantation, 101
symptoms attributable to, 14
and systemic disease, 96
systemic enquiry, 15
see also Hepatocellular cancer;
Leukaemia; Lymphoma;
Myeloma
Malpighian bodies, 10
MALT (mucosa-associated
lymphoid type) lymphoma,
60–61
Mantle cell lymphoma, 61
Marfan syndrome, 71
Marginal pool, neutrophils, 6

Marginal zone, spleen, 10
Marginal zone lymphoma, 61
Massive cervical lymphadenopathy,
16f
Mast cells, 7
May–Grünwald–Giemsa (MGG)
stain, 18–19
MDR1 (multi-drug resistance
gene), 54
Mean cell haemoglobin (MCH),
22, 25, 36–37
Mean cell haemoglobin
concentration (MCHC), 22
Mean cell volume (MCV), 22, 25,
36–37
Mean corpuscular haemoglobin
(MCH), 32
Mean corpuscular volume (MCV),
32
Medical history, 15
Mefloquine, 99
Megakaryocytes, increased in
thrombocytopenia, 69
Megaloblastic anaemia
B_{12} deficiency, 26–27
bone marrow aspirate in, 26f
clinical syndromes, 26–27
diagnosis, 27
folate deficiency, 26–27
in pregnancy, 88
treatment, 27
Melphalan, 54, 63
'Memory' B-cells, 9
Menstruation, iron deficiency,
24–25
Mercaptopurine, 43, 54
Merozoites, 98
Metabolism, red cell see Red cell
metabolism
Methicillin-resistant Staphylococcus
aureus (MRSA), 86
Methotrexate, 43, 54
Methylene blue stain, blood film,
18–19
Microangiopathic haemolytic
anaemia (MAHA), 31, 31f
Microarrays/gene profiling, 100
Microcytic anaemias, 22
Microcytosis, 22
Microthrombus formation, in DIC,
76
Minimal residual disease (MRD),
haematological malignancy,
21, 101
Mitoxantrone, 54
Molecular biology
acute lymphoblastic leukaemia,
43
acute myeloid leukaemia, 41
application in haematology, 101
blood tests, 82
DNA analysis techniques,
100–101
Monoclonal antibodies (MoAbs),
55
Monoclonal B-cell lymphocytosis,
46
in elderly people, 93
Monoclonal gammopathy of
uncertain significance
(MGUS)
elderly people, 93
myeloma, 62

Monocyte colony-stimulating
factor (M-CSF), 7
Monocytes, 7
Monocytopenia, 7, 48
Mononuclear phagocyte system, 7
Mononucleosis, infectious, 97
Monospot test, mononucleosis, 97
M-proteins, myeloma, 62
MRI scans see Magnetic resonance
imaging (MRI)
Mucosa-associated lymphoid type
(MALT) lymphoma, 60–61
Multi drug resistance, 54, 98
Multimer analysis, Von Willebrand
disease, 74f, 75
Multiple myeloma see Myeloma
Mutations see Genetic
abnormalities
MYC oncogene, non-Hodgkin's
lymphoma, 60
Myelodysplastic syndromes (MDS)
and acute myeloid leukaemia,
39, 50
and aplastic anaemia, 52–53
classification, 50
clinical features, 50
diagnosis, 50
in elderly people, 92
epigenetic therapies, 55
genetic factors, 50
high-risk, 51
hypocellular, 52–53
low-risk, 51
morphology, 50
and myelofibrosis, 67
platelet function disorders, 71
prognosis, 50–51
treatment, 51
Myelofibrosis
characteristics, 66–67
clinical features, 67
diagnosis, 67
essential thrombocythaemia,
progression from, 66
management, 67
polycythaemia, 64–65
prognosis, 67
'Myeloid' antigens, 41
Myeloma
asymptomatic ('smouldering'),
62
biology, 62
bisphosphonate, 63, 94
clinical features, 62
complications, 63
diagnosis, 62–63
humoral immunity defects, 86
hypogammaglobulinaemia, 87
management and outcome, 63
palliative treatment, 63, 95t
platelet function disorders, 71
proteasome inhibitors, 55
staging, 62–63
Waldenström's
macroglobulinaemia, 63
Myeloperoxidase
acute lymphoblastic leukaemia,
42
acute myeloid leukaemia, 40–41
Myeloproliferative disorders
and acute myeloid leukaemia,
39
basophilia, 7

chronic myeloid leukaemia, 44
JAK2 inhibitors, 55
and myelofibrosis, 67
platelet function disorders, 71
and thrombophilia, 79
Myocardial infarction,
thrombolytic therapy, 81

N

Natural killer (NK) cells, 9
Naturally occurring antibodies, 82
Nausea and vomiting, malignant
disease, 95
Neck, lymph nodes, 17f
Neisseria meningitidis, 11
Neonates/neonatal disorders *see*
Newborns
Neural tube defects, 88
Neutropenia
antibiotic treatment, 87t
aspergillosis, 86f
bacterial infection, 86
growth factors, 87
haematopoietic growth factor
therapy, 55
hairy cell leukaemia, 48
history taking, 14
immunosuppression, 86
infection, 7
isolated, causes of, 7t
prevention of infection, 87
pyrexial neutropenic patient, 87
systemic disease, 96
T-cell large granular lymphocyte
leukaemia, 48–49
Neutrophilia/neutrophil
leucocytosis, 6–7
Neutrophils, 6–7
dysfunction, 86
transfusion, 85
Newborns
anaemia of prematurity, 90
haemolytic disease of the
newborn, 90
iron deficiency in, 91
polycythaemia in, 90–91
RhD prophylaxis in RhD-
negative mothers, 90
sites of blood production in, 2f
thrombocytopenia, 91
venepuncture, 105
vitamin K deficiency, 77
see also Paediatric haematology;
Pregnancy
Next-generation sequencing, 101
Nicotinamide adenosine
dinucleotide phosphate
(NADPH), 5
Nilotinib, 45, 55
Nitroblue tetrazolium test, chronic
granulomatous disease, 7
Non-haemolytic transfusion
reactions, 84
Non-Hodgkin's lymphoma
aetiology, 60
classification, 60
clinical presentation, 60
diagnosis, 60–61
high- and low-grade tumours, 60
immunosuppression, 86
lymphocytosis, 9

management, 61
monoclonal antibodies, 55
nodal involvement, 60
proteasome inhibitors, 55
Sjögren's syndrome, 96
staging, 60–61
see also Hodgkin's lymphoma
(HL); Lymphoma
Nonsteroidal anti-inflammatory
drugs (NSAIDs), 94
Normochromic anaemias, 22
Normocytic anaemias, 22
Normocytosis, 22
Nose bleeds, thrombocytopenia,
14
Nucleoside analogues, hairy cell
leukaemia, 48

O

Observation of patient, 16
Ofatumumab, 55
Oligonucleotide microarrays, 100
Ondansetron, 95
Opiate analgesia, 94
Organelles, platelets, 12
Osmotic fragility, hereditary
spherocytosis, 28f
Oxygen, transport, 4–5
Oxygen dissociation curve, 5f

P

P₅₀ level, haemoglobin and oxygen
transport, 5
Packed cell volume (PCV), 22,
90–91
Paediatric haematology
acute lymphoblastic leukaemia,
43
anaemia, 22
bone marrow aspiration, general
anaesthesia, 106
congenital dyserythropoietic
anaemia, 91
Diamond–Blackfan anaemia, 91
haemoglobinopathies, 15–16
haemophilia, 15
iron deficiency in infancy, 91
neonatal disorders, 90–91
normal values, 90
red cell aplasia in children and
adolescents, 91
sickle cell syndromes, 35
spleen, absent, 11
transient erythroblastopenia of
childhood, 91
umbilical cord blood (UCB)
transplantation, 57
venepuncture, 105
Pain
bone, in myeloma, 62
malignant disease, 14, 62
management of in palliative
care, 94
splenic, 14, 67
vascular-occlusive crises, 35
Palliative treatment
chemotherapy and radiotherapy,
94
complementary therapy, 95
myeloma, 63, 95f

non-pain symptoms, control,
94–95
pain management, 94
psychosocial oncology, 95
see also Malignant disease
Pallor, anaemia, 22
Pancytopenia
aplastic anaemia, 52
chronic lymphocytic leukaemia,
47
hairy cell leukaemia, 48
hypersplenism, 11
and leukocytes, 7
myelodysplastic syndromes, 52f
non-Hodgkin's lymphoma, 60
Pappenheimer (siderotic) granules,
11
Paracetamol, 94
Parallel sequencing, 101
Paraproteins, myeloma, 62
Parasitic infection, 7
malaria, 98–99
Paroxysmal nocturnal
haemoglobinuria (PNH)
aplastic anaemia, 53
haemolytic anaemia, 31
Partial exchange transfusion, 91
Partial thromboplastin time with
kaolin (PTTK), 20
Parvovirus, aplastic anaemia, 52
Paul–Bunnel test, mononucleosis,
97
Pentamidine, 87
Pentostatin, hairy cell leukaemia,
48
Periarteriolar lymphatic sheath, 10
Periodic acid Schiff (PAS), acute
lymphoblastic leukaemia, 42
Peripheral blood
blood film, in AML, 39f
myelodysplastic syndromes, 50
Peripheral blood stem cells
(PBSC), 56–57
Peripheral T-cell lymphomas, 61
Peripheral venous cannulation,
105
Perls' stain, 19, 31f
Pernicious anaemia, 26–27, 27f
ethnic origin of patient, 16
in pregnancy, 88
Petechial haemorrhage,
thrombocytopenia, 68
PET scans *see* Positron emission
tomography (PET) scans
PFA-100 (platelet function
instrument), 70
P-glycoprotein, 54
Phagocytes, 6, 10
Phagocytosis, 6
Philadelphia (Ph) chromosome
acute lymphoblastic leukaemia,
43
chronic myeloid leukaemia,
38–39, 44, 44f
Phospholipids, red cells, 4
Piperacillin, 87
Plasma
fibrinogen *see* Fibrinogen,
plasma
transfusion, 85
viscosity, 21
volume expansion, in pregnancy,
88

see also Fresh frozen plasma
(FFP)
Plasmacytomas, 62
Plasma-derived factor VIII, 72–73
Plasma protein fraction (PPF), 85
Plasmin, 13
Plasmodium falciparum, 98–99
Plasmodium malariae, 98
Plasmodium ovale, 98
Plasmodium vivax, 98
Plasticity concept, 2
Platelet-derived growth factor
(PDGF), 66
Platelet function disorders
acquired, 70–71
causes of abnormal function, 71t
essential thrombocythaemia, 66
history taking, 14
inherited, 70–71
vascular purpuras, 71
Platelet function instruments, 70
Platelets
in acquired coagulation
disorders, 76–77
activation, 10, 12
adhesion, 12
role of vWF in, 74f
aggregation, 12, 70f
Von Willebrand disease, 75
blood transfusion, 71, 85
chronic renal failure,
abnormalities in, 96
clumping of, in
thrombocytopenia, 68f
count, 68–69
cytoplasm, 12
destruction, in
thrombocytopenia, 68
dilution, in thrombocytopenia,
68
essential thrombocythaemia, 66
hyposplenism, 11
intrinsic and extrinsic pathways,
12–13, 13f
laboratory testing of function, 70
loose plug, 12
low count *see*
Thrombocytopenia
organelles, 12
procoagulant action, 12
pro-thrombinase complex, 12
role, 12
transfusion of, 27, 85
and vasoconstriction, 12
Plummer–Vinson syndrome,
24–25
Pneumocystis jiroveci (carinii)
pneumonia, 86–87
PNH *see* Paroxysmal nocturnal
haemoglobinuria (PNH)
Polycythaemia
acute phase response, 20
apparent, 64–65
approach to patient with, 64
clinical syndromes, 64–65
essential thrombocythaemia,
progression from, 66
in newborn, 90–91
renal disease, 96
secondary, 65, 65f
smoking, 15
Polycythaemia vera (PV), 64–66,
65f

Polymerase chain reaction (PCR), 73, 90, 100–101
  real-time quantitative polymerase chain reaction (RQ-PCR), 45
Polymorphism, prothrombin gene, 78
Positron emission tomography (PET) scans, 59, 61
Posterior iliac crest, 106f–107f
Post-transfusion purpura, thrombocytopenia, 69
Precursor lymphoid neoplasms, 42
Prednisolone
  diffuse large B-cell lymphoma, 61
  follicular lymphoma, 61
  myeloma, 63
  thrombocytopenia, 69
  warm autoimmune haemolytic anaemia, 30
  see also Steroid treatment
Pre-eclampsia, 88–89
Pregnancy
  acute obstetric haemorrhage, 89t
  anaemia in, 22, 88
  antenatal detection of genetic disorders, 101
  coagulation abnormalities in, 89
  common haematological changes, 88f
  disseminated intravascular coagulation in, 88–89
  essential thrombocythaemia, 66
  haematological changes, 88
  HELLP syndrome, 89
  sickle cell anaemia (HbSS), 35
  thrombocytopenia in, 88–89
  thrombophilia in, 79
  see also Newborns; Paediatric haematology
Prematurity, anaemia of, 90
Prenatal diagnosis, 33, 35
Procoagulant action, platelets, 12
Proguanil, malaria, 99
Prolymphocytes, 48
Prolymphocytic leukaemia (PLL), 48
Prostatic carcinoma, bone marrow invasion, 97f
Protein C
  coagulation regulation, 13
  deficiency, familial thrombophilia, 78–79
Protein S
  coagulation regulation, 13
  deficiency, familial thrombophilia, 78–79
Proteolytic enzymes, 12
Proteasome inhibitors, 55
Prothrombin, 12–13
Pro-thrombinase complex, platelets, 12
Prothrombin complex concentrate, 77
Prothrombin G20210A, familial thrombophilia, 78
Prothrombin time (PT)
  disseminated intravascular coagulation, 76
  haemostasis, 12–13
  laboratory haematology, 20
  vitamin K deficiency, 77

and warfarin, 81
  see also Activated partial thromboplastin time (APTT)
Pseudomonas aeruginosa, 86
Pseudopolycythaemia, 64–65
Pseudoxanthoma elasticum, 71
Psoas muscle bleed, haemophilia A, 72f
Pulmonary arteriovenous malformations (PAVMs), 71
Pulmonary embolism (PE)
  main pulmonary trunk, 80f
  in pregnancy, 89
  thrombophilia, 78
Pure red cell aplasia (PRCA), 91
Purine analogues, hairy cell leukaemia, 48
Purpura fulminans, 79
Purpuric rash
  myelodysplastic syndrome, 50f
  thrombocytopenia, 68, 69f
Pyruvate kinase (pk) deficiency, 29

Q

Quantitative immunoassay, vWF antigen, 75
Quinine, 99
Quinolone antibiotic, 87

R

Radioimmunoassay, erythropoietin estimation by, 64
Radioimmunotherapy, follicular lymphoma, 61
Radiotherapy
  chronic lymphocytic leukaemia, 47
  follicular lymphoma, 61
  Hodgkin's lymphoma, 59
  myeloma, 63
  palliative, 94
  stem cell transplantation, 56–57
Rai system, Binet adaptation, 46
Rashes, purpuric
  myelodysplastic syndrome, 50f
  thrombocytopenia, 68, 69f
Raynaud's phenomenon, 30
Real-time quantitative polymerase chain reaction (RQ-PCR), 45
Recombinant activated protein C, acquired coagulation disorders, 76
Recombinant vWF, 75
Rectal examination, 16
Red cell aplasia, 91
Red cell distribution width (RDW), 25
Red cell indices, 22
Red cell metabolism, 5
  abnormalities, 29
  schematic diagram, 29f
Red cells, 4–5
  ageing and death, 5
  blood count, 18
  characteristic biconcave shape, 4f
  enlarged (macrocytosis), 15, 24
  erythropoietin, 4
  haemoglobin and oxygen transport, 5

high concentration in polycythaemia, 64
intrasplenic pooling, in hypersplenism, 11
membrane, 4f
  disorders, 29
'normochromic normocytic' indices, 28
premature destruction, in hypersplenism, 11
removal, where unwanted, 10
renal disease, increased production in, 96
structure, 4
transfusion, 84–85, 84t
Red pulp, spleen, 10, 11f
Reed–Sternberg cells, lymph node biopsy, in HL, 58f
Regulatory molecules *see* Growth factors
Renal disease, 96
Renal failure
  Burr cells, 96f
  chronic, 71, 96
  in elderly people, 92
  haemolytic transfusion reactions, 84
  platelet function disorders, 71
Resistance, multi-drug, 54
  malaria, 98
Respiratory burst, phagocytosis, 6
Reticulocytes
  haemolytic anaemia, 28
  increased, in warm AIHA, 30f
Reticulocytopenia, aplastic anaemia, 52
Rhesus (Rh) blood group system, 82–83
  clinical practice, 85
  paediatric haematology, 90
Rheumatoid arthritis, 37, 96
Richter syndrome, 46
Ristocetin, failure to aggregate with, 70
Rituximab, 55
  chronic lymphocytic leukaemia, 47
  diffuse large B-cell lymphoma, 61
  follicular lymphoma, 61
  prolymphocytic leukaemia, 48
  treatment advances, 102
  warm autoimmune haemolytic anaemia, 30
Rivaroxaban, 81, 102–103
Romanowsky's stain, 18–19, 28
Ruxolitinib, 55, 67

S

Schilling test, vitamin B$_{12}$ absorption, 27
Schizonts, 98
Scintigraphy, 11
Screening strategies, sickle cell syndromes, 35
SDS–PAGE multimer analysis, vW factor, 74f
Sedation, bone marrow aspiration and trephine biopsy, 106–107

Senile purpura, 71f
Sepsis, 14, 76
Septicaemia, 86
Sequestration, 34, 68
Serial analysis of gene expression (SAGE), 100
Severe aplastic anaemia (SAA), 53
Sézary syndrome, 49
Shock, blood transfusion, 84
Sickle cell syndromes
  counselling, 35
  dactylitis, 34f
  doubly heterozygous sickling disorders, 35
  inheritance, 34f
  pathophysiology, 34
  sickle cell anaemia (HbSS), 34–35, 34f
    ethnic origin of patient, 16
    in pregnancy, 88
    splenic atrophy, 10–11
  sickle cell trait (HbAS), 35
Side-effects
  bone marrow harvesting, 107
  cytotoxic drugs, 54
  interferon alfa, 48
  possible haematological, 15t
Signal transduction, 3
Silver impregnation, trephine biopsy, 19
Sjögren's syndrome, 96
Skin disorders
  infection, 86f
  sickle cell anaemia, 34
Smear cells, chronic lymphocytic leukaemia, 46
Smears, marrow aspirate, 106
Smoking, history taking, 15
Social history, 15
Southern blotting, factor VIII gene inversion in haemophilia, 73f
Spectrin, 4
Spectrophotometer, automated haematology counters, 18
Spindle poisons, 54
Spleen
  abnormal states, 10–11
  absent, 10–11
  and B-lymphocytes, 9
  enlargement, schematic view, 17f
  examination, 17, 17f
  function, 10
  Howell–Jolly bodies, 10–11
  light microscopy, 11f
  location of lymphocytes in, 8
  red and white pulp, 10, 11f
  structure, 10
Splenectomy, 10–11
  chronic lymphocytic leukaemia, 47
  hairy cell leukaemia, 48
  hereditary elliptocytosis, 29
  pyruvate kinase (pk) deficiency, 29
  thrombocytopenia, 69
  warm autoimmune haemolytic anaemia, 30
Splenic artery, 10
Splenic cords, 10
Splenic sinuses, 10

Splenomegaly
  chronic lymphocytic leukaemia, 46
  chronic myeloid leukaemia, 44
  common causes, 17t
  hypersplenism, 11
  myelodysplastic syndromes, 50
  myelofibrosis, 66–67, 67f
  pain in, 14
  polycythaemia, 64
  prolymphocytic leukaemia, 48
  thrombocytopenia, 68
  tropical splenomegaly syndrome, 99
Staging of malignant disease
  chronic lymphocytic leukaemia, 46
  Hodgkin's lymphoma, 58–59, 59f
  myeloma, 62–63
  non-Hodgkin's lymphoma, 60–61
Stains and dyes, blood films, 18–19
  see also specific stains, such as Sudan black stain
Staphylococcus epidermidis, 86
Stem cell hierarchy, haematopoiesis, 2, 3f
Stem cell mobilisation, 55
Stem cell transplantation (SCT)
  acute myeloid leukaemia, 41
  allogeneic see Allogeneic stem cell transplantation
  aplastic anaemia, 53
  autologous see Autologous stem cell transplantation
  chronic myeloid leukaemia, 45
  graft-versus-host disease, 56, 57f
  haematological malignancy, 101
  immunosuppression, 86–87
  leukapheresis, peripheral blood stem cells harvested by, 56, 57f
  non-myeloablative ('reduced intensity') allogeneic, 57
  sickle cell anaemia (HbSS), 35
  syngeneic, 56
  twin (allogeneic and syngeneic), 56
  umbilical cord blood, 57
  see also Blood transfusion
Stercobilinogen, faecal, 28
Steroid treatment
  chronic lymphocytic leukaemia, 47
  myeloma, 63
  thrombocytopenia, 69
  warm autoimmune haemolytic anaemia, 30
  see also Prednisolone
Stomach abnormalities, vitamin B_{12} deficiency, 27
Storage pool disorders, 70
Streptococcus faecalis, skin infection, 86f
Streptococcus pneumoniae, 11
Streptokinase, 81
Stromal cells, 2
Stylet, bone marrow aspiration and trephine biopsy, 106–107
'Subacute combined degeneration', 26

Submicroscopic mutations, leukaemia, 38
Sudan black stain, 40–42
Superior vena cava syndrome, 60
Supplementation
  folic acid, 27
  iron, 88
  vitamin K, 77, 81
Supportive care
  acute myeloid leukaemia, 41
  aplastic anaemia, 53
  haematopoietic growth factor therapy, 55
  myelodysplastic syndromes, 51
Supravital stain, blood film, 18–19
Surgery
  sickle cell anaemia (HbSS), 35
  splenectomy see Splenectomy
5q-syndrome, 50
Syngeneic stem cell transplantation, and allogeneic SCT, 56
Syringe drivers, continuous drug infusions, 95
Systemic disease
  basophilia, 7
  blood count, 18
  connective tissue, 71, 96
  infection, 97
  liver, 96
  malignancy, 96
  non-Hodgkin's lymphoma, 60
  renal, 96
  and thrombophilia, 78
  see also Infection; Liver disease; Malignant disease
Systemic lupus erythematosus (SLE), 79, 96

T

Tazobactam, 87
T-cell large granular lymphocyte leukaemia (T-LGL), 48–49
T-cell receptor (TCR), 8
Tear-drop poikilocytes, myelofibrosis, 67
Telangiectasia, 71
Telomeres, in aplastic anaemia, 52
Thalassaemias
  classification, 32
  clinical syndromes, 32–33
  gene therapy, 103
  prenatal diagnosis, 33
  spleen, absent, 11
α-Thalassaemias, 32
β-Thalassaemia intermedia, 33
β-Thalassaemia major, 32–33
β-Thalassaemia trait (minor), 33
Thalidomide, 55
  myelofibrosis, 67
  myeloma, 63
Third-generation recombinant factor VIII, 72–73
3-D confocal imaging, 102
Thrombin, 12–13
  inhibitors, 102–103
Thrombocytes see Platelets
Thrombocytopenia
  acute lymphoblastic leukaemia, 42
  alcohol misuse, 96

alloimmune, 91
autoimmune, 46
bleeding, 14, 68
bone marrow aspiration, 106
causes, 68
clinical presentation, 68
clinical syndromes, 68–69
heparin use, 80
hypersplenism, 11
incidental (gestational), 88
myelodysplastic syndromes, 50
myeloma, 62
in newborn, 91
in pregnancy, 88–89
symptoms attributable to, 14
T-cell large granular lymphocyte leukaemia, 48–49
  see also Immune thrombocytopenia (ITP)
Thrombocytosis, systemic enquiry, 15
Thromboembolism, anticoagulant therapy, 89
Thrombolytic therapy, 81
Thrombomodulin inhibitors, 102
Thrombophilia
  acquired forms, 79
  acute venous thrombosis, 79
  familial, 78–79
  genetic counselling, 79
  patients to be investigated, 78
  in pregnancy, 79
Thromboplastin, prothrombin time test, 20
Thrombopoeitin receptor (TPO-R), second generation agonists, 69
Thrombosis
  in elderly people, 92, 92f
  large vessel, in DIC, 76
  polycythaemia, risk in, 64
Thrombotic thrombocytopenic purpura (TTP), 31
Thymus
  destruction of T-lymphocytes by, 8
  location of lymphocytes in, 8
Tissue factor pathway inhibitor (TFPI), 13
Tissue hypoxia, anaemia, 22
Tissue necrosis, haemorrhagic, 76
Tissue plasminogen activator (t-PA), 13, 81
T-lymphocytes, 8
  acute lymphoblastic leukaemia, 42
  adult T-cell leukaemia lymphoma, 49
  interaction with antigen-presenting cells, 8f
  removal in stem cell transplantation, 56
  splenic structure, 10
Topoisomerase poisons/inhibitors, 54
Tourniquets, 104–105
Tranexamic acid, bleeding, 73
Transcranial Doppler ultrasonography, sickle cell syndromes, 35
Transcription factors, 2
Transforming growth factor-β, 66
Transfusion see Blood transfusion

Transfusion associated circulation overload (TACO), 84
Transfusion-related acute lung injury (TRALI), 84
Transient erythroblastopenia of childhood, 91
Treatment of conditions
  advances in, 102–103
  bleeding, in haemophilia A, 72–73
  chronic lymphocytic leukaemia, 46–47, 47f
  chronic myeloid leukaemia, 45, 55
  infection, 87
  megaloblastic anaemia, 27
  myelodysplastic syndromes, 51
  viral, 73
  see also Chemotherapy; Drug treatment; Surgery
Trephine biopsy, bone marrow
  acute lymphoblastic leukaemia, 42
  acute myeloid leukaemia, 40
  aplastic anaemia, 52–53
  chronic lymphocytic leukaemia, 46
  examination procedure, 19
  hairy cell leukaemia, 48
  human T-cell leukaemic lymphoma, 39f
  myelofibrosis, 67f
  polycythaemia, 64
  procedure, 107
  staining, 19
  and structure of bone marrow, 2
  systemic disease, 96
  thrombocytopenia, 69
  uses, 19
Tricyclic antidepressants, pain management, 94
Trilaminar platelet membrane, 12
Trophozoites, 98–99
Tropical splenomegaly syndrome, 99
Twin (allogeneic and syngeneic) stem cell transplantation, 56
Tyrosine kinase inhibitors (TKIs), 55
  acute myeloid leukaemia, 55
  chronic myeloid leukaemia, 45
Tyrosine kinase receptor gene mutation, acute myeloid leukaemia, 41

U

Ulceration, cold autoimmune haemolytic anaemia, 30
Ultrastructural studies, 2
Umbilical cord blood (UCB) transplantation, 57
Unfractionated heparin, 80, 89
Uraemia, 71
Urobilin, 5
Urobilinogen, 5, 28
Urokinase, 81

V

Variant Creutzfeldt-Jakob disease (vCJD), 84

Varicella zoster, 87
Vascular-occlusive crises, sickle cell anaemia, 34–35
Vascular purpuras, 71
Velocimetry, fetal middle cerebral artery, 90
Venepuncture, 104–105
Venesection, polycythaemia, 65
Venous access, 105
Venous thrombosis
    acute, 79
    in elderly people, 92f
    Factor V Leiden (FVR506Q), 78
    idiopathic, 81
    malignant disease, 96
    see also Deep vein thrombosis (DVT)
Vertebroplasty, myeloma, 63
Very severe aplastic anaemia (VSAA), 53
Vinblastine, 54
    Hodgkin's lymphoma, 59
Vincristine, 54
    diffuse large B-cell lymphoma, 61
    follicular lymphoma, 61

Viral infection
    adult T-cell leukaemia lymphoma, 49
    aplastic anaemia, 52
    haemophilia A, 73
    hepatitis *see* Hepatitis
    immunosuppression, 86–87
    systemic disease, 97
    thrombocytopenia, 68
Visceral leishmaniasis (kala-azar), 99
Vitamin B_{12} deficiency
    intramuscular injection, 24–25
    megaloblastic anaemia, 26–27
    in pregnancy, 88
Vitamin K
    deficiency, 76–77
    intravenous, 81
    platelets, 12
    supplementation, 77, 81, 92
    and warfarin, 76, 80f
Vitamin K derived clotting factor, 73
Von Willebrand disease (vWD)
    classification, 74
    clinical features, 74–75

    diagnosis, 74f
    laboratory diagnosis, 75
    management, 75
    types 1 and 2, 74
Von Willebrand factor (vWF)
    platelet function disorders, 70
    range of levels, 74
    role in platelet adhesion, 74f
    thrombotic thrombocytopenic purpura, 31
Voriconazole, 87

W

Waldenström's macroglobulinaemia, 63
Warfarin
    indications for use, 80–81
    method of action, 80
    in pregnancy, 89
    protein C and S deficiencies, 78–79
    side-effects, 79
    and vitamin K, 76, 80f

Warm autoimmune haemolytic anaemia, 30, 30f
White cell count (WBC)
    acute myeloid leukaemia, 40
    chronic myeloid leukaemia, 44
    laboratory haematology, 18
    reference values, 90
    see also Leukocytes
White cells, low count *see* Leucopenia
White pulp, spleen, 10, 11f
World Health Organization (WHO) classification systems
    acute lymphoblastic leukaemia, 42
    acute myeloid leukaemia, 40
    Hodgkin's lymphoma, 58
    non-Hodgkin's lymphoma, 60
Wright's stain, 18–19

Z

ZAP-70 (signalling molecule), 46
Zidovudine, 49

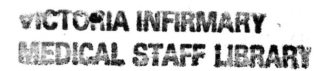